Liver Diseases

An essential guide for nurses and health care professionals

Edited by

Suzanne Sargent

MSc, PGC (TLHE), BSc (Hons), RGN

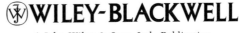
WILEY-BLACKWELL

A John Wiley & Sons, Ltd., Publication

This edition first published 2009
© 2009 Blackwell Publishing Ltd

Blackwell Publishing was acquired by John Wiley & Sons in February 2007. Blackwell's publishing programme has been merged with Wiley's global Scientific, Technical, and Medical business to form Wiley-Blackwell.

Registered office
John Wiley & Sons Ltd, The Atrium, Southern Gate, Chichester, West Sussex, PO19 8SQ, United Kingdom

Editorial offices
9600 Garsington Road, Oxford, OX4 2DQ, United Kingdom
2121 State Avenue, Ames, Iowa 50014-8300, USA

For details of our global editorial offices, for customer services and for information about how to apply for permission to reuse the copyright material in this book please see our website at www.wiley.com/wiley-blackwell.

Library of Congress Cataloging-in-Publication Data

Liver diseases : an essential guide for nurses and health care professionals / edited by Suzanne Sargent.
p. ; cm.
Includes bibliographical references and index.
ISBN 978-1-4051-6306-4 (pbk. : alk. paper)   1. Liver–Diseases–Nursing.   I. Sargent, Suzanne.
[DNLM: 1. Liver Diseases–Nurses' Instruction.   2. Adult. WI 700 L7835 2009]
RC845.L585 2009
616.3′620231–dc22
2008039838

A catalogue record for this book is available from the British Library.

Set in 10 on 12.5 pt Sabon by SNP Best-set Typesetter Ltd., Hong Kong
Printed and bound in Singapore by Ho Printing Singapore Pte Ltd

2   2012

Contents

13 Acute liver failure   214
Zebina Ratansi

14 Nutrition in liver disease   234
Susie Hamlin and Julie Leaper

15 Drug-induced liver injury   256
Suzanne Sargent

Colour plates appear after page 146

Contributors

Michelle Clayton MSc, PGC (Clin Teach), BSc (Hons), RGN
Lecturer in Liver Care
School of Healthcare
University of Leeds
Leeds

Teresa Corbani RN, BSc (Hons)
Practice Development Nurse
Liver Unit
Kings College Hospital NHS Foundation Trust
London

Tracey Dudley RN, BSc (Hons)
Post-transplant Hepatitis Clinical Nurse Specialist
The Liver Transplant and Hepatobiliary Surgery Unit
Queen Elizabeth Hospital
Birmingham

Danielle Fullwood RN, BSc (Hons)
Practice Development Nurse
Liver Intensive Care Unit
Kings College Hospital NHS Foundation Trust
London

Lynda Greenslade MSc, RGN
Clinical Nurse Specialist in Hepatology
Royal Free Hampstead NHS Trust
London

Susie Hamlin BSc (Hons), RD
Liver Specialist Dietician
St James's University Hospital
Leeds

Dr Michael Heneghan MD, MMedSc, FRCPI
Consultant Hepatologist
Kings College Hospital NHS Foundation Trust
London

Chris Hill RN, BSc (Hons)
Lecturer Practitioner Intensive Care
Royal Free Hampstead NHS Trust
London

Dr Sarah Hughes MA, MB, BCh, MRCP
Specialist Registrar in Hepatology
Institute of Liver Studies
Kings College Hospital NHS Foundation Trust
London

Catherine Houlston RGN, BSc (Hons), Critical Care Diploma, ENB 100
Practice Development Sister
Addenbrookes Hospital
Cambridge University Hospitals NHS Foundation Trust
Cambridge

Nikie Jervis RGN, ENB A09
Lead Hepatobiliary Oncology Clinical Nurse Specialist
Institute of Liver Studies
Kings College Hospital NHS Foundation Trust
London

Julie Leaper BSc, RD
Liver Specialist Dietician
St James's University Hospital
Leeds

Wendy Littlejohn RGN
Transplant Service Manager
Institute of Liver Studies
Kings College Hospital NHS Foundation Trust
London

Dr Antonis Nikolopoulos MBBS, MRCP
Specialist Registrar
Centre for Hepatology
University College London
Royal Free Hampstead NHS Trust
London

Dr Jude A. Oben BM, BCh(Oxon), PhD, MRCP
Wellcome Trust Senior Lecturer and Consultant Hepatologist
Centre for Hepatology
University College London
Royal Free Hampstead NHS Trust
London

Helen O'Neal RN, BSc (Hons), Dip HE A09
Practice Development Sister
John Farman Intensive Care Unit
Addenbrookes Hospital
Cambridge University Hospitals NHS Foundation Trust
Cambridge

Zebina Ratansi MSc, RGN
Senior Nurse Liver Intensive Care Unit
Kings College Hospital NHS Foundation Trust
London

Joanna Routledge RGN
Transplant Coordinator
Institute of Liver Studies
Kings College Hospital NHS Foundation Trust
London

Suzanne Sargent MSc, PGC (TLHE), BSc (Hons), RGN
Lecturer Practitioner
Institute of Liver Studies
Kings College Hospital NHS Foundation Trust
London

Dr Rachel Taylor RGN, RSCN DipRes, MSc, PhD
Visiting Research Fellow
FN School of Nursing & Midwifery
James Clerk Maxwell Building
Kings College
London

Kerry Webb MSc, RMN
Clinical Nurse Specialist in Addiction Psychiatry
Liver Unit
Queen Elizabeth Hospital
Birmingham
Honorary Lecturer
University of Birmingham

Dr Terence Wong MA, MD, FRCP
Consultant Gastroenterologist
Guys and St. Thomas' NHS Foundation Trust
London

Foreword

The British Liver Nurses Forum (BLNF) began in 1998 with a small group of nurses all with a common interest in caring for patients with liver disease. From this has grown a successful organisation which continues to be steered by nurses passionate about liver nursing. In 2008 the BLNF celebrated 10 years of being an active force in liver nursing, and continuing to strive to improve the quality of care for liver patients, highlight issues related to liver disease and empower liver nurses.

The prominence of liver disease has changed beyond recognition with some disease processes being highlighted both by the media and government. The government's national scoping exercise for liver disease has given the BLNF an opportunity to voice the concerns of nurses within this speciality and raise the profile of liver nursing in the public arena.

The impact of liver disease is rising across the whole of the UK and indeed globally; nurses and other health care professionals are encountering patients with liver disease not just on medical and gastroenterology wards, but in a number of clinical arenas. One of the key drivers that led to the development of the BLNF was to develop, expand and raise the profile of liver nursing; in executing this aim it became apparent that there was a lack of resources for nurses and allied health professionals and most of the available resources were written by eminent hepatologists. This book aims to address this void and provides a textbook that is aimed at nurses and other health care professionals caring for patients with liver disease, to furnish them with current and contemporary evidence and practice.

British Liver Nurses Forum
December 2008

Acknowledgements

I am grateful to all the chapter contributors for all the hard work, support and tolerance during the development of this book. Additionally I would like to offer thanks and appreciation to the following people for their reviews and expert feedback in some of the chapters: Dr Georg Auzinger, Michelle Clayton, Sarah Dunton, Danielle Fullwood, Dr William Gelson, Dr Kevin Gunning, Pauline Hood, Dr Gilbert Park, Zebina Ratansi, Dr Rachel Taylor, Ian Webzell, Dr Terry Wong.

And to the following people for kindly contributing illustrations and histological pictures and photographs: Dr Alberto Quaglia, Professor Bernard Portman, Dr Terry Wong, Mr Hector Vilca-Melendez.

I would personally like to thank both Terry and Michelle, for their unstinting advice and support. Finally I would like to thank my colleagues and family for their continual support, understanding and encouragement whilst preparing this book.

Anatomy and physiology

1

Chris Hill

Introduction

This chapter will provide a brief overview of the anatomy and physiology of the liver, examining the blood supply, internal structures and the most common hepatic functions. It will provide an overview of the pathophysiology of cirrhosis, subsequent chapters will provide more details on particular problems. This chapter is not an exhaustive guide to liver anatomy and physiology, but it is hoped that the reader will gain an appreciation of how complex and far reaching the liver's influence over health can be, and how this function is supported by the structure of the liver.

The liver

The liver is the largest solid organ in the body, weighing approximately 1500 g in adults, and comprises of one fiftieth of the total adult body weight. The liver lies in the right upper quadrant of the abdominal cavity covered by Glisson's capsule, and is therefore protected by the rib cage. The liver has two anatomical lobes (Figure 1.1), with the right being six times larger than the left. The right and left lobes are separated anteriorly by the falciform ligament, and inferiorly by the ligamentum teres. The left lobe also includes the caudate and quadrate lobes. It is

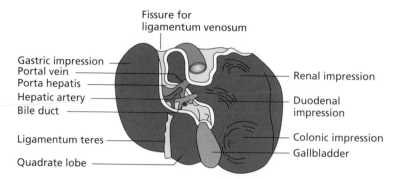

Figure 1.1 Inferior view of the liver. Reproduced from Sherlock S, Dooley J (2002) with permission from Blackwell Science.

separated from these two lobes by the attachment of the ligumentum teres, and the fissures for the ligumentum teres and the ligamentum venosum (Sherlock and Dooley, 2002). The hepatic artery, portal vein, afferent and efferent nerve supply bile ducts and lymphatics enter the liver at a central area known as the hilus. The liver performs many functions in both health and disease, though only the main ones will be described in this chapter. Its nerve supply plays a role in many of these functions (Tiniakos et al., 1996; Sherlock and Dooley, 2002).

The liver has both a venous and arterial blood supply. These provide a total of around 1350 mL/min of blood – around one quarter of the resting cardiac output. The portal vein drains the splanchnic circulation and provides 75% of the liver's blood supply, the hepatic artery supplies the remaining 25%. The venous outflow from the liver is through the hepatic vein into the inferior vena cava. The liver gives very little resistance to the flow of blood from the portal vein, with an average pressure of 9 mmHg (range 5–10 mmHg). This pressure is sufficient to drive 1 L of blood through the liver each minute.

Hepatic microstructure

The liver contains hepatocytes, endothelial cells, Kupffer cells, pit cells and hepatic stellate cells (HSCs). The latter are also called Ito cells, fat-storing cells, perisinusoidal cells and lipocytes. Hepatocytes are the liver parenchymal cells and comprise of approximately 60% of the liver; endothelial cells line the walls of sinusoids (see below); Kupffer cells are phagocytic cells found on the walls of sinusoids that were first observed by Karl Wilhelm von Kupffer in 1876 (Haubrich, 2004). Pit cells are a type of natural killer cell found in the liver, their name comes from their characteristic cytoplasmic granules resembling the pits in a grape (Wisse et al., 1976). HSCs are a major regulator of normal liver homeostasis (Li and Friedman, 2001) and are found in the space of Disse (see below).

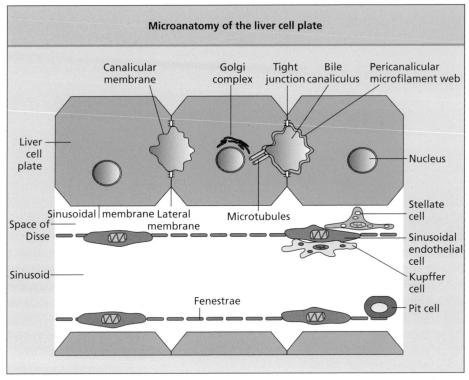

Microanatomy of the liver cell plate

© Elsevier 2006. Bacon, O'Grady, Di Bisceglie and Lake: Comprehensive Clinical Hepatology, 2nd edition

Figure 1.2 The microanatomy of the liver cell plate, showing the relationship of the four non-parenchymal cells to the hepatocytes. Kupffer cells and pit cells lie within the sinusoidal lumen. Endothelial cells separate the sinusoidal lumen from the space of Disse. Stellate cells (lipocytes) lie within the space of Disse. Reproduced from Bacon et al. (2006) with permission from Elsevier.

The portal vein and hepatic artery branch repeatedly until blood from the finest branches of the portal vein and hepatic artery flow into 'sinusoids'. These are lined with endothelial cells and are similar to capillaries in other tissues. The sinusoids drain into fine central veins which link up with other central veins before draining into the hepatic vein. The arterial and venous supplies are separate until they mix within the sinusoid.

Hepatocytes are arranged in thin layers (hepatic plates) as shown in Figure 1.2, giving a maximum surface area for exchange of substances with the blood. The hepatocytes are separated from the blood by the 'space of Disse' and the endothelial cells. The space of Disse contains microvilli projecting from the hepatocytes, HSCs and a low-density extracellular matrix (ECM). HSCs encircle the sinusoid within the space of Disse.

Liver endothelial cells have many holes (fenestrations), not possessed by other endothelial cells, which enable large molecules such as albumin to pass between the blood and the space of Disse. The low-density ECM in the space of Disse allows molecules to pass freely but still supports the overall structure, and the hepatocyte microvilli provide a large surface area for passage of substances into and out of the hepatocytes.

Bile canaliculi are minute channels between adjacent hepatocytes that deliver bile into bile ductules in the portal area. The bile is kept apart from the blood and the space of Disse.

Many organs have a 'functional unit' that is defined as the smallest section of the organ that can carry out the basic function of that organ. An example is the nephron – the functional unit of the kidney. The functional unit of the liver is not self-apparent, and has been extensively debated. The liver can be imagined as divided into 'classical' lobules with a central venule in the middle, and in some of the corners of the polygon (typically drawn as a hexagon) surrounding this is a 'portal triad' containing branches of the portal vein and the hepatic artery, and a bile duct.

Rappaport et al. (1954) also defined a functional unit for the liver, the 'liver acinus', a volume of liver between a distributory branch of the portal vein and the central vein(s) that it drains into. It is further divided into three zones: zone 1 nearest the liver vascular inflow; zone 3 nearest the central venule where blood leaves the hepatocytes; and zone 2 between them (Figure 1.3). Zone 3 suffers the most from injury whether viral, toxic or anoxic (Sherlock and Dooley, 2002). A slightly different concept was later proposed by Matsumoto and Kawakami (1982). In both concepts the different areas receive different levels of oxygenation and substrates (such as glucose) as blood flows through the liver. They also differ to some extent in the metabolic functions they carry out (Kietzmann and Jungermann, 1997).

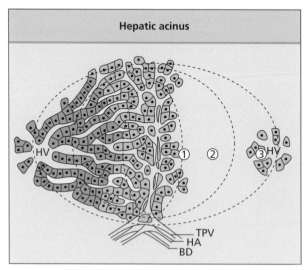

Elsevier 2006. Bacon, O'Grady, Di Bisceglie and Lake:
Comprehensive Clinical Hepatology, 2nd edition

Figure 1.3 Hepatic acinus. Reproduced from Bacon et al. (2006) with permission from Elsevier. (HV = hepatic venule; HA = hepatic artery; TPV = portal vein; BD = bile duct).

Carbohydrate metabolism

The liver has a central role in the maintenance of blood glucose levels. It supplies glucose when blood levels are low and takes it up when supply is plentiful.

Glucose is stored within hepatocytes by converting it to glycogen (glycogenesis). Glycogen is a branched polymer, essentially a long string of glucose molecules joined together, with one chain sometimes dividing into two. Storing glucose within the cell as glucose molecules would significantly alter osmotic pressure within the cell leading to problems with intracellular–extracellular fluid balance. Hepatocytes can store up to 5–8% of their weight as glycogen; the adult liver stores on average about 80 g.

Glycogen is readily broken down into glucose (glycogenolysis), so is a good source of energy for sudden, strenuous activity. Glycogenolysis involves enzymes 'chipping off' glucose molecules from the glycogen and can be triggered by glucagon (produced in response to a low blood sugar) and adrenaline.

During fasting around 11% of glycogen stores are used each hour. After a few hours the liver increasingly turns to gluconeogenesis to supply glucose. This is the production of new glucose from non-carbohydrates, mainly lactate, amino acids and glycerol (not fatty acids). The supply of glucose shifts between directly supplied dietary glucose, glucose from glycogenesis and glucose from gluconeogenesis over the day (Figure 1.4).

Glucose metabolism is controlled by hormones as described, but there is increasing recognition that it is also controlled by genes cycling in a circadian rhythm (Rudic et al., 2004; Pititsyn et al., 2006). The liver has its own circadian rhythm that is synchronised with the 'master' circadian rhythm clock in the suprachiasmatic nucleus in the brain by signals such as glucocorticoid release (Reddy et al., 2007).

Muscle cells can also store glycogen (up to 1–3% of their weight). The much larger total mass of muscle can store more glycogen than liver. However muscle

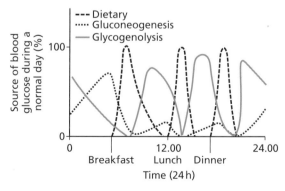

Figure 1.4 Glucogenesis. Reproduced from Baynes and Dominiczak (2005) *Medical Biochemistry*, 2nd edn, p 158, with permission from Mosby.

cells do not possess the enzyme necessary to enable release of glucose from the cell into the blood. A small amount of gluconeogenesis takes place in the kidneys.

Fat metabolism

The liver plays an essential role in the digestion of dietary fats. It produces bile salts which are essential for the emulsification of fats within the gut. Almost all fats in the diet are absorbed from the intestines into the lymphatic system. The fats are broken down into monoglycerides and fatty acids that are absorbed into the intestinal epithelial cells and then enter the lymphatic system as tiny, dispersed particles called chylomicrons.

Functions of the liver in the metabolism of fat can be summarised as:

- Oxidation of fatty acids to supply energy
- Synthesis of cholesterol, phospholipids and lipoproteins
- Synthesis of fats from proteins and carbohydrates

Fatty acids typically contain 16 carbon atoms. To use them for energy the liver splits them into acetyl coA (two carbon atoms long) by beta-oxidation. The acetyl coA can enter the tricarboxylic acid cycle and be used directly as an energy source. Beta-oxidation can take place in all cells in the body, but the liver is particularly efficient at it and can produce more than it needs. The excess acetyl coA is converted into the very soluble acetoacetic acid which can pass easily into other cells where it is converted back into acetyl CoA and used for energy.

Some of the acetoacetic acid is converted into beta-hydroxybutyric acid and very small amounts into acetone. These can also pass easily into other cells around the body where they can be used for energy. Their blood concentrations are normally very low. However in starvation and diabetic ketoacidosis the concentrations of these three substances can rise to many times normal and the presence of acetoacetic acid can be detected in the urine (usually called ketones on the dipstick). This implies that much fat is being metabolised to provide energy.

If an excess of carbohydrates and proteins are presented to the liver they will be converted into fatty acids. Some will be stored in the liver (5% of liver weight is due to fat), the rest will be released into the blood and taken up by adipocytes and stored as fat. Adipocytes can synthesise minute quantities of fat from carbohydrate but the majority takes place in the liver. Fatty acids are continually cycling between the liver and adipose tissue, half the fatty acid in the plasma is replaced every 2–3 minutes.

Protein metabolism

Dietary proteins are digested and broken down into amino acids over several hours. These enter the blood stream and are rapidly absorbed into cells all over the body. Subsequently there is a constant interchange and equilibrium between plasma amino acids, plasma proteins, amino acids in cells and cellular proteins. Plasma proteins can be rapidly degraded within the reticuloendothelial system. Liver and other cells can rapidly form and degrade proteins. Overall, in health, there is a constant state of equilibrium.

Amino acids can also be used for energy after removing nitrogen, but this leads to the release of the highly toxic substance ammonia (NH_3). The liver removes ammonia from the blood and converts it to urea (and a minor amount into glutamine). The biochemical process for doing this is known as the urea cycle. Some of the chemical steps in the urea cycle are present in other tissues and are important for removal of ammonia from those tissues, but the complete cycle is present only in the liver. Elevated levels of serum ammonia are seen in both acute and chronic liver disease. In acute liver failure this is linked to the impairment in the conversion of ammonia to urea due to hepatic necrosis. In chronic liver disease the rate of urea synthesis is markedly reduced, which is attributed to several factors such as portosystemic shunting and increased intestinal production (Luxon, 2006). Hyperammonaemia has been linked to hepatic encephalopathy and is discussed in depth in Chapter 6.

Protein synthesis

The liver can synthesise about 48 g of protein per day. Albumin is the major protein synthesised (approximately 12–15 g) and an important constituent of blood as it is the predominant cause of the oncotic pressure of blood. Albumin also acts as an acid–base buffer and binds drugs and electrolytes in the blood. Its synthesis by the liver is affected by nutritional status, and the blood albumin level is sometimes used as an indicator of nutritional status.

The acute phase response is a non-specific response to tissue injury or infection. This involves a change in the concentration of a number of proteins in the blood known as acute phase reactants. These are defined by having a change in concentration of larger than or equal to 25% by 1 week after the initial injury or infection. Some proteins increase: these *positive* acute phase reactants are predominantly synthesised by the liver and include alpha-1 antitrypsin, coagulation proteins and C-reactive protein (CRP). Substances whose concentration decreases as part of the acute phase response are known as *negative* acute phase reactants. These include albumin and transferrin.

CRP is a binding protein (opsonin) that binds to macromolecules released by infective agents or damaged tissue and enhances their phagocytosis. The blood level of CRP is often used as a marker of infection – although it can be raised as part of a general inflammatory response with no infection present.

Clotting factors

The liver is the site of synthesis of all clotting factors and their inhibitors (Amitrano et al., 2002). The prothrombin time (PT) is an index of clotting function, which depends on the production of clotting factors in the liver and can be used as a measure of the liver's synthetic ability. Liver failure will lead to a prolongation of the PT with the degree of prolongation related to the severity of liver failure. Liver disease can also cause problems with haemostasis in other ways such as causing a drop in platelet numbers and function.

Vitamin K is needed by the liver for the normal production of clotting factors II, VII, IX and X. Vitamin K deficiency will cause a reduction in the levels of these factors (which will be reflected in a prolonged PT). Liver disease does not directly cause a vitamin K deficiency, but vitamin K is a fat-soluble vitamin that needs biliary salts for its absorption. Thus cholestasis can cause reduced absorption of vitamin K.

Storage of vitamins/iron

The vitamin stored in greatest quantity in the liver is vitamin A (in hepatic stellate cells), but large quantities of vitamins D and B_{12} are normally stored as well. Sufficient quantities of vitamin A can be stored to prevent deficiency for as long as 10 months, vitamin D for 3–4 months, and vitamin B_{12} for over 1 year. The liver is also involved in storage of iron and copper.

Blood cleansing

An important non-metabolic function of the liver is the 'cleansing' of blood leaving the splanchnic circulation by Kupffer cells. The gut is heavily populated by large numbers of a multiplicity of bacteria and there is a potential for bacteria to be able to leave the gut and enter the vascular system. Any bacteria in the portal vein will pass into the liver and should be phagocytosed by Kupffer cells.

Processing of drugs and other xenobiotics

Xenobiotics are substances that are foreign to the body (e.g. drugs). They are potentially toxic and systems have evolved to eliminate them from the body. The most obvious is urinary excretion, though some substances are secreted into bile by the liver (but many are then reabsorbed from the intestine).

Most elimination takes place via the kidneys. These can efficiently eliminate water-soluble xenobiotics but less so lipophilic xenobiotics. The body first metabolises these to less lipophilic substances that can be more easily eliminated by the kidneys. This takes place predominantly in the liver.

Xenobiotic metabolism in the liver involves two kinds of biochemical reaction known as phase I and phase II reactions which often take place sequentially. Phase

I reactions generally involve a family of enzymes known as the hepatic cytochrome P450 system. Phase II reactions involve a chemical reaction in which a large molecule is added to the drug. Again this makes the drug more water soluble and easier to excrete from the body.

Enzymes are often thought of as being specific for a single substrate, but P450 enzymes may metabolise many different drugs. They can be clinically important in a number of ways. When multiple drugs are administered concurrently they can 'compete' for metabolism by the same enzyme and inhibit each other's metabolism. An example is cardiac arrythmias, or central nervous system (CNS) seizures, caused by an increased theophylline level when it is given with erythromycin. In enzyme induction the normal level of an enzyme is increased and drugs metabolised by that enzyme are metabolised faster then normal. Enzyme induction can be produced by some drugs, foods, alcohol and smoking. The levels of particular P450 enzymes can also be affected by genetics, leading to individual and racial differences in metabolism of drugs.

The portal vein delivers blood from the gut directly to the liver, enterally ingested substances are exposed to the enzymes in the liver before they get to the rest of the body. This is refered to as first-pass metabolism. Some drugs are metabolised so efficiently by the liver that little actually gets through to the rest of the body. The liver also plays a major role in the elimination of hormones and activated clotting factors.

Excocrine function

The liver also has an exocrine function. About 500 mL of bile is secreted each day, consisting of water, inorganic electrolytes and organic solutes such as bile salts. Bile salts are the sodium and potassium salts of bile acids and have a detergent-like effect in the gut lumen, emulsifying dietary fat to aid its digestion. Bile secretion is an excretory route for bile pigments, cholesterol, steroids, heavy metals and some drugs. Patients who have jaundice due to intra- or extrahepatic obstruction of the bile duct usually have raised blood levels of cholesterol and alkaline phosphatase. Bile is an alkaline solution containing bicarbonate (secreted by both hepatocytes and biliary duct cells) and aids in the neutralisation of acid chyme entering the duodenum from the stomach.

Two major primary bile acids are synthesised in the liver from cholesterol at the rate of 0.5 g/day (cholic acid and chenodeoxycholic acid). Secondary bile acids are produced within the gut by the action of bacteria on primary bile acids. Cholic acid is converted to deoxycholic acid and chenodeoxycholic acid to lithocholic acid.

Bile is continuously secreted by hepatocytes into biliary canaliculi. Between meals contraction of the sphincter of Oddi causes bile to accumulate in the gallbladder where the bile salts are concentrated. The most important trigger for relaxation of the sphincter of Oddi and release of bile is return of bile salts to the liver from the splanchnic circulation.

The majority of bile salts (90–95%) are reabsorbed from the small intestine, most from the terminal ileum (meaning that a large proportion remains throughout the small intestine to promote fat absorption). The remaining bile salts enter the colon where more are reabsorbed. Those lost in the stool are replaced by synthesis in the liver. The total pool of bile salts (approx 2.5 g) is recycled up to six to eight times in a day.

Bilirubin

The bile pigments bilirubin and biliverdin are produced from substances containing haem such as haemoglobin. Red blood cells have a life span of around 110 days, with aged red cells being destroyed mainly by the reticuloendothelial cells of spleen, lymph nodes, bone marrow and liver. The haemoglobin is first metabolised by the enzyme heme oxygenase into biliverdin, and then converted to bilirubin. Bilirubin is not soluble in water and in the blood it is transported attached to serum albumin (this is referred to as unconjugated bilirubin).

In the liver the bilirubin has two glucuronate groups attached (conjugated) to it. This conjugated bilirubin is then excreted into the bile canaliculi. Bacteria in the gut convert bilirubin to stercobilinogen, which then forms stercobilin. Most stercobilin is excreted in the faeces and is responsible for the colour of faeces. Some stercobilin is reabsorbed from the gut and can then be re-excreted by either the liver or kidneys.

Liver cirrhosis/fibrosis

Liver capacity for regeneration following a single insult is excellent. A hepactectomy may involve the removal of two thirds of the liver, but the remaining hepatocytes can reproliferate to restore the mass of the organ within days to weeks (Guangsheng and Steer, 2006). However chronic or repetitive injury results in fibrosis, which can develop into cirrhosis (Figure 1.5, Plate 1). Cirrhosis represents the end stage of many different liver disorders, such as alcoholism and chronic hepatitis. Fibrosis and cirrhosis are part of a continuous disease spectrum.

Liver fibrosis is characterised by the production of excess extracellular material in the space of Disse and a loss of fenestrations from the sinusoidal endothelial cells. This is referred to as capilliarisation. The microvilli of the hepatocytes disappear and overall there is a reduction in the ability to exchange substances between the blood and hepatocytes.

HSCs are the key cells in fibrosis. Inflammatory cells move into injured areas of liver and these, together with damaged and regenerating hepatocytes, release signalling molecules (cytokines) which 'activate' the HSCs. Activated HSCs

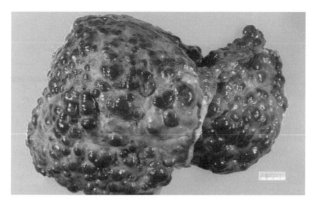

Figure 1.5 Photograph showing extensive liver cirrhosis. Used with permission from Bernard Portmann. For a colour version of this figure, please see Plate 1 in the colour plate section.

profilerate and secrete fibrillar collagens producing an increase in extracellular matrix in the space of Disse. Other changes that take place in HSCs when they become activated are the loss of the retinoid (vitamin A) droplets and the production of smooth muscle actin.

Cirrhosis is characterised by diffuse alteration of the normal liver architecture with nodules of regenerating hepatocytes surrounded by fibrous bands. Blood can be shunted along 'bypass' vessels avoiding hepatocytes, and so do not take part in the normal exchange of substances between blood and hepatoctye. There is also interruption of biliary channels which can prevent normal drainage of bile produced by the hepatocytes. Cirrhosis results from necrosis and then nodular regrowth of hepatocytes. It is a diffuse problem, not local to any part of the liver, and the ultimate pattern of damage is much the same regardless of cause. The Child-Pugh score is used to assess the prognosis and appropriate treatment in cirrhosis and is demonstrated in Table 1.1.

Table 1.1 The Child-Pugh score. Adapted from Bacon et al. (2006).

	Points scored for increasing abnormality		
Clinical and biochemical assessment criteria	1	2	3
Encephalopathy (grade)	None	1 and 2	3 and 4
Ascites	Absent	Slight	Moderate
Albumin (g/L)	>35	28–35	<28
INR	<1.7	1.7–2.2	>2.2
Bilirubin (μmol/L)	<34	34–50	>50
Bilirubin (for primary biliary cirrhosis) (μmol/L)	<69	69–170	>170
Top score	Grade A 5–6	Grade B 7–9	Grade C 10–15
Survival in chronic liver disease at 1 year	Grade A 84%	Grade B 62%	Grade C 42%

Table 1.2 Complications associated with liver cirrhosis.

Portal hypertension
  Ascites
  Varices
    Oesophagus
    Stomach
    Rectum (haemorrhoids)
    Abdominal vein distension (caput medusae)
  Splenomegaly
    Anaemia
    Thrombocytopenia
    Leucopenia
  Portopulmonary shunts
    Decreased blood oxygenation

Liver failure
  Deranged clotting
  Thrombocytopenia
  Elevated bilirubin
  Hepatorenal failure
  Hepatic encephalopathy
  Immune system dysfunction
  Hypoalbuminaemia
    Oedema
  Increased skin pigmentation
  Fetor hepaticus
  Decreased hormone metabolism
    Gynaecomastia
    Testicular atrophy
    Loss of body hair
    Spider angiomas
    Palmar erythema
    Menstrual dysfunction
    Increased antidiuretic hormone and aldosterone

Hepatocellular carcinoma

Cirrhosis can be classified as micronodular or macronodular. In micronodular cirrhosis the regenerating nodules are less than 3 mm in diameter and the fibrous bands separating the nodules are usually thin. In macronodular cirrhosis the nodules are over 3 mm in diameter. There is a tendency for nodules to increase in size over time, and micronodular cirrhosis can become macronodular. Cirrhosis is often classified by its presumed cause, histologically; early stages may show evidence of the cause, but this cannot be determined from the histology later on.

Many health problems are caused by cirrhosis (Table 1.2); some are the result of the development of portal hypertension – an increase in the blood pressure in the portal vein. The cause of this is complex and not completely understood. The disruption of vascular channels caused by alteration of normal liver vascular architecture predisposes to this pressure increase. Additionally, activated HSCs produce smooth muscle actin within the cell and also become sensitive to the powerful vasoconstrictor endothelin. Liver injury also results in a reduction in production of the vasodilator nitric oxide which would normally oppose the action of the endothelin (Groszmann et al., 2001). This results in the contraction of the HSCs which increase sinusoidal resistance and contribute to the development of portal hypertension.

Portal hypertension leads to further problems. Portosystemic shunts develop as the increased pressure leads to the development of collateral channels between the portal vein and systemic veins. One manifestation of this is varices, thin-walled varicosities that either form in the oesophagus, stomach or rectum. These are prone to rupture which can lead to fatal bleeding (see Chapter 4). Clotting problems caused by deranged liver function can make this complication even more difficult to deal with which is described further in Chapter 4.

Ascites refers to the development of larger than normal quantities of fluid in the peritoneal cavity; patients with severe ascites may have large volumes of fluid with consequent problems such as abdominal discomfort and dyspnoea. The development of ascites is still not completely understood, however Chapter 5 examines the proposed hypothesis. Hepatic encephalopathy is another manifestation of advanced liver disease. Again the pathogenesis is not fully understood, but is thought to be related to the inability of the liver to clear toxic substances from the blood. This is discussed in more depth in Chapter 6.

Fibrosis and cirrhosis can be asymptomatic; the majority of hepatic functional capacity must be lost before hepatic failure ensues. Clinically this is important as many patients do not present until after they have severe structural injury to their liver. Liver fibrosis and cirrhosis have traditionally been viewed as irreversible; however there is evidence now that fibrosis at least is reversible under some conditions (Friedman, 2003). Iredale (2003) looks forward to a future where fibrosis and cirrhosis are treatable.

Chapter summary

This chapter has reviewed the more important aspects of liver anatomy and physiology. It has shown how the normal structure of the liver superbly supports its physiological functions, and how the development of an abnormal structure in cirrhosis is detrimental. An understanding of the functions of the liver will help the health care professional appreciate how liver disease can affect people in so many different ways, and can improve the quality of care given to people with liver disease.

References

Amitrano L, Guardascione MA, Brancaccio V, Balzano A (2002) Coagulation disorders in liver disease. *Seminars in Liver Disease* **22**(1):83–96

Bacon BR, O'Grady JG, Di Bisceglie AM, Lake JR (eds) (2006) *Comprehensive Clinical Hepatology*, 2nd edn. Mosby Elsevier, Philadelphia

Baynes JW, Dominiczak MH (2005) *Medical Biochemistry*, 2nd edn. Mosby Elsevier, Philadelphia

Friedman SL (2003) Liver fibrosis – from bench to bedside. *Journal of Hepatology* 38:S38-S53

Groszmann RJ, Loureiro MR, Tsai M-H (2001) The biology of portal hypertension. In: Arias IM (ed) *The Liver: Biology and Pathobiology*, 4th edn. Lippincott Williams & Wilkins, London

Guangsheng G, Steer CJ (2006) Cellular biology of normal liver function. In: Bacon BR, O'Grady JG, Di Bisceglie AM, Lake JR (eds) *Comprehensive Clinical Hepatology*, 2nd edn. Mosby Elsevier, Philadelphia

Haubrich WS (2004) Kupffer of Kupffer cells. *Gastroenterology* 27:16

Iredale JP (2003) Cirrhosis: new research provides a basis for rational and targeted treatments. *British Medical Journal* 327:143–147

Kietzmann T, Jungermann K (1997) Metabolic zonation of liver parenchyma and its short-term and long-term regulation. In: Vidal-Vanaclocha F (ed) *Functional Hetererogeneity of Liver Tissue*. R.G. Landes Company, Austin

Li D, Friedman SL (2001) Hepatic stellate cells: morphology, function and regulation. In: Arias IM (ed) *The Liver: Biology and Pathobiology*, 4th edn. Lippincott Williams & Wilkins, London

Luxon BA (2006) Functions of the liver. In: Bacon BR, O'Grady JG, Di Bisceglie AM, Lake JR (eds) *Comprehensive Clinical Hepatology*, 2nd edn. Mosby Elsevier, Philadelphia

Matsumoto T, Kawakami M (1982) The unit-concept of hepatic parenchyma: a re-examination based on angioarchitectural studies. *Acta Pathologica Japonica* 32(suppl. 2):285–314

Pititsyn AA, Svonic S, Conrad SA, Scott LK, Mynatt RL, Gimble JM (2006) Circadian clocks are resounding in peripheral tissues. *PLoS Computational Biology* 2(3):e16

Rappaport AM, Borowy ZJ, Lougheed WM, Lotto WN (1954) Subdivision of hexagonal liver lobules into a structural and functional unit: role in hepatic physiology and pathology. *The Anatomical Record* 119(1):11–33

Reddy AB, Maywood ES, Karp NA, King VM, Inoue Y, Gonzalez FJ, Lilley KS, Kyriacou CP, Hastings MH (2007) Glucocorticoid signalling synchronizes the liver circadian transcriptome. *Hepatology* 45:1478–1488

Rudic RD, McNamara P, Curtis AM, Boston RC, Panda S, et al. (2004) BMAL1 and CLOCK, two essential components of the circadian clock, are involved in glucose homeostasis. *PLoS Computational Biology* 2(11):e377

Sherlock S, Dooley J (2002) *Diseases of the Liver and Biliary System*, 11th edn. Blackwell Publishing, Oxford

Tiniakos DG, Lee JA, Burt AD (1996) Innervation of the liver: morphology and function. *Liver* 16:151–160

Wisse E, van't Noordende JM, van der Meulen J, Deums WTh (1976) The pit cell: description of a new type of cell in rat liver sinusoids and peripheral blood. *Cell and Tissue Research* 173:423–443

Assessment of liver function and diagnostic studies

2

Lynda Greenslade

Introduction

This chapter looks at the different ways in which liver function is assessed and the various techniques used to diagnose liver disease. A complete medical history, complete physical examination, evaluation of liver function tests and further invasive and non-invasive tests are imperative to ensure an accurate diagnosis. Nurses in advanced and specialist roles have autonomy with decision making (RCN, 2002; McGee and Castledine, 2004), i.e. taking a comprehensive history, making a physical assessment and the ordering of investigations as a central part of their role. The key to making a diagnosis of liver disease is being able to take a comprehensive history with emphasis on the risk factors and linking of information gained to the ordering of relevant tests and diagnostic studies.

Patient history

A comprehensive history from a patient with liver disease is essential as many vague or non-specific symptoms may be of considerable significance but may not be apparent to the patient, e.g. lethargy, itch and malaise, and can occur in up to 60% of patients with both acute and chronic liver disease (Howdle, 2006). An important aspect of gaining information is to ask the patient directly, questions that may identify risk factors; sometimes these are of a sensitive nature which some patients may be guarded against. Patient history needs to be sensitively handled to ensure accuracy and highlight the need for further enquiry. Many patients will complain of general malaise and fatigue, particularly in primary biliary cirrhosis, autoimmune hepatitis and viral hepatitis, which will often have a detrimental effect on the patients' quality of life (Howdle, 2006).

Many patients presenting to their general practitioner (GP) with liver disease often have non-specific symptoms and are frequently frustrated at the delay in making a diagnosis or being referred to a gastroenterologist or hepatologist. Many GPs, for example, may not have seen a case of haemochromatosis (Emery and Rose, 2001) or primary biliary cirrhosis (PBC).

When gathering information it is important to ask in detail about the following predisposing risk factors for liver disease (Howdle, 2006):

- **Viral hepatitis** – history of any previous intravenous drug use however brief or remote (as the hepatitis C virus may have been latent for up to 30 years). Any sharing of needles or equipment used to take drugs, their sexual history and orientation and known high-risk factors such as haemodialysis
- **Alcohol consumption** – includes an accurate history of the quantity, strength of alcohol, pattern of alcohol consumption and age when drinking started. It is important to know if the patient drinks every day, at weekends only, first thing in the morning and when they had their last drink. Any previous admissions for alcohol-related reasons, drink–driving offences or a family history of alcohol-related liver disease are also significant
- **Careful medication history** – to identify any prescription, over-the-counter medications, herbal or Chinese remedies or recreational drugs, which may cause abnormal liver function tests. With an elderly or confused patient, contacting the GP will give a more accurate drug history, as it is not just recent medication used that can cause abnormal liver function tests
- **Past medical history** – previous episodes of jaundice may indicate a chronic viral hepatitis and previous blood transfusions/blood products either in the UK or abroad may increase the risk of hepatitis B or C. A history of ulcerative colitis may indicate primary sclerosing cholangitis (PSC) and previous gallstone disease can recur. Also previous biliary surgery may have caused a biliary stricture
- **Family history** – this may signpost a possible cause of liver disease, such as hereditary haemochromatosis or Wilson's disease where family links are revealed. A family history of heavy alcohol use or alcohol-related liver disease is also linked to a genetic cause and is often the most common familial condition that patients are aware of due to the impact on the family's life. Some patients with autoimmune disease may have a relative with the same or other autoimmune liver disease or a non-liver autoimmune condition such as rheumatoid arthritis or thyroid disease. Where a mother has hepatitis B this would be relevant to her children, as hepatitis B could have been acquired through

perinatal transmission. A family history of diabetes may also be linked to non-alcoholic steatohepatitis (NASH), autoimmune hepatitis or genetic haemochromatosis

■ **Occupational history** – to exclude causes of liver disease from working with industrial chemicals and toxins, or from working with or keeping animals. Any recent overseas travel where exposure to hepatitis A or E may have occurred is also pertinent

Signs of liver disease

There are many signs of liver disease, which vary according to the severity of the disease (Figure 2.1). A general examination of each body system may reveal signs of liver disease. Observations may reveal muscle wasting, loss of fat deposits and

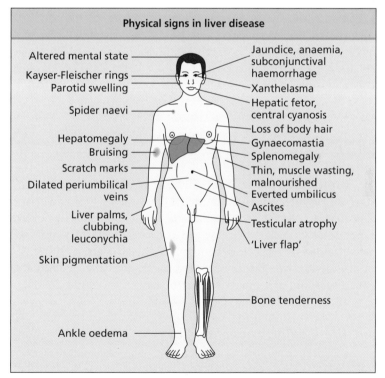

© Elsevier 2006. Bacon, O'Grady, Di Bisceglie and Lake: Comprehensive Clinical Hepatology, 2nd edition

Figure 2.1   Physical signs in liver disease. Reproduced from Bacon et al. (2006) with permission from Elsevier.

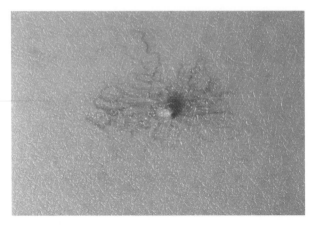

Figure 2.2   A spider naevus. The central arteriole resembles a spider's body and the radiating vessels the spider's legs. Reprinted with permission from eMedicine.com, 2007. Available at: http://www.emedicine.com/derm.topic293.htm. For a colour version of this figure, please see Plate 2 in the colour plate section.

thinning of the skin, which indicate malnutrition and severity of the liver disease. There may be jaundice, abdominal swelling and leg oedema, which would indicate severe liver disease; obesity may suggest NASH, and excessive spider naevi (Figure 2.2, Plate 2) may suggest cirrhosis due to alcohol abuse (Howdle, 2006).

Laboratory tests

Biochemical tests are used to detect liver diseases, to direct the diagnostic work-up, estimate the severity of liver disease and evaluate therapy (Sherlock and Dooley, 2002). Liver function tests (Table 2.1) are the first line of diagnosis of liver disease but there may be other reasons for any abnormal readings so an abnormality may need to be confirmed by repeating the test (Green and Flamm, 2002). The typical liver function tests provide information regarding synthetic function and cellular damage, but also about any biliary tree involvement (Stonesifer, 2004).

Tests which reflect liver hepatic injury

The aminotransferases, alanine aminotransferase (ALT) and aspartate aminotransferase (AST), are the most commonly used markers of hepatic injury and are often the first clue to practitioners that further investigations are warranted (Johnson, 1999; Stonesifer, 2004). Imperial and Keeffe (2006) suggest that different degrees of elevation are useful as diagnostic clues. For example, patients with cirrhosis often have slightly elevated AST or ALT levels, whereas patients with acute

Table 2.1 Normal values of common liver function tests and causes of derangement in liver disease. Adapted from Sherlock and Dooley (2002), Stonesifer (2004).

Test	Normal range	Basis of abnormality	Associated liver disease
Total bilirubin	<17 µmol/L (0.3–1.0 mg/dL)	Decreased hepatic clearance	Diagnosis of jaundice and assessment of severity
Conjugated (direct bilirubin)	<5 µmol/L (0.1–0.3 mg/dL)		Gilbert's syndrome, haemolysis
Alkaline phosphatase	35–115 U/L	Overproduction and leakage into serum	Modest elevation – many types of liver disease Marked elevation – cholestasis, hepatic infiltration, alcoholic hepatitis
Aspartate transaminase (AST/SGOT)	7–40 U/L	Leakage from damaged hepatocytes	Early diagnosis of hepatocellular disease; follow progress
Alanine aminotransferase (ALT/SGPT)	3–30 U/L	Leakage from damaged hepatocytes	ALT lower than AST in alcohol-induced liver disease
γ-glutamyl transpeptidase (GGT)	2–65 U/L	Overproduction and leakage into serum	Diagnosis of alcohol abuse, marker biliary cholestasis
5'-nucleotidase	0–17 U/L	Overproduction and leakage into serum	Modest elevation – many types of liver disease Marked elevation – cholestasis, hepatic infiltration, alcoholic hepatitis
Albumin	35–54 g/L	Decreased synthesis	Assesses severity of hepatic synthetic function
Prothrombin time (PT) after vitamin K	12–16 seconds	Decreased synthesis	Assesses severity of hepatic function

ischaemia or hyperacute liver injury, e.g. paracetamol (acetaminophen) hepatoxicity, have the highest peaks (Johnson, 1999).

Additionally the AST:ALT ratio can be useful for diagnostic purposes. An AST:ALT ratio of 2:1 can be suggestive of alcohol-related liver disease; this partly stems from the depletion of vitamin B_6 (Johnson, 1999; Imperial and Keeffe 2006).

- ALT (normal level 3–30 U/L) is an enzyme produced within the cells of the liver, and is the most sensitive marker for hepatocyte damage. The level of ALT abnormality is increased in conditions where cells of the liver have been inflamed or have undergone cell death. As the cells are damaged, ALT leaks into the bloodstream leading to a rise in the serum level. Any form of hepatocyte damage can result in an elevation in the ALT
- AST (normal level 7–40 U/L). This enzyme also reflects damage to the hepatic cell but is less specific for liver disease. AST may be elevated in other conditions such as myocardial infarction. Although AST is not as specific for the liver as the ALT, ratios between ALT and AST are useful to physicians in assessing the aetiology of liver enzyme abnormalities, for example where the ALT is lower than AST in alcohol-related liver disease

Tests that demonstrate cholestatic liver disease/injury

The tests that are usually used to define cholestasis are alkaline phosphatase (ALP) and gammaglutamyl transpeptidase (GGT), which in cholestasis typically become elevated in 90% of patients several days after bile duct obstruction or intrahepatic cholestasis (Johnson, 1999; Imperial and Keeffe, 2006):

- ALP (normal level 35–115 U/L) is an enzyme associated with, but not specific to, the biliary tract, as it is also found in bone and the placenta. Renal or intestinal damage can also cause an increase of ALP. If the ALP is elevated, biliary tract damage and inflammation should be considered. However, other aetiologies must also be ruled out which can be achieved by requesting isoenzymes. A common method to assess the aetiology of the elevated ALP is to determine whether the GGT is elevated or whether other liver function tests are abnormal (such as bilirubin). Because of its long half-life of 17 days, the serum ALP will remain elevated for more than 1 week after relief of biliary obstruction (Martin and Friedman, 2004). ALP may be elevated in primary biliary cirrhosis, alcoholic hepatitis, PSC and choledocholithiasis
- GGT (normal level 2–65 U/L) is also produced by the bile ducts. However, it is not very specific to the liver or bile ducts so levels can be increased in other diseases such as renal failure, myocardial infarction and pancreatitic disease. It can be used to confirm that the ALP is of hepatic aetiology (Martin and Friedman, 2004; Imperial and Keefe, 2006). Medications such as phenytoin and alcohol consumption of more than three drinks per day can induce increases in GGT. However, as the half-life of GGT is 26 days, its surreptitious

use as a marker for alcohol consumption is limited (Martin and Friedman, 2004)

- 5′-Nucleotidase (normal level 0–17 U/L) is more specific for liver injury than ALP and GGT, and therefore corresponds more closely with hepatobiliary injury (Stonesifer, 2004). It is a useful indictor in diagnosing liver disease in children and pregnancy

Tests of synthetic function

- Bilirubin (total bilirubin normal level <17 µmol/L). Bilirubin results from the enzymatic breakdown of haemoglobin (haem) released from red blood cells. The unconjugated bilirubin is conjugated with glucuronic acid in the hepatocyctes to increase its water solubility and this is then excreted into bile (Johnson, 1999). A more detailed description of the bilirubin metabolism pathway is given in Chapter 3. Bilirubin levels >35–50 µmol/L indicate jaundice. Bilirubin measurements are usually reported as total bilirubin, which represents both the conjugated and unconjugated fractions. Other laboratory measurements of bilirubin can be more specific, and can establish which fraction of bilirubin is raised. This allows the causes hyperbilirubinaemia to be differentiated. Direct serum bilirubin corresponds to the levels of conjugated bilirubin and indirect represents unconjugated bilirubin (value obtained by subtracting the conjugated value from total bilirubin) (Martin and Friedman, 2004). Different causes of hyperbilirubinaemia and the management of jaundice are discussed in Chapter 3
- Albumin (normal level 35–54 g/L) is one of many proteins synthesised by the liver, and accounts for 65% of serum protein (Martin and Friedman, 2004). Albumin has a half-life of 21 days and thus serum albumin concentrations are slow to change in response to alterations in protein synthesis (Johnson, 1999). In chronic liver disease the albumin may be low (hypoalbuminaemia), indicating a diminished synthetic function of the liver (normal rate 12–15 g/day). Such findings suggest a diagnosis of cirrhosis and are an indicator of the severity of chronic liver disease. Hence the use of albumin as one of the criteria for the Childs-Pugh classification used to grade the severity of cirrhosis (see Chapter 1). Hypoalbuminaemia is less commonly seen in acute liver failure because of the rapid onset of the disease and the long half-life of albumin. Measurements of pre-albumin are more sensitive due to the shorter half-life of 1.9 days (Imperial and Keeffe, 2006). Caution is required regarding hypoalbuminaemia as it may not be specific to liver disease; it is also seen in malnutrition, acute pancreatitis, and chronic inflammation or may reflect glomerular or gastrointestinal losses (Martin and Friedman, 2004)
- Prothrombin time (PT) (normal 12–16 seconds), international normalised ratio (INR) (normal 0.9–1.21). All blood clotting factors except factor VIII (which is produced by the endothelial cells) are synthesised within the hepatocytes.

The PT, however, does not become abnormal until more than 80% of the liver's synthetic capacity is lost (Johnson, 1999), and consequently may be normal in patients with cirrhosis. PT can be influenced by malabsorption, because factors ll, Vll and X are dependent on vitamin K. Therefore this may prohibit the PT from being a sensitive marker for patients with chronic liver disease (Imperial and Keefe, 2006). The elevation in PT due to vitamin K deficiency can be tested by the administration of vitamin K (10 mg) for 3 days. A PT that either improves by 30% or normalises within 24 hours, is indicative of normal hepatic function (Stonesifer, 2004). The PT is most useful for patients with alcoholic hepatitis or acute liver failure (ALF), and fulfils part of the prognostic criteria for ALF patients necessitating super-urgent liver transplantation (see Chapter 13). In the UK the international normalised ratio (INR) is used more frequently to assess hepatic function in ALF because of its standardised values; in France, factor V is more commonly used. As with an elevated INR, a factor V value of less than 20% of normal is indicative of poor outcome in the absence of liver transplantation (Gopal and Rosen, 2000)

■ Ammonia (normal level 8.8–26.4 µmol/L). Hyperammonaemia is commonly seen in patients with liver disease due to poor hepatic function. In patients with chronic liver disease it has been acknowledged that the level of ammonia does not necessary correlate with the level of hepatic encephalopathy. This is due to the ammonia concentrations being much higher in the brain than in the blood (Johnson, 1999). In patients with ALF, the study of ammonia levels has become increasingly important due to the association of hyperammonaemia (>88 µmol/L) with cerebral oedema and cerebral herniation (Clemmesen et al., 1999). Arterial samples are considered more accurate, as in venous samples the concentration of ammonia can be higher as a result of muscle metabolism of amino acids (Johnson, 1999)

Other laboratory tests used in liver disease

Immunoglobulins are synthesised by lymphocytes and are not a direct marker of liver function. However, elevation can be seen in patients with chronic liver disease which is possibly caused by impaired Kupffer cell function. Martin and Friedman (2004) suggest the pattern of elevation may suggest the aetiology of the underlying liver disease:

■ Elevated IgG – autoimmune hepatitis
■ Elevated IgM – primary biliary cirrhosis
■ IgA – alcoholic liver disease

Tests more specific to individual diseases such as viral hepatitis markers, caeruloplasmin (Wilson's disease), ferritin (hereditary haemochromatosis), alpha-1 antitrypsin (alpha-1-antitrypsin deficiency) and tumour markers, such as alphafetoprotein, are discussed within the relevant chapters.

Diagnostic studies

Liver biopsy

A needle biopsy of the liver was first performed by Paul Ehrlich in 1883 (Sherlock and Dooley, 2002). Since then it has become a key tool in confirming diagnosis suspected from abnormal blood tests, and is often considered the gold standard for the evaluation of liver disease.

A liver biopsy is where a small piece of liver tissue is removed and examined under a microscope to make a diagnosis, assess the amount of cellular damage, and to look for improvement after initiation of treatment, e.g. treating graft rejection in a post liver transplant patient. Liver biopsies can be accomplished through several different routes: percutaneous (blind or guided by ultrasound, computed tomography (CT) or magnetic resonance imaging (MRI)), transjugular and operative/laparoscopic, all of which are discussed below.

The indications for liver biopsy are varied (Table 2.2) and may change as new technologies which are not as invasive are developed, such as fibroscans. To reduce sampling error the amount of tissue required is usually 1–4 cm long and needs to include the four portal zones in order to make a histological diagnosis. Blood tests required before a liver biopsy are PT, INR and platelets usually within the week prior to performing the biopsy. Blood should be grouped and saved with the facility of compatible blood being available. Informed consent and a patient information sheet are essential for patients undergoing liver biopsy (BSG, 2004). Whether a patient should have an ultrasound scan before the biopsy to rule out any anatomical abnormalities and for patients whom the liver disease cannot be identified, remains an issue for debate (BSG, 2004). Pharmacological therapies, e.g. aspirin and non-steroidal anti-inflammatory drugs (NSAIDs), need to be discontinued a few days prior to the procedure.

Table 2.2 Indications for a liver biopsy. Adapted from British Society of Gastroenterology (2004) *Guidelines on the Use of Liver Biopsy in Clinical Practice.*

Chronic viral hepatitis – hepatitis B and hepatitis C
Raised serum ferritin
Suspected disorders of copper metabolism
Advanced disease in primary biliary cirrhosis (PBC) to stage the disease progression
Small duct primary sclerosing cholangitis (PSC)
Alcohol-related disease
Autoimmune hepatitis
Non-alcoholic liver disease (NAFLD)
Focal liver lesions
Infections and pyrexia of unknown origin
Following liver transplant
Occasionally for research purposes

Table 2.3   Contraindications to liver biopsy. Adapted from BSG (2004) *Guidelines on the Use of Liver Biopsy in Clinical Practice.*

Contraindications to liver biopsy	Incidence and rationale
Uncooperative patient	Patients need to remain still and hold their breath when biopsy needle inserted. Sudden movement may cause a tear in the liver. Consider sedation with midazolam
Extrahepatic biliary obstruction	In one study serious biliary complications were 2% and significant complications 4%. Should only be considered if doubt about diagnosis and benefit to patient outweighs the risk
Bacterial cholangitis	A relative contraindication due to the increased risk of inducing peritonitis and sepsis
Abnormal coagulation indices	If prothrombin time is prolonged by 4 seconds or more (or INR >1.4) despite vitamin K then other investigations should be considered Platelet count may have different threshold in different centres but a general rule would be above 80×10^9/L (80 000/mm^3) for a percutaneous biopsy
Ascites	Will make it difficult to obtain a biopsy sample due to the distance between the abdominal wall and liver percutaneously. However transjugular liver biopsy would not be contraindicated or the patient could have a total paracentesis prior to biopsy
Malignancy	There is a six to ten times higher incidence of bleeding so these patients should not be biopsied as outpatients
Obesity	May make it more difficult to identify the liver and should be considered for ultrasound-guided or transjugular biopsy
Cystic lesions	Modern imaging can more easily identify these so making liver biopsy unnecessary
Amyloidosis	High risk of bleeding and death after liver biopsy
Sickle cell disease	There is a higher risk of bleeding using the percutaneous route so transjugular route is used
Valvular heart disease	Prophylactic antibiotics should be used to minimise the risks of sepsis

A guide to contraindications of liver biopsy is shown in Table 2.3. However, many of these risk factors were established in the early days of liver biopsy before the advent of the Menghini technique, and the use of ultrasound and transvenous routes.

Percutaneous liver biopsy

A percutaneous liver biopsy may be performed in one of three different ways. It may be blind, guided (ultrasound/CT/MRI) or where the biopsy track is plugged afterwards.

The most common approach to liver biopsy is for the patient to lie supine; the edges of the liver are usually defined by percussion or by the use of ultrasound. After cleansing the skin, the biopsy site is then injected with local anaesthetic to minimise pain. This is done in the superficial and deep planes (Zaman et al., 2006). A small incision is made in the skin, to introduce the biopsy needle. The patient will need to hold their breath with the biopsy taken on expiration. The procedure for taking the biopsy is primarily dependent on the needle type (Grant and

Neuberger, 1999). The two types of biopsy needles most commonly used are Menghini and Tru-cut.

During the procedure patients may complain of a drawing feeling across the epigastrium, for the first 24 hours post procedure patients may have a slight right-sided ache, or a referred pain from the diaphgragm to the right shoulder (Sherlock and Dooley, 2002). Many clinicians ask patients to lie on their right side following liver biopsy for at least 2 hours; however there is no evidence for this practice (Hyun and Beutal, 2005).

Observation for a percutaneous liver biopsy is usually quarter-hourly pulse and blood pressure (BP) for 2 hours, then half-hourly pulse and BP for 2 hours, then hourly pulse and BP for 2 hours. Six hours of observation, vital sign recording and bed rest is the minimal duration of care. Patients can usually be discharged the same day. This is primarily due to the fact that most complications are seen within the first 3 hours post procedure. Complications post biopsies are rare but potentially fatal and include pain, bleeding into the peritoneum, haemobilia and sepsis (Stonesifer, 2004).

Transvenous (transjugular) liver biopsy

Sherlock and Dooley (2002) propose the following indications for transjugular liver biopsy:

■ Coagulation defects
■ Pretransplant ALF
■ Massive ascites
■ Small liver
■ Measurement of wedged hepatic venous pressure
■ Uncooperative patients
■ Also following any liver transplant whilst still an inpatient

The biopsy is performed in a vascular laboratory with video-fluoroscopy equipment and cardiac monitoring due to the risk of cardiac arrhythmias as the catheter passes through the right atrium (BSG, 2004). After cannulation of the internal jugular vein, a sheath is inserted into the right atrium and passed to the right vena cava. A catheter containing a biopsy needle is then advanced into the hepatic vein where, after checking the position by the injection of contrast medium, the needle is advanced and the biopsy taken (Grant and Neuberger, 1999). If the transjugular route is not possible, then a transfemoral route may be used.

Laproscopic liver biopsy

This is performed under direct vision and is suitable for patients with a degree of abnormal clotting, as direct haemostasis can be applied should there be any bleeding. It is often used when transjugular liver biopsy is not available and in patients where it is important to have a histological diagnosis in order to make further management plans, for instance in a patient with a focal lesion. Likewise a liver biopsy can be obtained during surgery if liver disease or tumour is suspected.

Complications in laproscopic liver biopsy include those of the laparotomy itself (BSG, 2004).

Ultrasonic transient elastography (Fibroscan®)

Due to the non-invasive technique, fibroscans are being more commonly used as an alternative to liver biopsy for the staging of liver fibrosis (Figure 2.3). The ultrasonic transient elastography technique is based on the assessment of tissue elasticity. A probe is placed perpendicularly against the skin between the liver and then triggered; the rate of sheer progression is measured by ultrasound. The speed of travel correlates with the degree of liver fibrosis. After ten readings, results are expressed in Kpa.

Imaging

Imaging of the liver and surrounding organs is paramount when diagnosing liver disease and increasingly sophisticated interventional radiology plays an important

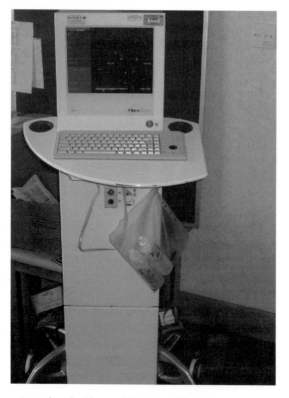

Figure 2.3 Fibroscan. Reproduced with permission from Echosens.

role in the diagnosis and sometimes treatment of liver disease. This section will look at the different imaging techniques available, and discuss both their applications and limitations.

Radiography

Plain radiography has a limited role in the investigation of liver disease (Beckingham and Ryder, 2001). However, a plain radiograph of the abdomen may show:

- Gallstones – 10% may have enough calcium to be seen
- Air in the biliary tree owing to recent invasive therapy, surgery or a fistula between the intestine and the gallbladder
- Pancreatic calcification
- Calcification of the gallbladder (rare)

Ultrasonography

An ultrasound scan is the initial imaging study of choice in liver disease, as it is quick, easy to use, readily available, cost effective, done in real time and is non-invasive. An ultrasound scan involves the analysis of the reflected ultrasound beam detected by a probe which is moved across the abdomen and can detect masses as small as 1 cm (Martin and Friedman, 2004). The normal liver appears as a relatively homogeneous structure and ultrasonography allows the gallbladder, common bile duct, pancreas, portal vein and other structures in the liver to be visualised. A disadvantage to ultrasonography is that there can be numerous artefacts when visualising the abdomen so an experienced operator is essential. Restrictions of sound wave penetration through certain tissues, such as bowel gas, bone and fatty tissues, can impair views.

Doppler ultrasound scans demonstrate the blood flow direction and velocity, and therefore are used to assess the patency of the hepatic artery and portal veins (Martin and Friedman, 2004).

Computed tomography

CT was first introduced in 1998 and works by rotating an ionising radiation source around the patient and reconstructing the images based on the attenuating differences of X-ray beams (Bieneman and Bisceglie, 2006). The liver is displayed as a series of adjacent cross-sectional slices, and typically 10–12 images are required to examine the whole liver. In addition to detecting masses, CT can imply the presence of cirrhosis, portal hypertension, as well as changes commonly seen in patients with haemochromatosis or fatty liver disease.

Contrast can be given to increase the anatomical definition. For patients with hepatocellular carcinomas (HCC) lipiodol is used instead of contrast, as this is taken up and retained by the HCC allowing the detection of neoplastic lesions of less than 5 mm (Sherlock and Dooley, 2002; Martin and Friedman, 2004).

Spiral or helical CT is a more recent modification, and provides faster imaging at the peak of contrast. Further advances include multidetector CT, which allows imaging from a single breath hold and three-dimensional constructions of the liver vasculature and biliary tree (Martin and Friedman, 2004).

CT portography is a process where intravenous contrast is injected into the superior mesenteric artery; this increases sensitivity in the detection of hepatic lesions. It is estimated that CT portography can detect 75% of HCCs of less than 2 cm, and 88% of primary or secondary lesions. However as this is an invasive procedure it is generally reserved for patients who are candidates for hepatic resection (Sherlock and Dooley, 2002).

The disadvantages of CT are the cost, the lack of portability, renal dysfunction secondary to the contrast in patients with cirrhosis and the patient's exposure to radiation.

Magnetic resonance imaging

An MRI scan places the patient in a magnetic field which applies radiofrequency waves to produce cross-sectional images; it is dependent on the magnetic properties of protons present in various parts of the body, which are then translated into images (Martin and Friedman, 2004). The detection of hepatic lesions is comparable to CT, and MRI is deemed an excellent technique for evaluation of hepatic blood flow and hepatic iron overload. The advantage of MRI is that it requires no contrast to visualise blood vessel or bile ducts (Sherlock and Dooley, 2002). The disadvantages are primarily cost, non-portability and the exclusion for patients with pacemakers or metallic devices (Martin and Friedman, 2004).

Hepatic angiography

This is used less often than in the past in hepatology practice but still has a role to play in visualising the blood supply of tumours and to pinpoint bleeding sites where they can be embolised with coils.

Endoscopic investigations are discussed in Chapter 4 and in the individual chapters in relation to specific liver diseases and diagnostic findings.

Complications and considerations

In investigation of liver disease many of the investigations require a sample of blood or imaging and have few complications. The more invasive tests such as liver biopsy have been discussed. One of the main nursing considerations with a patient undergoing investigation is patient anxiety. Often the patient has been feeling unwell for some time and may have been referred from a GP to a local district general hospital or specialist centre without a diagnosis and then may be diagnosed with a rare liver disease such as primary biliary cirrhosis or autoimmune hepatitis. Consequently support and information about investigations are important to help to make the patient's journey an informed one.

Chapter summary

The chapter has reviewed the assessment of liver function and the more common diagnostic studies used to diagnose, monitor and treat patients with liver disease. It introduced the key investigations and laboratory tests that will be explored further in other chapters when discussing individual liver diseases and their complications. The case study illustrates the investigative pathway of the patient to a diagnosis and the importance of investigating persistently raised liver function tests.

Illustrative case study

The patient is a 54-year-old married man with two teenage sons, who works as a senior civil servant. He noticed that he was becoming increasing tired with a loss of concentration. He had no previous medical history and was fit and well, he travelled abroad three times a year for holidays and enjoyed sport as well as about 14 units of alcohol a week. He thought his grandmother had died of liver cancer but there was no other history of liver disease in the family.

The GP's routine examination and blood tests revealed he had raised blood glucose; he commenced treatment for type 2 diabetes with oral hypoglycaemics. His liver function tests were not checked at this point and over the next 6 months his blood glucose remained high and poorly controlled, he also remained tired. His GP rechecked his bloods and found mildly abnormal liver function tests but did not refer him for further investigation, and instead elected to repeat the liver function tests in 3 months with the patient abstaining from alcohol. After they remained elevated the patient was referred to a hepatologist who found mildly elevated bilirubin 23 μmol/L, AST 66 U/L, ALT 134 U/L, GGT 86 U/L. His full blood count was normal apart from a low platelet count of 133×10^9/L, serum ferritin was 4400 μg/L (normal range 40–340 μg/L) and a transferrin saturation 105% (normal range 20–40%); his glucose remained high despite optimal oral medication.

A percutaneous liver biopsy showed cirrhosis with mild inflammatory activity and marked siderosis in keeping with haemochromatosis. Eighteen months later with weekly venesection and no alcohol his ferritin was now 222 μg/L with a transferrin saturation of 78.2%. He had normal liver function tests and his blood sugar was within normal limits and he has been able to reduce his oral hypoglycaemic medication. Both his sons and siblings have been genetically tested for the gene for haemochromatosis. One of his sons carries the gene for it and now has regular screening of his ferritin and liver function tests in order prevent any future damage to his major organs.

References

Bacon BR, O'Grady JG, Di Bisceglie AM, Lake JR (eds) (2006) *Comprehensive Clinical Hepatology*, 2nd edn. Mosby Elsevier, Philadelphia

Beckingham IJ, Ryder SD (2001) ABC of diseases of liver, pancreas, and biliary system: Investigation of liver and biliary disease. *British Medical Journal* 322:33–36

Beineman BK, Bisceglie AM (2006) Imaging of the liver. In: Bacon, BR, O'Grady JG, Di Biscegile AM, Lake JR (eds) *Comprehensive Clinical Hepatology*, 2nd edn. Mosby Elsevier, Philadelphia

British Society of Gastroenterology (BSG) (2004) *Guidelines on the Use of Liver Biopsy in Clinical Practice*. Available at www.bsg.org.uk (accessed 11/02/08)

Clemmesen JO, Larsen FS, Kondrup J, Hansen BA, Ott P (1999) Cerebral herniation in patient with acute liver failure is correlated with arterial ammonia concentrations. *Hepatology* 29:648–653

Emery J, Rose P (2001) Hereditary haemochromatosis: never seen a case? Editorial. *British Journal of General Practice* 51(446):347–348

Gopal DV, Rosen HR (2000) Abnormal findings in liver function tests: interpreting the results to narrow the diagnosis and establish prognosis. *Postgraduate Medicine* 107(2):100–114

Grant A, Neuberger J (1999) Guidelines on the use of liver biopsy in clinical practice. *Gut* 45(suppl IV): IVl-IVll

Green RM, Flamm S (2002) AGA technical review on the evaluation of liver chemistry tests. *Gastroenterology* 123(4):1367–1384

Howdle PD (2006) History and physical examination. In: Bacon, BR, O'Grady JG, Di Biscegile AM, Lake JR (eds) *Comprehensive Clinical Hepatology*, 2nd edn. Mosby Elsevier, Philadelphia

Hyun CB, Beutal VJ (2005) Prospective trial of post liver biopsy recovery positions. Does positioning really matter? *Journal of Clinical Gastroenterology* 39:328–332

Imperial JC, Keeffe EB (2006) Laboratory tests. In: Bacon, BR, O'Grady JG, Di Biscegile AM, Lake JR (eds) *Comprehensive Clinical Hepatology*, 2nd edn. Mosby Elsevier, Philadelphia

Johnson D (1999) Special considerations in interpreting liver function tests. *American Family Physician* 59(8). Available at http://www.aafp.org/afp/990415ap/2223.html (accessed 10/02/08)

Martin P, Friedman LS (2004) Assessment of liver function and diagnostic studies. In: Friedman LS, Keefe EB (eds) *Handbook of Liver Disease*, 2nd edn. Churchill Livingstone, Philadelphia

McGee P, Castledine G (2004) *Advanced Nursing Practice*, 2nd edn. Blackwell Publishing, Oxford, p 10

Royal College of Nursing (2002) *Maxi Nurses: Nurses Working in Advanced and Extended Roles Promoting and Developing Patient-Centred Health Care*. Royal College of Nursing, London

Sherlock S, Dooley J (2002) *Diseases of the Liver and Biliary System*, 11th edn. Blackwell Publishing, Oxford

Stonesifer E (2004) Common laboratory and diagnostic testing in patients with gastrointestinal disease. *AACN Clinical Issue: Advanced Practice in Acute and Critical Care* **15**(4):582–594

Zaman A, Ingram K, Flora KD (2006) *Diagnostic Liver Biopsy*. eMedicine. Available at http://www.emedicine.com/med/topic2969.htm (accessed 09/08/06)

Jaundice

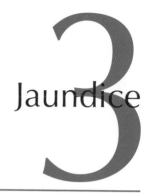

Michelle Clayton

Introduction

This chapter will discuss jaundice and consider the implications of both medical and nursing management. It will additionally review the pathophysiology of the formation of bilirubin from haem through conjugation and the enterohepatic circulation after excretion in bile. Investigations, physical examination and history taking will be discussed. Specific diseases will also be reviewed, including gallbladder disease, intrahepatic cholestasis of pregnancy and how drugs can cause jaundice.

Jaundice is one of the commonest presentations in patients with liver and biliary disease. It occurs when there is a raised level of bilirubin in the body, pigmenting the skin, sclera and mucous membranes (Figure 3.1, Plate 3). Raised bilirubin levels are known as hyperbilirubinaemia, where levels rise above 30 µmol/L; the higher the level of bilirubin, the deeper the jaundice. Visible jaundice is not usually detected until the bilirubin level exceeds 50 µmol/L (Lidofsky, 2006). Jaundice can be confirmed by a number of simple investigations including patient history, physical examination and biochemical screening; however determining the cause of the jaundice may require further investigation.

Classification of jaundice

There is no clear consensus on a definitive classification for jaundice. Some literature suggests three categories of jaundice: prehepatic, hepatic and posthepatic

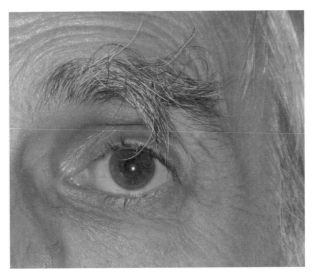

Figure 3.1   The jaundiced patient. For a colour version of this figure, please see Plate 3 in the colour plate section.

(Beckingham and Ryder, 2001); other literature uses different terminology, e.g. cholestatic instead of posthepatic (Sherlock and Dooley, 2002). Cholestasis refers to 'static bile' and in terms of classification of jaundice should not be confused with cholestatic liver disease which includes primary biliary cirrhosis. Other terminology suggested is that jaundice results either from an increase in bilirubin production or a decrease in the hepatobiliary elimination of bilirubin. This second category is subdivided into isolated disorders of bilirubin metabolism, liver diseases and obstruction of the bile ducts (Lidofsky, 2006).

Prehepatic

Prehepatic jaundice occurs due to an increase in bilirubin production. There are several causes, including: increased haemolysis, for example spherocytosis, homozygous sickle cell disease or thalassaemia major (Beckingham and Ryder, 2001); ineffective erythropoiesis; reabsorption of a haematoma; and massive blood transfusion (transfused erythrocytes have a shortened life-span) (Lidofsky, 2006). These causes lead to the production of excessive amounts of unconjugated bilirubin, which is produced faster than the liver can conjugate it. Bilirubin levels will be raised but serum transaminases and alkaline phosphatase remain normal (Sherlock and Dooley, 2002).

Hepatic

This is due to failure of the hepatocytes to effectively excrete conjugated bilirubin into the bile canaliculi. Serum transaminases also tend to be raised due to the underlying disease process (Sherlock and Dooley, 2002). The most common hepatic causes are viral hepatitis, alcohol-related liver disease, primary biliary cirrhosis, drug-induced jaundice and alcoholic hepatitis (Beckingham and Ryder, 2001).

Posthepatic or cholestatic

This is often due to biliary obstruction where bile does not reach the duodenum in sufficient amounts. The most common obstruction of the biliary tree occurs due to gallstones or choldocholithiasis, other causes can be attributed to biliary strictures, trauma, inflammatory processes, malignancy and extrinsic compression such as carcinoma of the pancreas.

Bilirubin formation

To be able to understand jaundice, it is necessary to understand the metabolism of haem and formation of bilirubin. Bilirubin is the end-product of haem degradation. Haem undergoes a number of complex chemical reactions where it is converted to bilirubin. The majority of haem is derived from the breakdown of old red blood cells (80–85%) and a small proportion comes from other haem-containing proteins such as cytochrome P450 (Figure 3.2).

The first chemical process involves the release of iron and carbon monoxide from the haem molecule due to the action of haem oxygenase; this takes place in the macrophages of the spleen, liver and bone marrow for haem that is derived from red blood cell haemoglobin. The resulting iron portion is sent for recycling and carbon monoxide is carried as carboxyhaemoglobin and excreted via the lungs. Biliverdin is created by this enzymatic process.

Biliverdin is then converted to bilirubin by the cytosolic enzyme, biliverdin reductase. The bilirubin created at this point is unconjugated bilirubin. Unconjugated bilirubin has a chemical structure of a tetrapyrole and, due to the internal hydrogen bonds, it is highly water insoluble.

Due to this water insolubility, unconjugated bilirubin binds to albumin and circulates in the plasma. The unconjugated bilirubin is then taken up by the hepatocytes that line the sinusoids. Unconjugated bilirubin is released from the albumin molecule and transported across the hepatocyte membrane into the cell. This is thought to occur with the help of organic anion transporting polypeptide (OATP). The unconjugated bilirubin is then picked up by ligandins and fatty acid binding proteins which transport it across the cytosol into the endoplasmic reticulum within the hepatocyte for conjugation to take place. Ligandin is a soluble hepatic

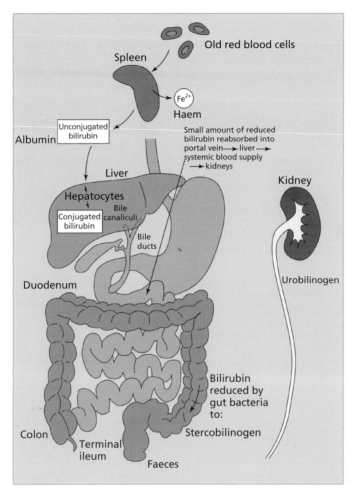

Figure 3.2   Bilirubin pathway. Reproduced with permission from Beckingham IJ and Ryder S (2001) *British Medical Journal* **322**:33–36.

protein that binds to bilirubin and other organic anions and is important in the uptake, retention and flux of bilirubin from the plasma into the liver (Litwack et al., 1971; Listowsky et al., 1978).

The hepatocytes then convert the unconjugated bilirubin, which is highly water insoluble, into conjugated bilirubin, which is water soluble. The microsomal enzyme uridine diphosphate glucuronosyl transferase (UGT) is responsible for this process of changing the bilirubin to a water-soluble form. Conjugated bilirubin is then converted into two forms: monoglucuronide bilirubin and diglucuronide bilirubin. Diglucuronide bilirubin accounts for 80% and monoglucuronide bilirubin 20%. Changes in this balance can occur; for example, if there is a large amount of haemolysis, the amount of monoglucuronide bilirubin will increase (Sherlock and Dooley, 2002).

The conjugation of the bilirubin to a water-soluble form allows the excretion of the bilirubin out of the hepatocytes into the bile canaliculi where it forms bile with a number of other substances. Bile formation is an osmotic process; there is active secretion of solutes followed by water through osmotic attraction (Oude Elferink, 2003). Bile formation is considerable, with adults producing 400–800 mL of bile per day.

Bile is a greenish bitter-tasting fluid that contains bilirubin, bile salts, cholesterol, phospholipids, electrolytes and water. Bile passes down the small bile canaliculi into the larger hepatic ducts which form at the porta hepaticus as the common bile duct. The gallbladder is the storage device for bile where it is concentrated and stored until required as part of the digestive process. Bile can bypass the gallbladder and pass straight down the common bile duct and into the intestine via the sphincter of Oddi. The common bile duct sits in close proximity to the pancreatic duct which is also encircled by the sphincter of Oddi.

Bile functions

Bile has two important functions, one is to facilitate the excretion of bilirubin as described and the other is important in digestion and absorption of fats by the body. Bile itself contains no enzymes; it does, however, contain bile salts, these are important in assisting the action of lipases on fats in the duodenum and small intestine. These are derivates of cholesterol and are made in the hepatocytes. Cholesterol is synthesised into cholic acid and chenocholic acid, which are known as bile acids; these are conjugated with glycine or taurine and then secreted. At this point of conjugation they are termed bile salts, due to the change in ionic form (Kullak-Ublick et al., 2004). Bile salts are transported out of the hepatocytes by the bile salt export pump (BSEP). The bile salts help to emulsify fats due to their composition; one side of the molecule is lipophilic (fat attracting) and the other side is hydrophilic (water attracting). They can therefore emulsify fat by breaking the fat down into minute droplets. This increases the surface area and makes it easier for digestion by lipases. The emulsification of fats is important in releasing the fat-soluble vitamins A, D, E and K, all of which have important roles within the body. Ninety percent of bile salts are reabsorbed in the ileum and returned to the liver to be recycled and utilised again; this can be up to six to ten times daily (Jansen and Sturm, 2003).

Once bilirubin enters the bowel as part of bile it undergoes further changes due to bacterial action within the intestine. Bacterial β-glucuronidase deconjugates the bilirubin in the terminal ileum and colon. This converts bilirubin into urobilinogen. Some of this urobilinogen is reabsorbed by the small intestine and is taken back to the liver via the hepatic portal vein. It is mostly excreted into the bile, whilst some of it leaves by the systemic circulation and is excreted via the kidney. The urobilinogens that are not reabsorbed are called stercobilinogens; they remain in the bowel and are then converted to stercobilin, which gives faeces their brown colouration.

Diseases of bilirubin metabolism

Diseases of bilirubin metabolism are generally associated with a disruption in the bilirubin pathway usually due to a genetic defect. Many diseases come to light during infancy with the signs and symptoms of chronic liver disease and with treatment many patients survive into adulthood. Some diseases such as progressive familial intrahepatic cholestasis (PFIC), an autosomal recessive disorder, may require liver transplantation in childhood (Jansen and Sturm, 2003). High levels of bilirubin are known to be toxic to other cells in the body.

Diseases such as Gilbert's syndrome, Crigler–Najjar syndrome and Dubin-Johnson syndrome produce hyperbilirubinaemia either in unconjugated or conjugated forms and are known as familial non-haemolytic hyperbilirubinaemia diseases.

Gilbert's syndrome rarely manifests itself unless it is found during biochemical screening or the individual is suffering from an illness that induces a fasting state, e.g. nausea and vomiting. The condition is benign and is believed to be present in up to 10% of the Caucasian population; it is usually detected during or after adolescence (Lidofsky, 2006). There is a partial deficiency in hepatic bilirubin glucuronidation (Sherlock and Dooley, 2002), which means higher levels of unconjugated bilirubin are detected particularly when unwell; the levels do not usually exceed 68 µmol/L (Lidofsky, 2006). No treatment is necessary; however patients with this condition require education and reassurance regarding their disease.

Crigler–Najjar syndrome types I and II are also related to unconjugated hyperbilirubinaemia. In type I large amounts of unconjugated bilirubin, in excess of 340 µmol/L, affect the infant in the neonatal period as the bilirubin crosses the blood–brain barrier and enters the basal ganglia leading to kernicterus (Lidofsky, 2006). This is due to the infant lacking the enzymes required for conjugation of bilirubin. Many die or suffer irreversible brain damage although liver transplantation may be an option.

Patients with Crigler–Najjar syndrome type II also have unconjugated hyperbilirubinaemia at lower levels which can be controlled by using phenobarbital and phototherapy. Patients may spend up to 16 hours a day under phototherapy to keep the bilirubin levels from becoming harmful.

Dubin-Johnson syndrome relates to conjugated hyperbilirubinaemia which does not impair liver function but does lead to jaundice. It is a relatively uncommon condition although a high incidence has been reported in Iranian Jews (Sherlock and Dooley, 2002). Liver biopsy in these patients reveals a greenish black colouration of the parenchyma.

Physical examination and history taking

Patients with jaundice may exhibit very obvious signs in terms of skin and sclera discolouration, however it is important to consider other indicators, which include pale stools and dark urine. The skin should also be observed for scratch marks,

Table 3.1 Physical signs in hepatic jaundice. Adapted from Travis et al. (2005).

Acute	Chronic	Either
Well nourished	Leuconychia/telangiectasia	Palmar erythema
Tender hepatomegaly	Loss of muscle bulk	Bruising
	Splenomegaly	Splenomegaly
	Ascites	
	Peripheral oedema	
	Loss of axillary/pubic hair	
	Testicular atrophy	
	Small or large liver	

excoriation, bruising and bleeding. The level of pruritis (from Latin *prurine* meaning to itch), and distribution of itch should be documented and how it affects the patient's quality of life. Other manifestations of liver disease can be found in jaundiced patients as shown in Table 3.1.

There is a close affiliation between jaundice and pruritus. It is well documented that pruritus not only interferes with everyday life but also can cause deterioration in the individual's quality of life, sleep deprivation and in some cases suicidal ideation due to the relentless itching (Jones and Bergasa, 1996; Mela et al., 2003). Pruritus is intrinsically subjective in nature due to the individual's perception of the itch. Therefore it cannot be objectively quantified or evaluated (Mela et al., 2003); however the main treatment aim is to relieve the pruritus. Further discussion of treatment and care considerations regarding pruritus can be found in Chapter 11.

Anorexia is particularly pronounced in jaundiced patients. Nausea and vomiting are common with gallstones and vomiting is particularly associated with obstructive biliary disease (Howdle, 2006).

Investigations

A number of different investigations can be used to assess jaundice, its severity and cause.

Laboratory

Blood tests are the simplest and cheapest in establishing a baseline for further investigation:

- Serum bilirubin indicates the depth and severity of jaundice. A raised serum bilirubin can indicate increased production, reduced hepatic uptake and/or conjugation of bilirubin, or decreased biliary excretion. The normal range for bilirubin is 5–17 µmol/L (Sherlock and Dooley, 2002). Bilirubin can also be calculated in its conjugated and unconjugated fractions; this is known as a split bilirubin and can be a useful test in paediatric patients and adults with a disease of bilirubin metabolism

■ Serum alkaline phosphatase (normal range 35–115 U/L) can be a useful indicator in relation to biliary tract involvement. Alkaline phosphatase is increasingly synthesised by the hepatocytes when there is biliary damage. An increase in bile acid concentrations may promote this synthesis (Friedman and Keeffe, 2004). Serum alkaline phosphatase has a half-life of 17 days; therefore levels may remain raised up to 1 week post resolution of a biliary obstruction

■ Serum bile acids are a less frequently undertaken blood test. Bile acids are synthesised from cholesterol in the liver, where they are conjugated with glycine or taurine and then excreted into the bile. Elevated bile acids can be a sensitive marker of hepatobiliary dysfunction and are useful in intrahepatic cholestasis of pregnancy as levels greater than 40 µmol/L are associated with a higher risk of fetal complications (Friedman and Keeffe, 2004)

■ Prothrombin time (PT) or international normalised ratio (INR) is an important aspect to consider in relation to the jaundiced patient, particularly jaundice arising from a biliary obstruction. PT is a vitamin K dependent test. Vitamin K is a fat-soluble vitamin that requires bile to emulsify fat within the intestine to release it for absorption. Patients with biliary involvement tend to have a deranged PT due to the lack of vitamin K provided from a nutritional source

Radiological and endoscopic investigations

■ Ultrasonography is particularly useful in evaluation of the extrahepatic biliary tree and also revealing intrahepatic dilatation of the biliary tree. Gallstones may also be visualised, however stones sitting in the common bile duct are more difficult to see (Lidofsky, 2006)

■ Computed tomography (CT) can be utilised particularly with intravenous contrast. This investigation is useful in obese patients and where the biliary tree is obscured by gas (Lidofsky, 2006)

■ Endoscopic ultrasonography (EUS) (Figure 3.3) is a technique where an ultrasonography probe is fitted to the endoscope which is then held against the wall of the stomach or oesophagus to visualise the liver and biliary tree due to their close proximity. Results suggest that EUS is comparable with magnetic resonance cholangiopancreatography (MRCP) in the diagnosis of biliary stones or strictures (Lidofsky, 2006)

■ Endoscopic retrograde cholangiopancreatography (ERCP) allows direct visualisation of the biliary tree. ERCP is highly accurate in the diagnosis of biliary obstruction and allows the physician to undertake biopsies and brushings for cytology. Biliary stents can be introduced to help relieve the obstruction and sphincteromy may allow the extraction of gallstones

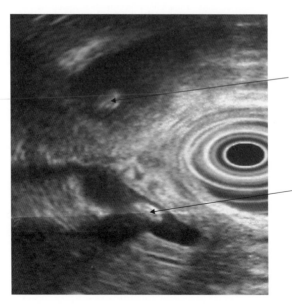

Figure 3.3 Gallstones (arrows) found on endoscopic ultrasonography.

- Percutaneous transhepatic cholangiography (PTC) is an invasive investigation that allows the visualisation of the biliary tree using radio-opaque contrast. A needle is advanced through the skin and penetrates the hepatic parenchyma; cannulation of a bile duct is then sought. Another important feature of the investigation is the ability to place an internal stent or external biliary drain. External biliary drainage can be a useful adjunct to decompressing the bilary system, though it does leave the patient at greater risk of infection by having the drain in place. A PTC is technically more difficult if the intrahepatic bile ducts are not dilated (Lidofsky, 2006)
- MRCP is a newer diagnostic test which images the biliary system. It has the benefits of being non-invasive and not requiring contrast medium, however cost and availability are precluding factors. Vaishali et al. (2004) found that MRCP was highly diagnostically accurate in patients with obstructive jaundice

All of the above investigations can assist the health care professional in their assessment of the severity and cause of jaundice. This will then guide further therapeutic options. Jaundice caused by biliary tree obstruction may be resolved by interventions such as ERCP or PTC, however if the cause of the jaundice is due to hepatocellular failure then treatment of the underlying disease process may ameroliate symptoms.

Malabsorption

When bile does not flow adequately then there is a risk of malabsorption of fats which manifests itself as steatorrhoea. In addition fat-soluble vitamins are not absorbed leading to potential problems with neurological and visual impairment (vitamins A and E), bone density (vitamin D) and coagulopathy (vitamin K). Further discussion on this can be found in Chapter 14.

Administration of vitamin K

Vitamin K is a co-factor in the synthesis of clotting factors II, VII, IX and X. It is important to establish if coagulopathy is due to deteriorating hepatic function, cholestasis or bile duct obstruction. Administration of vitamin K is integral in identifying the cause. Parental administration will differentiate between a synthetic and cholestatic cause or bile duct obstruction. An improvement in prothrombin time of >30% within 24 hours of administration suggests a cholestasis or bile duct obstruction (Luxon, 2006) rather than deteriorating synthetic function. There is no clear consensus of opinion on the amount of vitamin K administered and number of doses required.

Gallbladder disease

Gallstone disease has become more prevalent in the last 50 years due to an ageing population, changes in diet and the rise in obesity (Bateson, 1999). Gender and race also play a part, with females being more susceptible to gallstones, as are Native American and Hispanic populations.

There are two major types of gallstones, cholesterol and pigment gallstones. Cholesterol gallstones occur due to soluble cholesterol precipitating out of solution and developing into a crystal formation (Johnson, 2001). Pigmented stones can be either black or brown in colour and are formed from calcium bilirubinate and other substances. Black stones are usually found solely in the gallbladder, whereas brown stones tend to be located in the bile ducts and are associated with biliary stasis and infection (Friedman and Keeffe, 2004). Some patients will have a mixture of both types of stones. Fifteen percent of gallstones can be identified on a plain abdominal film, however the majority (95%) are found using ultrasound (Johnson, 2001).

The majority of patients who have gallstones tend to be asymptomatic and treatment in these cases is not advocated. Pain from bile duct stones is typically characterised by its location in the right upper quadrant or epigastrium and may radiate around or through to the back or into the right shoulder. Pain can be mild through to severe with nausea at times and can last a short amount of time (up to 6–8 hours, although 3–4 hours is most common) (Malet, 2004). Severe pain that exceeds 12 hours should be investigated as acute cholecystitis should be suspected in these cases. A calculous biliary pain relates to the same presentation of pain but in the absence of gallstones.

Treatment for symptomatic gallstones is elective cholcystectomy with many being performed laproscopically. Some patients may still require open cholestectomy but this approach has been reduced considerably by favourable results, including rapid recovery, less time off work and less scarring, from laparoscopic treatment (Johnson, 2001).

Gallbladder cancer is rare and difficult to detect as it is usually asymptomatic prior to its advanced stages, where it presents with weight loss, anaemia, persistent vomiting and a palpable mass in the right upper quadrant (Johnson, 2001).

Drug-induced jaundice

A number of drugs have been implicated in causing liver damage which may or may not involve the biliary ducts. These include prescribed drugs and non-prescribed medication such as herbal remedies and illegal drugs (McCarthy and Wilkinson, 1999). A number of drugs have the ability to damage the bile ducts leading to ductopenia (loss of the bile ducts) or vanishing bile duct syndrome. Other drugs can inhibit the bile salt export pump leading to an accumulation of bile salts in the hepatocytes and subsequent liver damage due to their toxicity (Kullak-Ublick et al., 2004). Cholestasis tends to be an integral factor in the disease process. Symptoms may be relatively benign, through to profound anorexia, fatigue and pruritis developing over a number of months (Geubel and Sempoux, 2000). Further discussion can be found in Chapter 15.

Intrahepatic cholestasis of pregnancy

Intrahepatic cholestasis of pregnancy (ICP) usually affects women in the last trimester of pregnancy (80%), with pruritus affecting the palms of the hands, soles of the feet and, in some cases, generalised itching all over the body. It also leads to fetal distress, premature delivery and stillbirth if untreated (Kroumpouzos, 2002). Increased antenatal surveillance and early delivery of the fetus at 36–37 weeks are required to reduce the incidence of stillbirth (Van Dyke, 2006).

Both oestrogen and progesterone play a part in ICP. Oestrogens interfere with bile acid secretion across the hepatocyte membrane (this is why pruritus can also occur in some women talking oral contraceptives). Progesterone is implicated due to its metabolites which inhibit hepatic glucuronyltransferase; this in turn reduces the ability to clear oestrogens from the hepatocytes, thus intensifies the effects

(Kroumpouzos, 2002). The symptoms will subside on the resolution of pregnancy. Further discussion can be found in Chapter 16.

Additional considerations

Jaundice has a number of implications for the psychological health of the individual. Stigma from the general public surrounding why the individual is jaundiced can mean that patients are labelled inappropriately as being alcoholics or drug abusers. Patients may exhibit skin discolouration ranging from a light yellow tinge through to a deep greenish hue. This, combined with scratches from pruritus and bruises and bleeding due to coagulopathy, can be distressing for the patient having to cope with a change in body image.

Health care professionals should be integral in helping patients to cope with these changes through listening, being supportive, giving information and educating patients. Patients require education to understand that scratching can lead to impaired skin integrity and a subsequent route for infection. It is important for the nurse to understand the patient's desire to itch due to the underlying pathophysiology. Patients require information on the importance of avoiding injury which may lead to further bruising or bleeding. Health care interventions and treatment options in relation to pruritus can be found in Chapter 11.

Chapter summary

This chapter has considered why jaundice occurs and reviewed the pathway that is integral for bilirubin to be produced and excreted. Jaundice can be a result of either liver or biliary involvement so it is important for health care professionals to be able to differentiate this through investigation and treat accordingly. Jaundice is a distressing symptom not only for the patient but also for family and friends; and can leave patients feeling not only ill but vulnerable due to changes in body image. Pruritus goes hand in hand with jaundice; this chapter needs to be read in conjugation with Chapter 11 which reviews pruritus and treatment options.

Illustrative case study

A 45-year-old male presented to his local accident and emergency department with a 2-week history of painful abdominal distension, reduced appetite with mild weight loss. He had no fever, nausea or vomiting or changes in his bowel habits. He was a non-smoker, with no previous relevant medical or family history and only consumed alcohol socially (approximately 15 units per week). He was not taking any current medication or herbal remedies. Physical examination revealed

Table 3.2   Illustrative case study laboratory results.

Laboratory results	Normal range	On presentation
Biluribin (mmol/L)	5–17	61
Serum albumin (g/L)	35–54	42
ALT (U/L)	3–30	100
AST (U/L)	7–40	99
ALP (U/L)	35–115	187
GGT (U/L)	2–65	78
INR	0.9–1.2	1.45
Platelets (×10^9/L)	130–400	864
Alpha-fetoprotein (µg/L)	<6.7	<1.0

mild jaundice, ascites and splenomegaly; and gross lower limb oedema. He was alert and orientated with no evidence of hepatic encephalopathy and no other stigmata of chronic liver disease.

Initial laboratory investigation demonstrated deranged liver function tests, an INR of 1.45 and raised platelet count as shown in Table 3.2.

An abdominal ultrasound scan showed moderate amounts of ascites, with a normal liver with no focal lesions. There was normal blood flow noted in the portal vein. There were no intra- or extrahepatic biliary tree dilatation or gallstones. The spleen was enlarged at 13.5 cm, as the physical examination initially suggested.

Results from a diagnostic ultrasound-guided paracentesis excluded spontaneous bacterial peritonitis with a polymorphonuclear leucocytes (PMN) <250 mm^3. A high gradient SAAG (serum albumin – ascitic fluid) of 17 g/L (serum albumin 42 g/L – ascites albumin 25 g/L) and a high protein (>2.0 g/L) suggested the cause of ascites was related to portal hypertension (see Chapter 5 for further information).

With the patient's history, physical examination, investigations and laboratory results, a diagnosis of Budd-Chiari syndrome was suspected which was confirmed with an abdominal CT scan which demonstrated occlusion to the hepatic vein, with normal portal venous flow.

The patient was commenced on anticoagulation therapy and was subsequently referred and transferred to a tertiary hepatology unit for further management, where he underwent a successful liver transplantation. The underlying pathophysiology of the patient's Budd-Chiari syndrome was attributed to a haematological condition.

References

Bateson M (1999) Gallbladder disease. *British Medical Journal* 318:1745–1748

Beckingham IJ, Ryder S (2001) ABC of diseases of liver, pancreas, and biliary system: investigations of liver and biliary disease. *British Medical Journal* 322:33–36

Friedman L, Keeffe E (2004) *Handbook of Liver Disease*, 2ⁿᵈ edn. Churchill Livingstone, Philadelphia

Geubel A, Sempoux C (2000) Drug and toxin-induced bile duct disorders. *Journal of Gastroenterology and Hepatology* 15:1232–1238

Howdle P (2006) History and physical examination. In: Bacon BR, O'Grady JG, Di Bisceglie AM, Lake JR (eds) *Comprehensive Clinical Hepatology*, 2ⁿᵈ edn. Mosby Elsevier, Philadelphia

Jansen P, Sturm E (2003) Genetic cholestasis, causes and consequences for hepatobiliary transport. *Liver International* 23:315–322

Johnson C (2001) ABC of the upper gastrointestinal tract: upper abdominal pain: gall bladder. *British Medical Journal* 323:1170–1173

Jones E, Bergasa N (1996) Why do cholestatic patients itch? *Gut* 38(5):644–645

Kroumpouzos G (2002) Intrahepatic cholestasis of pregnancy: what's new. *Journal of the European Academy of Dermatology and Venereology* 16:316–318

Kullak-Ublick G, Steiger B, Meier P (2004) Enterohepatic bile salt transporters in normal physiology and liver disease. *Gastroenterology* 126:322–342

Lidofsky S (2006) Jaundice. In: Bacon BR, O'Grady JG, Di Bisceglie AM, Lake JR (eds) *Comprehensive Clinical Hepatology*, 2ⁿᵈ edn. Mosby Elsevier, Philadelphia

Listowsky I, Gatmaitan Z, Arias I (1978) Ligandin retains and albumin loses bilirubin binding capacity in liver cytosol. *Proceedings of the National Academy of Science* 75(3):1213–1216

Litwack G, Ketterer B, Arias I (1971) Ligandin: a hepatic protein which bonds steroids, bilirubin, carcinogens and a number of exogenous organic anions. *Nature* 234:466–467

Luxon B (2006) Functions of the liver. In: Bacon BR, O'Grady JG, Di Bisceglie AM, Lake JR (eds) *Comprehensive Clinical Hepatology*, 2ⁿᵈ edn. Mosby Elsevier, Philadelphia

Malet PF (2004) Cholelithasis and cholecystitis. In Friedman L, Keeffe E (eds) *Handbook of Liver Disease*, 2ⁿᵈ edn. Churchill Livingstone, Philadelphia

McCarthy M, Wilkinson M (1999) Hepatology. *British Medical Journal* 318:1256–1259

Mela M, Mancuso A, Burroughs K (2003) Review article: pruritus in cholestatic and other liver disease. *Alimentary Pharmacology & Therapeutics* 17:857–870

Oude Elferink R (2003) Cholestasis. *Gut* 52(Suppl II):ii42–ii48

Sherlock S, Dooley J (2002) *The Liver and Biliary System*, 11ᵗʰ edn. Blackwell Publishing, Oxford

Travis SP, Ahmad T, Collier J, Steinhart AH (2005) *Pocket Consultant Gastroenterology*, 3ʳᵈ edn. Blackwell Publishing, Oxford

Vaishali M, Agarwal A, Upadhyaya D, Chauhan V, Sharma O, Skukla V (2004) Magnetic resonance cholangiopancreatography in obstructive jaundice. *Journal of Clinical Gastroenterology* 38(10):887–890

Van Dyke R (2006) Liver diseases in pregnancy. In: Bacon BR, O'Grady JG, Di Bisceglie AM, Lake JR (eds) *Comprehensive Clinical Hepatology*, 2ⁿᵈ edn. Mosby Elsevier, Philadelphia

Portal hypertension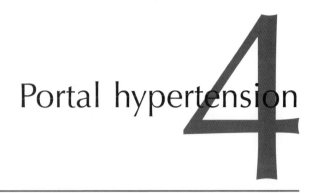

Terence Wong

Introduction

Portal hypertension is an important complication of liver cirrhosis leading to the formation of varices and contributing to the occurrence of ascites and hepatic encephalopathy. Portal hypertension is the cause of one of the most devastating complications of liver cirrhosis: variceal haemorrhage. This chapter will examine the underlying pathophysiology of portal hypertension in liver disease and the current management strategies used for variceal haemorrhage.

Definition

Portal hypertension is defined as an increased pressure in the portal vein. Normally the pressure of the blood in the portal vein is 7 mmHg. When this pressure rises to greater than 12 mmHg above the pressure in the hepatic vein then the patient is at an increased risk of bleeding from varices.

Causes

The portal vein transports approximately 1500 mL/min of blood from the small intestine, spleen and colon into the liver. From there blood flows through the hepatic sinusoids into the hepatic vein, and from there into the inferior vena cava (IVC) and heart. Any cause of obstruction of this flow will lead to portal hypertension. The main cause of portal hypertension is liver cirrhosis. Other intrahepatic conditions besides cirrhosis may lead to an obstruction to this flow of blood (such as certain toxins, infection with schistosomiasis). Portal hypertension may also be caused by extrahepatic causes, such as portal vein thrombosis and portal vein compression (e.g. from a tumour). Any cause of increased pressure in the hepatic veins will lead to increased pressure in the portal vein, so constrictive pericarditis, and hepatic vein thrombosis (Budd-Chiari syndrome) can also cause portal hypertension.

Consequences

Varices

The increases in the portal pressure lead to the diversion of blood into alternative routes from the portal venous circulation into the IVC. These are termed the portosystemic collateral circulation (Figure 4.1). These include oesophageal varices, gastric varices, rectal varices, abdominal wall varices, spleno-renal varices and lumbar varices. Portal hypertension can also cause venous congestion of the small vessels of the stomach (portal hypertensive gastropathy), which is a rare cause of bleeding.

Ascites

Portal hypertension is a contributory factor in the pathogenesis of ascites (see Chapter 5).

Portosystemic encephalopathy

In patients with portal hypertension the portal venous blood from the intestines is diverted into the systemic circulation and towards the brain without passing through the liver. This contributes towards the aetiology of portosystemic encephalopathy as described in Chapter 6.

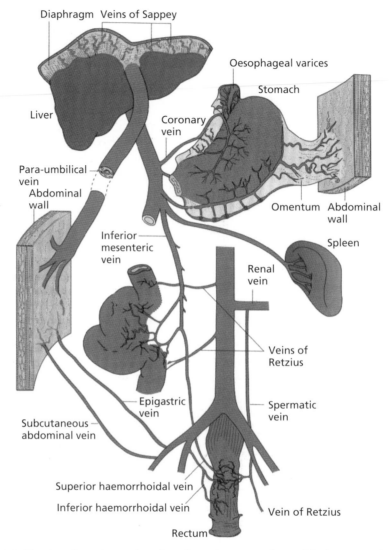

Figure 4.1 The sites of portal systemic collateral circulation in cirrhosis of the liver. Reproduced from Sherlock S, Dooley J (2002) *Diseases of the Liver and Biliary System*, 11th edn, with permission from Blackwell Science.

Clinical features

History

A history of upper gastrointestinal haemorrhage is the commonest presentation of portal hypertension. This manifests as either melaena or haematemesis. In the history some clues as to the cause of the portal hypertension should be sought, including any history of intravenous drug usage (past or present), blood transfusions, tattoos and alcohol intake.

Examination

The patient may have stigmata of chronic liver disease (see Chapter 2). In addition there may be dilated abdominal wall veins (or *caput medusa*), as these are a site of portosystemic collateral circulation. An enlarged spleen (splenomegaly) may be palpable as the increased portal pressure increases the pressure of blood within the spleen, causing it to become congested and enlarged. Ascites may be present (see above).

Investigations

Blood investigations

Haematology

Splenomegaly may lead to increased sequestration in the spleen, and therefore there may be a pancytopenia: the haemoglobin, white cell count and platelet count may all be reduced. In addition the haemoglobin may be low due to blood loss from varices.

The reduced synthetic function of the liver may lead to a reduction in the synthesis of clotting factors. This would cause a prolonged prothrombin time (PT) and international normalised ratio (INR).

Biochemistry

There may be changes consistent with liver cirrhosis on serum biochemistry. The serum sodium may be reduced due to reduced renal free water excretion, or diuretic usage. The urea and albumin may be reduced due to decreased hepatic synthesis; the creatinine may be raised due to hepatorenal syndrome, or pre-renal failure due to a hypotensive bleeding episode.

Imaging investigations

Ultrasonography

An ultrasound investigation of the abdomen and liver may show signs of portal hypertension. Splenomegaly can be accurately measured with ultrasound and is present in the majority of patients with portal hypertension. The portal vein may be dilated, and Doppler ultrasound measurements show a reduced portal vein blood flow. Ultrasonography is also useful in the detection of hepatocellular carcinoma that may complicate cirrhosis and cause portal hypertension by invasion of the portal vein.

Computed tomography scan

This is more accurate than ultrasonography in the detection of portal vein occlusion and focal liver lesions such as hepatocellular carcinoma. Retroperitoneal varices can also be detected on CT scanning.

Magnetic resonance imaging

MRI is more accurate than CT scanning in the detection of hepatocellular carcinoma and intra-abdominal varices. It does, however, require the patient to take a prolonged breath hold and some patients cannot tolerate MRI.

Hepatic venography

Hepatic venography and pressure studies are the 'gold standard' in the measurement of portal hypertension. A balloon catheter is passed into the hepatic vein by either an internal jugular venous, or femoral venous approach under radiographic guidance. Contrast is then injected into the hepatic vein and the pressure in the hepatic vein is measured. The balloon is then inflated to occlude the hepatic vein. The pressure then measured (the hepatic venous wedge pressure) is then the same as the portal venous pressure. The hepatic venous pressure gradient (HVPG) is calculated by subtracting the hepatic vein pressure from the hepatic venous wedge pressure. The HVPG is an excellent marker of portal hypertension severity. A HVPG of <12 mmHg correlates with a reduced risk of bleeding from varices, a good response to pharmacological therapy of portal hypertension and increased survival.

Endoscopy

Portal hypertension may cause many changes which can be seen with upper gastrointestinal endoscopy. Endoscopy is the gold standard in the assessment of oesophagogastric varices (Figure 4.2, Plate 4). Portal hypertensive gastropathy is caused by congestion of the blood vessels in the gastric wall and has a mosaic-like appearance. Varices may be present in the oesophagus, in the fundus of the stomach, on the lesser curve, or in the body of the stomach; all of these may bleed. Oesophageal varices are graded according to size (grade 1 varices can be depressed by the endoscope, grade 2 varices cannot be depressed by the endoscope, grade 3 are confluent). Various other signs at endoscopy (red spots, red wheal markings) confer an additional bleeding risk.

The major role of endoscopy in portal hypertension is in the treatment of bleeding varices (see below).

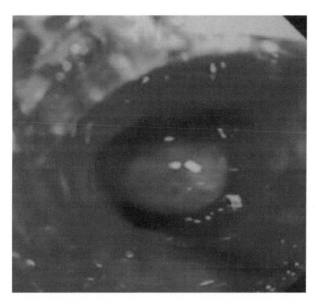

Figure 4.2 Endoscopic view of an oesophageal varix. For a colour version of this figure, please see Plate 4 in the colour plate section.

Management of variceal haemorrhage

Upper gastrointestinal haemorrhage (UGIH) is a common medical emergency with an incidence of 50–170 per 100,000 adults per year in the UK (Blatchford et al., 1997). In a UK audit, the overall mortality was 14%, with a higher mortality in older patients, or those with severe co-morbidity (Rockall et al., 1995). This mortality has not declined recently, probably due to the increasing age and co-morbidity of patients. Variceal haemorrhage is associated with a particularly high mortality of 50% in patients with bleeding varices compared with 11% in all patients with gastrointestinal bleeding. Patients who have had a variceal bleed have a 70% chance of bleeding again.

Initial assessment

The initial management of the patient should include a risk assessment of the severity of the bleed, and fluid resuscitation. Table 4.1 illustrates the immediate investigations required in patients with variceal haemorrhage.

Resuscitation

The immediate management is to resuscitate the patient (Jalan and Hayes, 2000). Multiple wide-bore venous access should be inserted in large veins (e.g. 16-gauge

Table 4.1 Immediate investigations in patients with variceal haemorrhage.

Haematology
Full blood count
Clotting screen
Blood group and cross-match

Biochemistry
Urea and electrolytes
Liver function tests
Blood glucose
Chest radiograph
ECG
Arterial blood gases

Other blood investigations to determine cause of cirrhosis
Hepatitis C antibody
Hepatitis Bs antigen
Serum ferritin
Antinuclear, anti-mitochondrial, anti-smooth muscle, anti-liver kidney microsomal antibodies
Serum immunoglobulins (IgG, IgM, IgA)
Serum alpha-fetoprotein
Serum alpha-1-antitrypsin
Serum caeruloplasmin

Imaging investigations in variceal haemorrhage
Ultrasound scan with Doppler ultrasound of the hepatic and portal veins
Contrast-enhanced CT in selected cases
Magnetic resonance imaging in selected cases
Hepatic portography in selected cases

peripheral cannula into the antecubital fossa). The severity of the bleed can be stratified according to signs of haemodynamic compromise. A severe bleed is normally indicated by a patient with a pulse >100 beats/min, a systolic blood pressure <100 mmHg, or a haemoglobin <100 g/L.

The most effective resuscitation fluid is cross-matched blood, followed by group-compatible blood, O-negative blood, then plasma expanders (e.g. Haemaccel® or Gelofusine®). In the majority of patients with variceal bleeding the patient can be resuscitated with plasma expanders whilst cross-matched blood is awaited. In some severe cases of variceal haemorrhage O-negative blood maybe required whilst cross-matching is performed. Central venous access may be necessary in patients with a severe bleed as patients with variceal haemorrhage are commonly complicated with systemic sepsis, and may be hypotensive due to sepsis rather than hypovolaemia. Central venous access with large-bore cannulae can also be used to rapidly transfuse fluids (e.g. a rapid infusion catheter into the femoral vein).

Fluid resuscitation should be commenced. In severe cases of haematemesis an endotracheal tube may be required, especially if the conscious level is impaired (e.g. in hepatic encephalopathy), to prevent pulmonary aspiration.

Endoscopy

Endoscopy can be undertaken either as a semi-elective, or urgent procedure. The timing of endoscopy has to be taken on an individual case basis, but fluid resuscitation takes priority over endoscopy. Endoscopy should be undertaken when the patient is haemodynamically stable, but this is not always possible in cases of severe bleeding. Endoscopy is associated with the risk of pulmonary aspiration, especially if the patient is having a large haematemesis, and therefore airway protection is often necessary prior to endoscopy, especially in the context of a large haematemesis, or if the patient's conscious level is impaired from encephalopathy. Ideally every acute hospital should have arrangements for out-of-hours endoscopy by appropriately trained clinicians (British Society of Gastroenterology Endoscopy, 2002), however there is wide variation in the provision of emergency endoscopy within the UK and a recent National Confidential Enquiry into Patient Outcome and Death (NCEPOD) reported that 62% of units had no out-of-hours endoscopy rota. Endoscopy can define the cause of bleeding, aid in risk stratification and enable endoscopic haemostasis to be performed. Specific endoscopic, pharmacological and surgical therapy can then be tailored towards individual causes of bleeding.

The mortality of bleeding after a variceal haemorrhage is related to the severity of the liver disease. A commonly used classification in assessing the severity of liver disease is the Child-Pugh score and is strongly predictive with mortality (Jalan and Hayes, 2000).

Treatment of acute variceal bleeding

Endoscopic therapy

Prior to endoscopy the patient must be well resuscitated and stable from the respiratory and cardiovascular perspectives (see above). If endoscopy is performed under conscious sedation a benzodiazepine (e.g. midazolam), and sometimes opiate (e.g. fentanyl), is used as a sedative agent. These are associated with respiratory depression and hypotension, and therefore the patient's oxygen saturation, pulse and blood pressure are continually monitored. ECG monitoring is recommended if there is any history of cardiac disease. Oxygen supplementation should be administered routinely. If the patient has had a prosthetic heart valve replacement, or a history of endocarditis, endocarditis prophylaxis should be administered in the form of pre- and postprocedural antibiotics. During the procedure itself there is a high risk of pulmonary aspiration, especially if the patient is having an active haematemesis. Adequate mouth suction should therefore be performed during the procedure to avoid inhalation of blood. In view of this risk many patients have their airway protected by endotracheal intubation.

After the procedure the patient should be recovered in an environment appropriate to nurse a sedated patient. Oxygen saturation, pulse and blood pressure should be continued to be monitored until the patient is fully conscious. Specific antagonists to benzodiazepines (e.g. flumazenil) and opiates (e.g. naloxone) should be to hand in both the procedural area and recovery in case the patient suffers respiratory failure due to the sedatives.

The main endoscopic treatment modalities for the treatment of oesophageal varices are endoscopic variceal band ligation (EVL) and endoscopic variceal sclerotherapy. Endoscopic sclerotherapy (ES) involves the injection of a sclerosant (e.g. ethanolamine) into the varix at the time of endoscopy. ES has been used for many decades, but its use has largely been superseded by EVL. EVL was first described in humans in 1988, and involves the application of a rubber band around the oesophageal varix. A specialised suction chamber is placed on the endoscope; at endoscopy the varix is sucked into this chamber and the rubber band applied (Figure 4.3, Plate 5). Subsequent studies have shown that EVL is superior to sclerotherapy both in the setting of the acute bleeding (Lo et al., 1997), and also in secondary prophylaxis of variceal haemorrhage (Gimson et al., 1993). EVL results in higher initial haemostasis rates, lower rebleeding rates and lower complication rates compared with ES. The newer multiband variceal banding devices are also superior to the first generation techniques that required an oesophageal overtube (Wong et al., 2000), as the overtube required the use of higher doses of sedation and was associated with oesophageal haemorrhage, haematoma and even

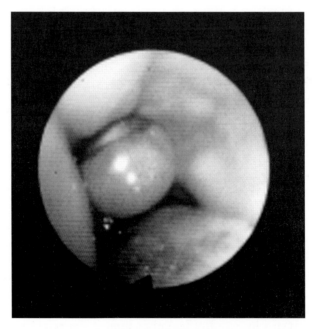

Figure 4.3 Band ligation on an oesophageal varix. Reproduced with permission from Krige JE, Beckingham IJ (2001) ABC of diseases of liver, pancreas, and biliary system. Portal hypertension – 1: varices. *British Medical Journal* **322**:348–351. For a colour version of this figure, please see Plate 5 in the colour plate section.

perforation. Side effects from EVL and ES are the formation of oesophageal ulceration and strictures; proton pump inhibitors (e.g. omeprazole) are therefore routinely administered after endoscopic therapy of varices.

Gastric varices are present in approximately 30% of patients with portal hypertension, and pose a challenge to the endoscopist due to the difficulties in achieving endoscopic haemostasis either with endoscopic sclerotherapy or band ligation. Recent studies using the injection of tissue adhesives such as N-butyl-cyanoacylate (Lo et al., 2001), and human thrombin (Heneghan et al., 2002) into the gastric varix at endscopy have shown high initial haemostasis rates.

Pharmacological therapy

Terlipressin, vasopressin, somatostatin and octreotide have all been shown to be of some benefit in initial haemostasis and reducing early rebleeding. Terlipressin is a synthetic analogue of vasopressin which causes splanchnic vasoconstriction, reduces portal blood flow and variceal pressure. Terlipressin reduces mortality and in the UK is the only licensed vasoactive agent in variceal haemorrhage (Ioannou et al., 2003). Earlier treatment with vasoactive agents (Levacher et al., 1995; Nidegger et al., 2003) seems to be associated with a better outcome, and therefore should be used before endoscopy when a variceal haemorrhage is clinically suspected. The optimal duration of therapy has not fully been established, but many of the studies continued vasoactive drugs for 5 days (de Franchis, 2005). In view of the vasoconstrictive effects of terlipressin, side effects include ischaemia of the small intestine, peripheral vasculature and myocardium. A baseline electrocardiogram (ECG) should therefore be performed prior to starting terlipressin, and the patient observed for any signs or symptoms of small bowel ischaemia (e.g. abdominal pain), myocardial ischaemia (e.g. chest pain) or peripheral vascular ischaemia.

Prophylactic antibiotics have been shown in multiple meta-analyses to reduce mortality in cirrhotic patients with gastrointestinal haemorrhage (Soares-Weiser et al., 2002). Quinolones (e.g. ciprofloxacin) or third-generation cephalosporins should therefore be routinely administered.

Combining endoscopic and pharmacological therapy improves initial haemostasis rates and reduces rebleeding rates when compared with endoscopic haemostasis alone (Banares et al., 2002).

Balloon tamponade

The use of balloon tamponade (Figure 4.4) is now reducing with effective endoscopic therapy and vasoactive drugs. The most commonly used balloon is the Sengstaken-Blakemore tube. This four-lumen balloon has a gastric and oesophageal balloons, and gastric and oesophageal aspiration channels. The tube is inserted per-orally into the stomach and the gastric balloon inflated with 250 mL of 10% radio-opaque contrast. The tube is then withdrawn, and the balloon held tight against the gastro-oesophageal junction by firm skin traction. Weight traction is

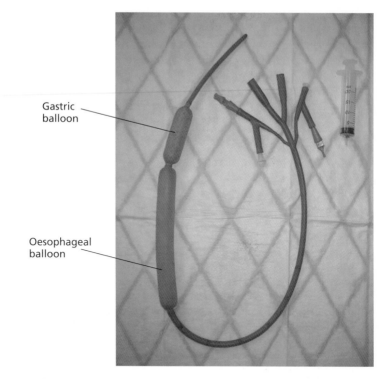

Gastric balloon

Oesophageal balloon

Figure 4.4 Balloon tamponade tube. Photograph reproduced with permission from Bard®, Urology and Surgical Specialities.

no longer recommended due to its lack of consistent traction maintenance. The position of the tube is then checked by radiograph, where the gastric balloon can easily be identified by the radio-opaque contrast; in particular it is important to confirm that the balloon has not been inflated in the oesophagus as this is associated with a high risk of oesophageal perforation. The oesophageal balloon should only rarely be inflated as it is associated with a high risk of oesophageal necrosis and perforation, and its use confined to bleeding refractory to other measures. If the oesophageal balloon is inflated it should be deflated every 4 hours.

Balloon tamponade is associated with the risk of oesophageal perforation, oesophageal necrosis and pulmonary aspiration; it is also unpleasant for the patient. In view of the discomfort it is normally used in ventilated and sedated patients. In view of the risk of oesophageal perforation it should only be used for a maximum of 24 hours.

Balloon tamponade is, however, highly effective in the temporary control of active bleeding, but is associated with 50% rebleeding after deflation of the balloon. It is associated with the risks of oesophageal rupture, ulceration and aspiration pneumonia, but is valuable in torrential bleeding as a temporising manoeuvre whilst awaiting definitive treatment (Jalan and Hayes, 2000; de Franchis, 2005).

Transjugular intrahepatic portosystemic shunt

Transjugular intrahepatic portosystemic shunt (TIPS) is a procedure placing a self-expanding metal stent radiologically between the portal vein and hepatic vein. This directly forms a shunt between the portal vein and hepatic vein. This procedure is highly effective in reducing portal pressures, which reduces blood flow through varices. TIPS is highly effective in reducing rebleeding, and in controlling acute haemorrhage (Jalan and Hayes, 2000). TIPS is, however, associated with a risk of encephalopathy, as the blood from the intestines is diverted directly into the systemic circulation, and shunt stenosis, although the latter is reduced with the use of the newer PTFE-covered stents (Bureau et al., 2004). Its use is currently limited to variceal haemorrhage refractory to endoscopic and pharmacological therapy.

Secondary prophylaxis of variceal haemorrhage

Beta-blockers

Non-selective beta-blockers reduce cardiac output, and cause splanchnic vasoconstriction reducing portal venous inflow and pressure. Beta-blockers are contra-indicated in patients with asthma. Patients on beta-blockers should have their pulse and blood pressure monitored. The target pulse rate is 50 beats per minute, or a reduction in the rest pulse rate by 25%. Several randomised controlled studies comparing propanolol or nadolol with placebo have shown a reduction in rebleeding and mortality with beta-blockers (Jalan and Hayes, 2000).

Endoscopic therapy

Initial studies comparing endoscopic sclerotherapy with no therapy showed a reduction in rebleeding in patients with endoscopic sclerotherapy, and subsequent studies comparing EVL with sclerotherapy indicated that EVL is associated with a lower rebleeding rate, complication rate and mortality when compared with endoscopic sclerotherapy (Gimson et al., 1993). EVL should be performed at regular (2-weekly) intervals until variceal eradication, with oral proton pump inhibitor prophylaxis against EVL-induced ulceration.

The combination of beta-blockers with endoscopic variceal band ligation has recently been shown to reduce rebleeding when compared with band ligation alone (de la Pena et al., 2005).

Chapter summary

Variceal haemorrhage is a serious complication of portal hypertension associated with a high mortality. Prompt recognition, fluid resuscitation, pharmacological therapy and prevention of complications are crucial in the management of this devastating complication of liver cirrhosis, and these measures, in conjunction with advances in pharmacological therapy, intensive care management and endoscopic therapy, have resulted in a reduction in mortality over the past decades.

Illustrative case study

A 50-year-old Chinese man was admitted with a large haematemesis. On examination he was minimally jaundiced, and had multiple spider naevi. His pulse was 120 bpm and blood pressure 120/80 mmHg, on admission. No ascites or splenomegaly was clinically apparent, and he was not encephalopathic. His haemoglobin was 80 g/L, INR 1.3, bilirubin 60 µmol/L, and albumin 30 g/L.

Two large-bore (16-gauge) intravenous cannulae were inserted and he was fluid resuscitated with intravenous colloid and blood transfusions. After a baseline ECG, intravenous terlipressin was commenced and he was started on prophylactic ciprofloxacin. He was nursed in a high dependency unit. His blood pressure and pulse were monitored every 30 minutes. His oxygen saturation and ECG were continually monitored.

Despite this the patient suffered a further large haematemesis in association with a drop in his blood pressure to 80/40 mmHg and in view of this he underwent endotracheal intubation to protect his airway and a large-bore central venous rapid infusion catheter was inserted. He was fluid resuscitated with a further four units of blood and fresh frozen plasma as a repeat haemoglobin was 60 g/L and INR 2.0. His blood pressure stabilised to 120/80 mmHg and pulse 80 bpm, and therefore he was transferred to the intensive care unit where he underwent upper gastrointestinal endoscopy.

At upper gastrointestinal endoscopy four grade II oesophageal varices were found, one of which was actively bleeding. These were treated at the time with EVL. Over the subsequent 24 hours he suffered no further bleeding, was extubated and transferred from the intensive care unit. Intravenous terlipressin and ciprofloxacin were continued for 5 days.

Subsequently his hepatitis serology taken on admission revealed that he was hepatitis B sAg positive with a high viral DNA level. His alpha fetoprotein was 30 kU/L. An ultrasound scan revealed a 5 cm hypervascular mass within the right lobe of the liver, and a contrast-enhanced CT scan confirmed a 5 cm hepatocellular carcinoma without invasion of the portal vein.

This case illustrates many key points as to the management of a patient with variceal haemorrhage. Firstly, the prompt recognition of a patient with cirrhosis due to his stigmata of chronic liver disease led to initial immediate treatment with terlipressin and antibiotics. The patient was then nursed in an environment appropriate to a condition with a high mortality and prompt endotracheal intubation on initial rebleeding enabled subsequent fluid resuscitation and endoscopy to be performed in a controlled manner without risk of pulmonary aspiration. Finally, the identification of the cause of cirrhosis and complicating hepatocellular carcinoma is important as the major causes of mortality in patients with variceal haemorrhage are complications of the patient's underlying liver disease, rather than uncontrolled bleeding.

References

Banares R, Albillos A, Rincon D, Alonso S, Gonzalez M, Ruiz-del-Arbol L, et al. (2002) Endoscopic treatment versus endoscopic plus pharmacologic treatment for acute variceal bleeding: a meta-analysis. *Hepatology* 35(3):609–615

Blatchford O, Davidson LA, Murray WR, Blatchford M, Pell J (1997) Acute upper gastrointestinal haemorrhage in west of Scotland: case ascertainment study. *British Medical Journal* 315(7107):510–514

British Society of Gastroenterology Endoscopy Committee (2002) Non-variceal upper gastrointestinal haemorrhage: guidelines. *Gut* 51(Suppl 4):iv1–6

Bureau C, Garcia-Pagan JC, Otal P, Pomier-Layrargues G, Chabbert V, Cortez C, et al. (2004) Improved clinical outcome using polytetrafluoroethylene-coated stents for TIPS: results of a randomized study. *Gastroenterology* 126(2):469–475

de Franchis R (2005) Evolving consensus in portal hypertension. Report of the Baveno IV consensus workshop on methodology of diagnosis and therapy in portal hypertension. *Journal of Hepatology* 43(1):167–176

de la Pena J, Brullet E, Sanchez-Hernandez E, Rivero M, Vergara M, Martin-Lorente JL, et al. (2005) Variceal ligation plus nadolol compared with ligation for prophylaxis of variceal rebleeding: a multicenter trial. *Hepatology* 41(3):572–578

Gimson AE, Ramage JK, Panos MZ, Hayllar K, Harrison PM, Williams R, et al. (1993) Randomised trial of variceal banding ligation versus injection sclerotherapy for bleeding oesophageal varices. *The Lancet* 342(8868):391–394

Heneghan MA, Byrne A, Harrison PM (2002) An open pilot study of the effects of a human fibrin glue for endoscopic treatment of patients with acute bleeding from gastric varices. *Gastrointestinal Endoscopy* 56(3):422–426

Ioannou G, Doust J, Rockey DC (2003) Terlipressin for acute esophageal variceal hemorrhage. *Cochrane Database of Systematic Reviews* (1):CD002147

Jalan R, Hayes PC (2000) UK guidelines on the management of variceal haemorrhage in cirrhotic patients. British Society of Gastroenterology. *Gut* 46(Suppl 3–4):III1–III15

Levacher S, Letoumelin P, Pateron D, Blaise M, Lapandry C, Pourriat JL (1995) Early administration of terlipressin plus glyceryl trinitrate to control active upper gastrointestinal bleeding in cirrhotic patients. *Lancet* 346(8979):865–868

Lo GH, Lai KH, Cheng JS, Chen MH, Chiang HT (2001) A prospective, randomized trial of butyl cyanoacrylate injection versus band ligation in the management of bleeding gastric varices. *Hepatology* 33(5):1060–1064

Lo GH, Lai KH, Cheng JS, Lin CK, Huang JS, Hsu PI, et al. (1997) Emergency banding ligation versus sclerotherapy for the control of active bleeding from esophageal varices. *Hepatology* 25(5):1101–1104

Nidegger D, Ragot S, Berthelemy P, Masliah C, Pilette C, Martin T, et al. (2003) Cirrhosis and bleeding: the need for very early management. *Journal of Hepatology* **39**(4):509–514

Rockall TA, Logan RF, Devlin HB, Northfield TC (1995) Incidence of and mortality from acute upper gastrointestinal haemorrhage in the United Kingdom. Steering Committee and members of the National Audit of Acute Upper Gastrointestinal Haemorrhage. *British Medical Journal* **311**(6999):222–226

Rockall TA, Logan RF, Devlin HB, Northfield TC (1996) Risk assessment after acute upper gastrointestinal haemorrhage. *Gut* **38**(3):316–321

Soares-Weiser K, Brezis M, Tur-Kaspa R, Leibovici L (2002) Antibiotic prophylaxis for cirrhotic patients with gastrointestinal bleeding. *Cochrane Database of Systematic Reviews* (2):CD002907

Wong T, Pereira SP, McNair A, Harrison PM (2000) A prospective, randomized comparison of the ease and safety of variceal ligation using a multiband vs. a conventional ligation device. *Endoscopy* **32**(12):931–934

Ascites, spontaneous bacterial peritonitis, hyponatraemia and hepatorenal failure

Suzanne Sargent

Introduction

Ascites is the most common complication of liver cirrhosis, and marks the transition from compensated to decompensated liver disease, which without liver transplantation is associated with 50% mortality over 2 years (Fernandez-Esparrach et al., 2001). Patients may additionally develop other complications associated with ascites, such as spontaneous bacterial peritonitis, dilutional hyponatraemia and hepatorenal syndrome, which are associated with a poor prognosis. This chapter will examine the underlying pathogenesis and current medical and nursing management of ascites, and the associated complications.

Definition

Ascites is the excessive accumulation of extracelluar fluid within the peritoneal cavity and is a major complication of liver cirrhosis, occurring in 50% of patients over a 10-year period (Gines et al., 1987). Whilst the most common cause of ascites is liver cirrhosis (85%), other causes have been attributed to malignancy, cardiac disease, tuberculosis, pancreatitis and other rare miscellaneous causes.

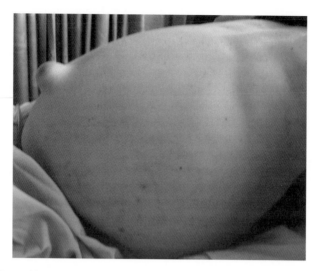

Figure 5.1   Patient with tense ascites with an umbilical hernia. For a colour version of this figure, please see Plate 6 in the colour plate section.

Table 5.1   Diagnostic criteria for refractory ascites proposed by the International Ascites Club (Cardenas et al., 2006).

- Treatment duration – patients must be on intensive diuretic therapy (spironalactone 400 mg/day and frurosemide 160 mg/day) for at least 7 days and on a restricted diet of less than 80 mmol/L salt per day
- Lack of treatment response – mean weight loss of <0.8 kg over 4 days and urinary sodium output of less than sodium intake
- Early ascites recurrence: reappearance of grade 2 or 3 ascites within 4 weeks of initial mobilisation
- Diuretic-induced complications:
  - Diuretic-induced hepatic encephalopathy is the development of encephalopathy in the absence of any precipitating cause
  - Diuretic-induced renal impairment is an increase of serum creatinine by 100% to a value of 176.8 µmol/L (2 mg/dL) in patients with ascites responding to treatment
  - Diuretic-induced hyponatremia is defined as a serum sodium decreased by >10 mmol/L to a serum sodium of <125 mmol/L
  - Diuretic-induced hypo- or hyperkalemia is defined as a change in serum potassium to <3 mmol/L or >6 mmol/L despite appropriate measures

Classification

Ascites is graded on the amount of abdominal distension and ascitic fluid detection, therefore grade 1 ascites is mild and only detectable by ultrasound examination, grade 2 ascites is moderate ascites with a moderate symmetrical distension of the abdomen and grade 3 ascites is classed as either large or gross ascites with marked abdominal distension (Figure 5.1, Plate 6) (Moore et al., 2003).

Refractory ascites occurs in 5–10% of patients with cirrhotic ascites, and is defined by the International Ascites Club (IAC) (Table 5.1) as ascites that cannot be mobilised, or early recurrence that cannot be satisfactorily prevented by medical therapy (Arroyo et al., 1996).

Pathogenesis of ascites formation

The pathophysiology underlying the formation of ascites is complex, with several proposed hypotheses. However the most widely accepted theory to explain the pathogenesis of sodium retention and the formation of ascites is the arterial vasodilation theory as shown in Figure 5.2 (Schrier et al., 1988). However, the

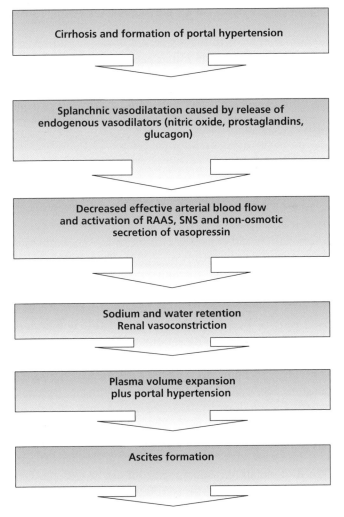

Figure 5.2 Pathogenesis of ascites in cirrhosis. As proposed by the arterial vasodilatation theory.

reduction in cardiac output seen in advanced cirrhosis is now currently being considered as a contributing factor.

According to the arterial vasodilation hypothesis, portal hypertension (portal pressure >12 mmHg) is the initial event (see Chapter 4) that results in the development of a collateral circulation, portosystemic shunting and arterial vasodilation. Arterial vasodilation is thought to occur secondary to the overproduction of vasodilators such as nitric oxide, prostaglandins and glucagons. In the early stages of cirrhosis, splanchnic arterial vasodilation is moderate and has only a small effect on the effective arterial blood volume, which is maintained within normal ranges by increases in both plasma volume and cardiac output (Schrier et al., 1988). However, in advanced cirrhosis splanchnic vasodilation becomes more pronounced causing a decrease in effective arterial blood volume, thereby increasing the stimulation of arterial and cardiopulmonary receptors, which include the sympathetic nervous system (SNS), renin–angiotensin–aldosterone system (RAAS) and the secretion of non-osmotic vasopressin (arginine). This results in both renal sodium and water retention and renal vasoconstriction. Increased lymph production from the splanchnic capillaries leads to the formation of ascites; however it is proposed that changes in peritoneal membrane and its permeability in controlling the passage of fluid may additionally contribute to ascites formation (Sherlock and Dooley, 2002). The arterial vasodilation theory also supports the underlying pathophysiology of both hepatorenal failure and dilutional hyponatraemia, which are discussed later in this chapter.

Diagnosis

A diagnosis of new-onset ascites is suspected on the basis of the patient's history and physical examination and is usually confirmed by successful abdominal paracentesis and/or ultrasonography (Runyon, 2004). Even if the cirrhosis is obvious from the history and examination it is imperative that other causes of ascites are excluded.

Because of the associated complications seen in patients with cirrhosis and ascites, an assessment of liver and renal function, full blood count (FBC) and international normalised ratio (INR) should be undertaken with an additional assessment of circulatory function (Gines et al., 2004a). On physical examination, patients may present with numerous stigmata of chronic liver disease suggesting portal hypertension, e.g. spider naevi, palmar erythema, splenomegaly, caput medusa and hepatic encephalopathy. If ascites is suspected, the presence of dullness on abdominal percussion and the demonstration of 'shifting dullness' will normally detect ascites providing at least 1.5 L of fluid are present. However, detection of ascites by physical examination in patients with obesity can be problematic (Runyon, 2004). Abdominal ultrasonography should be undertaken in all patients with ascites as this can detect as little as 100 mL of ascitic fluid and can provide additional data such as size of the liver and spleen, pancreas, lymph nodes, and

Table 5.2 Evaluation of ascitic fluid.

Diagnostic test	Values and indications

Ascitic fluid total protein (AFTP)	Exudates ascitic protein >25 g/L (2.5 g/dL)
	Transudate ascitic protein <25 g/L (2.5 g/dL)
	    AFTP concentration is usually low (<10 g/L) in 60% of cirrhotic patients
	    Protein concentration <10 g/L predicts a higher risk of developing SBP, and shorter life expectancy

Ascitic fluid cell count	Polymorphonuclear leucocyte (PMN) count ≥250 cells/mm³ is diagnostic of SBP
Serum ascites–albumin gradient (SAAG). Calculated as serum albumin concentration – ascitic fluid albumin concentration	Values >11 g/L (1.1 g/dL) suggest that ascites is related to portal hypertension, indicative of cirrhosis Values <11 g/L (1.1 g/dL) suggest causes other than portal hypertension such as malignancy, pancreatitis, tuberculosis *Accuracy of 97% in patients with portal hypertension*
Cultures in blood culture bottles	Detects both Gram-positive and Gram-negative pathogens
Amylase	Pancreatic ascites
Cytology	Carcinoma *Sensitivity of up to 96.7% has been demonstrated in peritoneal carcinoma but not routinely used for investigations of hepatocellular carcinoma*
Acid-fast smear	Indicative of tubercular ascites
Glucose	Indicative of abscess/peritonitis
Lactate dehydrogenase	Indicative of abscess/secondary peritonitis

exclude conditions such as portal vein thrombosis and hepatocellular carcinoma (Moore and Aithal, 2006).

The essential investigations other than those already discussed, should include diagnostic paracentesis with measurement of ascitic fluid protein, serum ascites albumin gradient (SAAG), neutrophil count, culture and amylase (Moore and Aithal, 2006). Details of further laboratory investigations, values, and the significance of findings are shown in Table 5.2.

Treatment

In addition to the discomfort and unwanted side effects of ascites, the accumulation of ascitic fluid may strongly affect the quality of life in patients, and this may present the rationale for treatment (Angeli and Gatta, 2005). Patients with grade 1 ascites, whilst not normally needing treatment, should still refrain from excessive salt intake as this can cause both a positive sodium balance and fluid retention (Cardenas and Gines, 2005a). In moderate (grade 2) or large (grade 3) ascites, the treatment is initially based on diet and diuretic therapy. For patients with refractory ascites, management options firstly include large-volume paracentesis,

paracentesis with diuretic therapy (providing there are no contraindications) or the radiological insertion of a transjugular intrahepatic portosystemic shunt (TIPS). In view of the 50% mortality over 2 years (Gines et al., 1987), patients with ascites should be evaluated for the suitability of a liver transplantation.

Sodium restriction

The principle of restriction is that the amount of fluid retained in the body depends on the balance between sodium ingested in the diet and sodium excreted in the urine. Therefore, if the sodium excreted is less than that ingested, patients accumulate ascites and oedema. Equally if sodium excreted is greater than the intake, then ascites and oedema decrease (Arroyo et al., 2000). A typical UK diet contains approximately 150 mmol of sodium per day of which 15% is from added salt and 70% is from manufactured foods (Moore and Aithal, 2006). Compliance is poor with very low sodium restrictions, which may exacerbate any protein malnutrition, therefore a sodium intake of 90 mmol (5.2 g) per day is advocated (Moore and Aithal, 2006). A dietetic referral is essential for all patients commencing or undertaking a low-sodium diet to provide patients and relatives or carers with appropriate dietetic advice and is discussed further in Chapter 14.

Diuretic therapy

The goal of diuretic therapy is to induce a slow and gradual diuresis without any undesirable side effects, especially dehydration and prerenal failure.

The initial diuretic of choice for single therapy is spironolactone. Plasma aldosterone concentrations increase in patients with cirrhosis and ascites, which play an important role in increasing renal tubular sodium reabsorption (Cardenas et al., 2006). Spironolactone, an aldosterone antagonist, therefore acts mainly on the aldosterone-sensitive sodium channels in the distal nephron to increase natriuresis and to conserve potassium (Moore and Aithal, 2006). Spironolactone is initially commenced at a dose of 100–200 mg/day, titrated to a maximum dose of 400 mg/day. The prolonged half-life of spironolactone and its metabolites (up to 5–7 days) allows once-daily dosing (Friedman and Keeffe, 2004). A therapeutic response is seen in 75% of patients, normally within 48 hours. Gynaecomastia is the main side effect, but hyperkalemia, metabolic acidosis and long drug half-life have also been noted (Runyon, 2004). Other diuretics acting in the distal tubes, such as amiloride, are less effective, but can be used in patients with severe side effects of spironolactone therapy (Cardenas et al., 2006).

Loop diuretics, such as furosemide, are commonly used as an adjunct to spironolactone therapy. The initial dose is 20–40 mg/day titrated to a maximum dose of 160 mg/day. However furosemide must be given with caution due to the associated side effects such as excessive diuresis and hypovolaemia, renal failure, hyponatraemia, hypokalaemia, muscle cramps and hepatic encephalopathy (Cardenas et al., 2006).

The response to diuretic therapy can be measured by weight loss, urine volume, sodium excretion and physical examination (Gines et al., 2004a). As the rate of ascitic fluid reabsorption is limited to 700–900 mL/day, the goal is to achieve a weight loss of 0.3–0.5 kg/day in patients without oedema and 0.8–1.0 kg/day in patients with oedema (until resolution of oedema) (Cardenas et al., 2006). If the weight loss exceeds this, it is usually at the expense of removing fluid from the intravascular space.

To ensure precision, patients should ideally be weighed before breakfast, with the patient wearing the same amount of clothing. Accurate documentation with weight charts is essential to plot and gauge the overall weight loss (Sargent, 2006). The principles of daily weighing also apply to outpatients, whereby bathroom scales should be used. Patients should be educated to maintain a daily record, which should be brought to the physician at outpatient clinics (Sherlock and Dooley, 2002).

Serum electrolytes, creatinine, urea and liver function tests should be monitored regularly. In the outpatient setting these should be examined a week after discharge, to allow for any treatment adjustments, however in stable outpatients these should be monitored every 4 weeks (Sherlock and Dooley, 2002).

Therapeutic paracentesis

Patients with large or refractory ascites are usually treated with repeated large-volume paracentesis (>5 L), as its combined use with colloid replacement has been demonstrated in several large clinical trials to be a rapid, safe and effective treatment (Moore and Aithal, 2006). On average, patients with refractory ascites require a therapeutic paracentesis every 2–4 weeks, which can be performed in an outpatient setting (Cardenas and Gines, 2005a).

Ascitic fluid is drained with a specially designed peritoneal needle under strict aseptic technique. For paracentesis of greater than 5 L, human albumin solution is usually administered intravenously at a rate of 6–8 g/L of ascitic fluid removed (e.g. 100 mL of 20% albumin for each 2–3 L drained) (Moore and Aithal, 2006). It is essential to record a baseline of vital signs prior to commencing large-volume paracentesis. During the procedure vital signs need to be initially recorded every 15–30 minutes, reducing the frequency if cardiovascular stability is maintained. Monitoring and recording strict fluid balance and administering the correct volume of albumin replacement therapy are vital, as circulatory dysfunction caused by ineffective intravascular volume can result in hypovolaemia, increased activation of the RAAS and hepatorenal failure. Patients also need to be observed for signs of other associated complications such as increased hepatic encephalopathy or infection. Whilst the use of human albumin solution remains the colloid of choice, the use of other synthetic plasma expanders has been advocated but is less effective at maintaining haemodynamic stability (Cardenas et al., 2006). Whilst there is no consensus on the overall length of time, paracentesis catheters should be removed as soon as possible, which is commonly between 4–6 hours, to minimise the risk of infection. Encouraging patients to lie on their side will reduce ascitic fluid leakage, and it may be necessary for the insertion of a purse string suture around the drainage site (Moore and Aithal, 2006). The temporary use of stoma collection bags can be useful to maintain skin integrity in patients with persistent leakage.

Transjugular intrahepatic portosystemic shunt

As an elevated portal pressure is one of the main factors contributing to the pathogenesis of ascites, achieving portal decompression with the use of a self-expanding portosystemic shunt is considered a successful treatment option for both oesophageal varices and refractory ascites (Moore et al., 2003). Under intravenous conscious sedation or general anaesthesia, a flexible metal prosthesis is inserted radiologically via the internal jugular vein to create a bridge between a branch of the hepatic vein and portal vein (Figure 5.3); this induces a decrease in portal pressures and subsequent improvement in renal function, and the reduction of ascites by reducing RAAS and increasing sodium excretion. TIPS is a recognised treatment option for patients with refractory ascites who need more than three large-volume paracenteses per month (Moore et al., 2003).

Whether TIPS is superior to repeated large-volume paracentesis for patients with refractory ascites remains contentious. A systematic review of five randomised control trials comparing TIPS with paracentesis supported that TIPS is more effective at removing ascites, but showed that there are no significant differences in mortality, gastrointestinal bleeding, infection and acute kidney injury (Saab et al.,

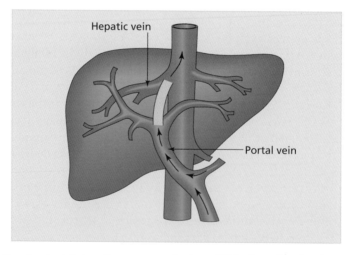

Figure 5.3 Transjugular intrahepatic portosystemic shunt (TIPS). Reproduced with permission from Krige JE, Beckingham IJ (2001) ABC of diseases of liver, pancreas, and biliary system. Portal hypertension – 1: varices. *British Medical Journal* **322**:348–351.

2006). The main contraindications for TIPS insertion are pre-existing hepatic encephalopathy, age greater than 70 years, pre-existing cardiac dysfunction and a Child-Pugh score greater than 12 (Moore et al., 2003).

Immediate postprocedure complications can be a consequence of intravenous sedation or general anaesthesia, capsular puncture and intrahepatic bleeding, or bruising around the puncture sites (Moore et al., 2003). TIPS is associated with a 25–30% incidence of hepatic encephalopathy and a high prevalence of stunt stenosis/obstruction (Sanyal et al., 2003), although stents with a polyurethane covering may reduce this. Ultrasound scans are routinely carried out 24 hours post procedure, and at 3, 6 and 12 months post insertion to assess the stent patency.

This chapter has primarily focused on the medical management of ascites, however, secondary complications such as pleural effusions, cardiovascular instability, peripheral and genital oedema, umbilical hernia, reduced mobility and loss of appetite may additionally impede on the patient's quality of life and independence. The psychological needs of these patients are vital and yet often overlooked by prioritising the medical needs. Patients with ascites are dealing with vast changes in body image, loss or a reduction in independence, as well as an awareness of deterioration in health and shortened life expectancy. Therefore, it may be necessary to refer patients for counselling or appropriate psychiatric support. If alcohol is the cause of liver disease then patients should be advised to abstain and referred to an appropriate health care professional for advice or treatment referral.

Spontaneous bacterial peritonitis

Bacterial infections are one of the most feared problems that complicate the course of patients with advanced liver disease (Cardenas and Gines, 2005a). Spontaneous bacterial peritonitis (SBP) occurs in 10–30% of patients with ascites and is characterised by the spontaneous infection of ascitic fluid in the absence of any intra-abdominal source of infection (Gines et al., 2004a). The mortality rate is estimated to be 20% with early diagnosis and the initiation of prompt treatments (Garcia-Tsao, 2001).

The underlying pathogenesis of SBP is thought to be the translocation of bacteria from the intestinal lumen to the lymph nodes, with subsequent bacteraemia and infection of ascitic fluid (Gines et al., 2004a). Aerobic Gram-negative organisms account for 72% of infections, principally *Escherichia coli* and *Klebsiella*. *Streptococcus* species are the most frequently found Gram-positive aerobes.

Although some patients with SBP may be asymptomatic, a significant number of patients will have some symptoms such as fever, mild abdominal pain, vomiting or confusion (Moore and Aithal, 2006). Additionally SBP should be excluded in patients who present with clinical deteriorations such as hepatic encephalopathy, hypotension, gastrointestinal bleeding or renal impairment (Moore et al., 2003).

The diagnosis of SBP is based upon the microscopic examination of the ascitic fluid. The presence of at least 250 polymorphonuclear leucocyte (PMN) cells/mm^3

of ascitic fluid is diagnostic of this condition, and should initiate treatment with broad-spectrum antibiotics (Gines et al., 2004a). Despite the use of sensitive methods of ascitic fluid culture, concentrations of bacteria in ascitic fluid are low in SBP. Consequently 20–40% of patients diagnosed with SBP with a high PMN count are culture negative (Cardenas et al., 2006). Nonetheless it is strongly recommended that 10 mL of ascitic fluid collected under sterile conditions should be directly inoculated into each culture bottle with media for both anaerobic and aerobic bacteria.

The treatment of choice for SBP is 5 days of third-generation non-nephrotoxic cephalosporins such as cefotaxime or quinolones. This is due to their broad antibiotic coverage, high efficiency and few side effects. Additionally, treatment with these antibiotic regimes has an incidence of 90% SBP resolution (Cardenas et al., 2006). As the incidence of SBP recurrence during the subsequent year is 40–70%, all patients with SBP should be considered for referral for liver transplantation (Moore and Aithal, 2006). Due to the associated high mortality of SBP, the use of long-term prophylactic antibiotics has been suggested to reduce the rate of recurrence, however this has been linked to the development of antibiotic-resistant organisms (Gines et al., 2004a).

The rapid onset of type 1 hepatorenal syndrome (HRS) in patients with SBP is associated with a hospital mortality of between 40–78% (Fasolato et al., 2007). Therefore as the underlying pathogenesis is linked to worsening circulatory disturbances and increased ineffective circulatory volume, the use of human albumin solution (1.5 g/kg on diagnosis of infection and 1 g/kg at 48 hours) in addition to antibiotic therapy has been shown to reduce the incidence of HRS from above 30% to 10% (Moore and Aithal, 2006).

Hyponatraemia

Dilutional hyponatraemia in cirrhosis is defined as a serum sodium concentration <130 mmol/L in the setting of an expanded cellular fluid volume. This is usually substantiated by the presence of ascites and/or oedema (Cardenas and Gines, 2005a). The prevalence of hyponatraemia in hospitalised patients with cirrhosis and ascites is estimated to be 30–35%, and is attributed to either diuretic therapy or haemodilution. In the absence of diuretic therapy dilutional hyponatraemia is indicative of a reduced survival (Porcel et al., 2002).

Dilutional hyponatraemia occurs as a result of the inability of patients to adjust the amount of water excreted in urine to that taken in (Sherlock and Dooley, 2002). The underlying pathophysiology is related to arterial vasodilation seen in patients with portal hypertension and liver cirrhosis which leads to arterial underfilling and the activation of the body's compensatory systems: the RAAS, SNS and baroreceptor stimulation of the non-osmotic release of arginine vasopressin (AVP). Control of the volume of water passed in the urine depends on the amount of water reabsorbed in the renal tubules and collecting ducts which is under the direct control of AVP. Therefore water retention in cirrhosis and ascites is due to excess vasopressin, stimulated by baroreceptors as a consequence of arterial vasodilation and arterial underfilling (Sherlock and Dooley, 2002).

The management of hyponatraemia secondary to diuretic therapy is primarily dependent on the patient's serum sodium levels and includes both fluid restriction to 1000 mL/day and the discontinuation of diuretics. Moore and Aithal (2006) suggest that patients with a serum sodium >126 mmol/L, can be managed without both water restriction and continuation of diuretic therapy, providing that renal function is neither deteriorating nor has significantly deteriorated during diuretic therapy. In patients with serum sodium of 121–125 mmol/L the opinions regarding treatments are at variance, with support for both discontinuation and continuation of diuretic therapy. However most experts unanimously support stopping diuretics if the serum sodium is <120 mmol/L. If the serum creatinine is >150 µmol/L the use of colloid plasma expanders has been advocated to preserve renal function (Moore and Aithal, 2006). Imposing fluid restriction on patients with hyponatraemia prevents further increases in total body water. Nevertheless, whilst this prevents a further decrease in serum sodium levels, fluid restrictions are not very effective in increasing serum sodium levels (Cardenas and Gines, 2005a).

Pharmacological therapies for dilutional hyponatraemia in cirrhosis have primarily focused on AVP inhibition (Cardenas and Gines, 2005a). Preliminary aquaretic therapies of vasopressin 2 receptor antagonists in the use of hyponatraemia look promising and are probably safe at low doses. Whether these improve overall mortality or morbidity is not yet known (Moore and Aithal, 2006).

Cirrhotic patients do not usually have symptoms from hyponatraemia until the sodium is <110 mmol/L or unless the decline in sodium is very rapid (Runyon, 2004). As a rapid correction of serum sodium poses a threat of producing pontine and extrapontine myelinolysis, the correction of hyponatraemia must be done slowly, avoiding increasing serum sodium >12 mmol/L over 24 hours (Cardenas and Gines, 2005b; Moore and Aithal, 2006).

Hepatorenal syndrome

Hepatorenal syndrome (HRS) is a unique form of functional renal failure without an identifiable renal pathology, that develops in 10% of patients with advanced cirrhosis or acute liver failure (Cardenas et al., 2006). Once patients develop HRS, spontaneous recovery of renal function without treatment is less than 5% (Sherlock and Dooley, 2002).

There are no specific tests for the diagnosis of HRS. Therefore the diagnosis is primarily based on excluding any other common causes of renal failure found in liver cirrhosis such as acute kidney injury secondary to hypovolaemia, volume depletion due to diuretics, vomiting or diarrhoea, or nephrotoxicity associated with both non-steroidal anti-inflammatory drugs (NSAIDs) and aminoglycoside antibiotic therapy or glomerulonephritis associated with hepatitis B and C (Cardenas

Table 5.3 International Ascites Club diagnostic criteria for HRS. Adapted from Moore (2000).

Major criteria

Low glomerular filtration rate, as indicated by serum creatinine >130 µmol/L (1.5 mg/dL) or 24-hour creatinine clearance <40 mL/min

Absence of shock, ongoing bacterial infection, fluid losses and current treatment with nephrotoxic drugs

No sustained improvement in renal function (decrease in serum creatinine <130 µmol/L (1.5 mg/dL) or increase in creatinine clearance >40 mL/min) following diuretic withdrawal or an expansion of plasma volume with 1.5 L of plasma expander

Proteinuria lower than 500 mg/day and no ultrasonographic evidence of obstructive uropathy or parenchymal renal disease

Additional/minor criteria

Urine volume <500 mL/day

Urine sodium <10 mmol/L (10 mEq/L)

Urine osmolarity greater than plasma osmolarity

Urine red blood cells less than 50 per high power field

Serum sodium concentration <130 mmol/L

et al., 2006). The International Ascites Club (IAC) proposes both major and additional diagnostic criteria for the diagnosis of HRS (Table 5.3). All the major criteria must be present for the diagnosis of HRS; the additional criteria, whilst not necessary for a diagnosis, can be beneficial in providing some supporting evidence (Arroyo et al., 1996).

The International Ascites Club have categorised HRS into types 1 and 2. Patients with type 1 HRS have a rapid progression (less than 2 weeks) of renal failure with doubling of the initial serum creatinine to >220 µmol/L (2.5 mg/dL), or a 50% reduction of the initial clearance to less than 20 mL/min (Cardenas et al., 2006). Until the recent advances in therapeutic treatments, the median survival of patient with type 1 HRS was only 1.7 weeks, with only 10% surviving more than 3 months (Gines et al., 2003). Patients who have a slower decline in renal function are classed as type 2 HRS.

The underlying pathogenesis of HRS is related to vasoconstriction of the renal circulation (Figure 5.4). However the precise mechanisms are unclear and are believed to be multifactoral, involving disturbances of circulatory function and the systemic and renal vasoactive mechanisms (Marik et al., 2006). Renal perfusion is dependent on adequate arterial blood pressure which is already reduced in cirrhosis. Consequently the RAAS, SNS and AVP are already stimulated in 80% of patients with cirrhosis, and are further elevated in HRS as hepatic function declines (Moore, 2000). These result in a reduction of renal function due to renal vasoconstriction, renal hypoperfusion and reduced glomerular filtration rate (GFR), and increased sodium and water absorption (Gines, 2003). Conversely, recent clinical data suggest that type 1 and type 2 HRS are different syndromes and not different expressions of a common underlying disorder. This is primarily due to the fact that renal failure in HRS type 1 is severe and progressive, mimicking acute kidney

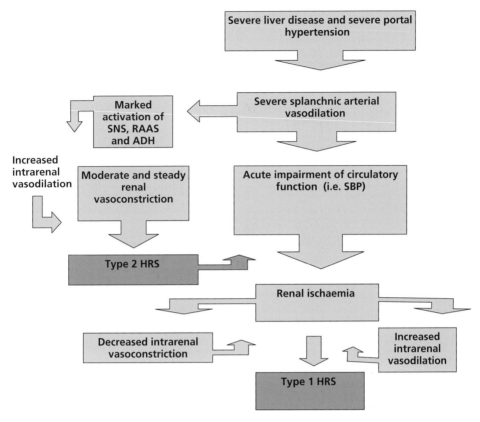

Figure 5.4 Pathogenesis of type 1 and 2 HRS. Reprinted from Friedman L, Keeffe E (2004) Pathogenesis of hepatorenal syndrome. *Handbook of Liver Disease* 2nd edn. p.166 with permission from Elsevier. (SNS = sympathetic nervous system; RAAS = renin–angiotensin–aldosterone system; ADH = antidiuretic hormone; SBP = spontaneous bacterial peritonitis).

injury seen in other conditions, e.g. sepsis. In contrast renal impairment seen in type 2 is moderate and steady (Arroyo et al., 2007).

Treatment of HRS

The initial management of these patients requires an exclusion of reversible or treatable conditions such as bacterial infection, gastrointestinal bleeding, and aggressive paracentesis leading to post-paracentesis circulatory dysfunction. The benefits of administering human albumin solution in conjunction with antibiotic therapy in SBP have already been described. Established treatment therapies for HRS primarily aim at reversing the splanchnic vasodilation and subsequent renal vasoconstriction, and include vasoconstrictors with additional plasma expansion, TIPS or liver transplantation.

Terlipressin (glypressin), a synthetic analogue of vasopressin, is the most frequently used and studied vasoconstrictor employed in the treatment of HRS. Used in combination with human albumin as a volume expander, terlipressin has demonstrated an improvement of renal function and normalisation of serum creatinine (Cardenas et al., 2006). Whilst there are no standard treatment guidelines, terlipressin is usually administered intravenously at a dose of 0.5–2 mg every 4–6 hours. The end point of therapy is usually a maximum of 15 days of treatment, or a serum creatinine <130 μmol/L (1.5 mg/dL). Terlipressin is usually given in conjunction with 20–40 g/day of intravenous human albumin solution.

Whilst urine volume tends to increase within 12–24 hours of terlipressin administration, improvement in GFR occurs slowly over several days. HRS recurrence is uncommon in patients responding to terlipressin therapy (Gines et al., 2003). Patients receiving terlipressin should have daily ECGs and regular monitoring of their limbs, neurological status and for abdominal pain to assess for potential ischaemic side effects. Discontinuation of therapy due to ischaemic side effects occurs in 5–10% of patients (Gines et al., 2003).

Other pharmacological agents such as α-adrenergic agonists noradrenaline (norepinephrine) and midodrine have demonstrated some success in the treatments of HRS (Alessandria et al., 2007). The use of oral tumour necrosis factor (TNF) inhibitor pentoxfylline has been shown to reduce the incidence of HRS in patients with acute alcoholic hepatitis (Cardenas et al., 2006).

Transjugular intrahepatic portosystemic shunt

Portal decompression following TIPS insertion results in a reduction in RAAS and SNS activity, consequently this reduces renal vasoconstriction and improves renal function. Although uncontrolled studies suggest that TIPS improves prognosis in HRS type 1 and type 2, the real impact of survival remains to be assessed (Cardenas et al., 2006).

Until comparative studies are undertaken, vasoconstrictors appear to be the treatment of choice in type 1 HRS because of the similar efficiency, wider availability and lower costs than TIPS (Gines et al., 2003). Additionally vasoconstrictor drugs can be given to most patients with HRS, regardless of the severity of the liver failure and can be used in all clinical settings (Gines et al., 2004b).

Renal replacement therapy

The efficiency of haemodialysis or continuous renal replacement therapy has not been adequately assessed in patients with HRS, therefore renal support should only be offered when there is a real chance of hepatic regeneration, hepatic recovery or a realistic chance of a liver transplant; as it only serves to prolong the terminal illness (Moore, 2000). Whilst newer treatments, such as extracorporeal albumin dialysis, have been shown to improve systemic haemodynamics and reduce the plasma levels of renin in type 1 HRS, due to the ability to remove albumin-bound substances, further research is needed to validate these findings.

Liver transplantation

Whilst the other outlined treatment options may improve short-term survival the only effective and permanent treatment for HRS in patients with end-stage liver disease is liver transplantation, as this allows both the disease and the associated liver disease to be cured. The main problem in the use of liver transplantation for type 1 HRS in patients with liver cirrhosis is that many patients die before transplantation is possible either because of their short-term survival expectancy or current long waiting lists for a suitable organ; consequently liver transplantation is more commonly seen in patients with type 2 HRS (Gines et al., 2003).

Chapter summary

This chapter has examined the pathogenesis and management of ascites in liver cirrhosis and the allied complications of spontaneous bacterial peritonitis, hyponatraemia and hepatorenal syndrome. Whilst the understanding of the underlying pathogenesis and management strategies have vastly improved over the last few decades, liver transplantation remains the only viable treatment option for long-term survival.

Illustrative case study

A 37-year-old man presented with a 4-week history of jaundice (serum bilirubin 212 µmol/L), INR of 1.38, with abdominal tenderness, a recent loss of appetite with unquantifiable weight loss, and fatigue. He had no previous medical history, but reported drinking heavily over the last 6 months due to stress and financial problems. His alcohol intake had increased from 20 to 140 units per day. His physical examination revealed hepatosplenomegaly, with a soft palpable abdomen. There were no other stigmata of chronic liver disease noted. The patient was diagnosed with decompensated alcoholic liver disease and acute alcoholic hepatitis. The discriminate function was calculated at 41.8 (please refer to Chapter 7 for further details).

A full liver disease aetiology screen was negative for any other causes of liver disease, and an abdominal ultrasound scan ruled out any obstructive causes of jaundice and confirmed his hepatosplenomegaly. The patient's remaining liver function tests of AST, ALT, alkaline phosphatase and GGT were consistent with the diagnosis of acute alcoholic hepatitis.

The patient's renal profile on admission was deranged with a serum creatinine of 196 µmol/L (normal value 35–135 µmol/L) and urea 28.9 mmol/L (normal value <7 mmol/L). His urine output was poor and he continued to become anuric, despite 2 L of intravenous colloid. The patient was cardiovascularly stable and had

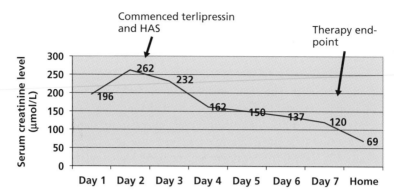

Figure 5.5　Demonstrating improvement in renal function after commencing terlipressin and HAS therapy.

no other risk factors for renal impairment. However, over the next 24 hours his renal function continued to decline and his serum creatinine increased to 262 µmol/L.

With an additional diagnosis of type 1 HRS the patient was commenced with intravenous terlipressin 0.5 mg q6h with an adjunct of 20 g of intravenous human albumin solution daily, and was transferred to a regional liver centre. For his severe alcoholic hepatitis he commenced on oral pentoxfylline 400 mg q8h and oral prednisolone. The patient continued on intravenous terlipressin therapy for 5 days until his serum creatinine was below 130 µmol/L. His serum creatinine continued to normalise and he was discharged home with normal renal function 10 days later (Figure 5.5).

As this case study demonstrates, type 1 HRS was once considered a terminal illness due to the high mortality, but recent advances in pharmacological therapies have enabled the reversal of HRS, allowing patients to regain normal renal function, without necessitating renal replacement therapies.

References

Alessandria C, Ottobrelli A, Debernardi-Venon W, Todros L, Torrani Cerenzia M, Martini S, Balzola F, Morgando A, Rizzetto M, Marzano A (2007) Noradrenaline vs terlipressin in patients with hepatorenal syndrome: a prospective; randomised, unblended, pilot study. *Journal of Hepatology* 47:499–505

Angeli P, Gatta A (2005) Medical treatment of ascites in cirrhosis. In: Gines P, Arroyo V, Rodes J, Schrier RW (eds) *Ascites and Renal Dysfunction in Liver Disease*, 2nd edn. Blackwell Publishing, Oxford

Arroyo V, Bataller R, Gines P (2000) Ascites and spontaneous bacterial peritonitis. In: O'Grady J, Lake J, Howdle P (eds) *Comprehensive Clinical Hepatology*. Mosby, London, pp. 2.7.1–2.7.14

Arroyo V, Gines P, Gerbes A, Dudley FJ, Gentilini P, Laffi G, Renyolds TB, Ring-Larsen H, Schomerich J (1996) Definition and diagnostic criteria of refractory ascites and hepatorenal syndrome in cirrhosis. International Ascites Club. *Hepatology* 23:164–176

Arroyo V, Terra C, Gines P (2007) Advances in the pathogenesis and treatment of type-1 and type-2 hepatorenal syndrome. *Journal of Hepatology* 46:935–946

Cardenas A, Gines P (2005a) Management of complication of cirrhosis in patients awaiting liver transplantation. *Journal of Hepatology* 42:S124–S133

Cardenas A, Gines P (2005b) Management of hyponatremia in cirrhosis. Gines P, Arroyo V, Rodes J, Schrier RW (eds) *Ascites and Renal Dysfunction in Liver Disease*, 2nd edn. Blackwell Publishing, Malden, MA, pp. 315–326

Cardenas A, Gines P, Arroyo V (2006) Ascites, hyponatremia, hepatorenal syndrome and spontaneous bacterial peritonitis. In: Bacon BR, O'Grady JG, Di Bisceglie AM, Lake JR (eds) *Comprehensive Clinical Hepatology*, 2nd edn. Elsevier-Mosby, Philadelphia, pp. 153–176

Fasolato S, Angeli P, Dallagnese L, Maresio G, Zola E, Mazza E, Salinas F, Dona S, Faqiuali S et al. (2007) Renal failure and bacterial infections in patients with cirrhosis; epidemiology and clinical features. *Hepatology* 45(1):223–229

Fernandez-Esparrach G, Sanchez-Fueyro A, Gines P, Uriz J, Quinto L, Ventura PJ et al. (2001) A prognostic model for predicting survival in cirrhosis with ascites. *Journal of Hepatology* 34:46–52

Friedman L, Keeffe E (2004) *Handbook of Liver Disease*, 2nd edn. Churchill Livingstone, Philadelphia

Garcia-Tsao G (2001) Current management of the complications of cirrhosis and portal hypertension, variceal haemorrhage, ascites and spontaneous bacterial peritonitis. *Gastroenterology* 120:726–748

Gines P, Cardenas A, Arroyo V, Rodes J (2004a) Management of cirrhosis and ascites. *The New England Journal of Medicine* 350(16):1646–1654

Gines P, Guevara M, Arroyo V, Rodes J (2003) Hepatorenal syndrome. *The Lancet* 362:1819–1827

Gines P, Quintero E, Arroyo V, Teres J, Bruguera M, Rimola A, Caballeria J, Rodes J, Rozman C (1987) Compensated cirrhosis: natural history and prognostic factors. *Hepatology* 7(1):122–128

Gines P, Torre A, Terra C, Guevara M (2004b) Review article: pharmacological treatments of hepatorenal syndrome. *Alimentary Pharmacology & Therapeutics* 20(suppl 3):57–62

Krige JE, Beckingham IJ (2001) ABC of diseases of liver, pancreas, and biliary system. Portal hypertension – 1: varices. *British Medical Journal* 322:348–351

Marik PE, Wood K, Starlz TE (2006) The course of type 1 hepato-renal syndrome post liver transplantation. *Nephrology, Dialysis, Transplantation* 21:478–482

Moore K (2000) Hepatorenal syndrome and other renal diseases. In: O'Grady J, Lake J, Howdle P (eds) *Comprehensive Clinical Hepatology*. Mosby, London, pp. 2.8.1–2.8.16

Moore KP, Aithal GP (2006) Guidelines on the management of ascites in cirrhosis. *Gut* **55**; 1–12

Moore KP, Wong F, Gines P, Bernardi M, Ochs A, Salerno F, Angeli P et al. (2003) The management of ascites in cirrhosis: Report on the consensus conference of the International Ascites Club. *Hepatology* **38**(1):258–266

Porcel A, Diaz F, Rendon P, Macias M, Martin-Herrera L, Giron-Gonzalez JA (2002) Dilutional hyponatremia in patients with liver cirrhosis and ascites. *Archives on Internal Medicine* **162**(3):323–328

Runyon BA (2004) Practice guidelines committee, American Association for the Study of Liver Disease (AASLD) Management of adult patients with ascites due to cirrhosis. *Hepatology* **39**(3):1–16

Saab S, Nieto JM, Lewis SK, Runyon BA (2006) TIPS versus paracentesis for cirrhotic patients with refractor ascites. *Cochrane Database of Systemic Reviews Issue 4*, art No CG004889 DOI: 10.1002/14651858.CD004889. pub.2

Sanyal A, Gennings C, Reddy KR, Wong F, Kowdley K, Benner K, McCashland T et al. (2003) A randomised control study of TIPS vs. large volume paracentesis in the treatment of refractory ascites. *Gastroenterology* **124**:634–643

Sargent S (2006) The management and care of cirrhotic ascites. *British Journal of Nursing* **15**(4):212–219

Schrier RW, Arroyo V, Bernardi M, Epstein M, Henriksen JH, Rodes J (1988) Peripheral arterial vasodilation hypothesis: a proposal for the initiation of renal sodium and water retention in cirrhosis. *Hepatology* **8**:1152–1157

Sherlock S, Dooley J (2002) *Diseases of the Liver and Biliary System*, 11th edn. Blackwell Publishing, Oxford

Hepatic encephalopathy

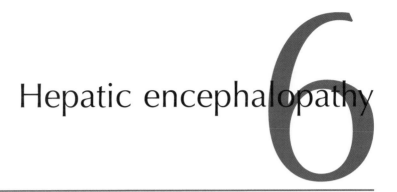

Catherine Houlston and Helen O'Neal

Introduction

Hepatic encephalopathy is the neurological impairment seen as a complication of acute and chronic liver disease. The three main theories of its pathophysiology will be discussed whilst others are summarised. The commonly recognised classification score for hepatic encephalopathy is described highlighting how the clinician may use it in their assessment of the disorder. The current treatments of encephalopathy are discussed. Specific considerations for the critical care management of hepatic encephalopathy secondary to acute liver failure are described in Chapter 13.

Definition

Hepatic encephalopathy has been described as a reversible impairment of cognitive function or level of consciousness in patients with liver disease or portosystemic shunts (Voigt and Conn, 1995). Ferenci et al. (2002) add that it occurs after exclusion of other brain disease in patients with both neuropsychiatric disorders and liver disease.

When liver function deteriorates the detoxification processes become impaired and shunting of blood occurs around the liver. This metabolic derangement results in an accumulation of neurotoxic products, primarily from the gut. These neurotoxins leak into the systemic circulation, reaching the brain and causing damage to the nervous system, which precipitates hepatic encephalopathy.

Pathophysiology of hepatic encephalopathy

Three main theories have been proposed to explain the development of hepatic encephalopathy in patients with liver failure. These are:

- Ammonia theory
- Gamma-amino butyric acid (GABA)/benzodiazepine theory
- False neurotransmitter theory

   Each of these has been examined as a cause for hepatic encephalopathy; however they may work synergistically to produce the effect of disordered consciousness. Other theories have been proposed (Table 6.1); these will not be reviewed due to limited evidence.

Ammonia hypothesis

This is the most popular hypothesis and is based on the accumulation of ammonia as a direct consequence of liver dysfunction. Evidence reinforcing this includes the

Table 6.1   Summary of the proposed hypotheses for the pathogenesis of hepatic encephalopathy.

Proposed hypotheses	Pathogenesis
Ammonia	Increased levels arise due to failure to be eliminated through the urea cycle within the dysfunctional liver. Hyperammonaemia has neurotoxic effects
GABA/benzodiazepines	Increased levels of GABA (the main inhibitory neurotransmitter in the brain) are found in liver dysfunction. Receptor sites for GABA are competed for by increased endogenous benzodiazepines causing neuroinhibition
False neurotransmitter theory (dopamine/norepinepherine)	In liver dysfunction weak neurotransmitters are produced from increased activity of gut bacteria on protein and production of aromatic amino acids. These replace true transmitters such as dopamine
Glutamate	Increased ammonia levels bind with glutamate and this saturation causes glutamate neurotransmitter dysfunction
Serotonin	Serotonin synthesis is increased by tryptophan levels in the plasma of patients with liver disease and influences the control of sleep–wake cycle
Manganese	The liver fails to excrete manganese effectively in cirrhosis. Raised levels cause a decrease in dopamine receptors which may illicit Parkinsonian features

clinical observation that treatments decreasing blood ammonia levels can improve hepatic encephalopathy symptoms. This theory has been contested, because 10% of patients with significant encephalopathy have normal serum ammonia levels (Sherlock and Dooley, 2002). Furthermore many patients with cirrhosis and elevated ammonia levels do not have encephalopathy (Nicolao et al., 2003). Many studies have been performed to prove this theory as a cause for hepatic encephalopathy, but they remain inconclusive (Faint, 2006).

The elimination of ammonia is a normal hepatic metabolic process using gut-derived enzymes to cleave it from proteins such as amines, amino acids, purines and pyrimidines. These enzymes are produced by normal gastrointestinal tract flora and catalyse deamination. In the liver, ammonia is either converted to urea or consumed in the conversion from glutamate (an excitatory neurotransmitter and precursor for GABA synthesis) to glutamine during the urea cycle. When hepatocyte function is impaired, ammonia and glutamine accumulate causing hyperammonaemia.

The effect of hyperammonaemia is exacerbated in liver dysfunction as portosystemic shunting diverts the ammonia into the systemic circulation. The skeletal muscle and kidneys metabolise and excrete ammonia to an extent by forming glutamine with the enzyme glutamine synthetase. In liver impairment the activity of this enzyme in muscle increases. However, in chronic cirrhosis muscle wasting is common so the amount of enzyme is less.

Increasing alkalosis contributes to rising ammonia levels (Yurdaydin, 2003) as hyperammonaemia stimulates the respiratory centre, resulting in respiratory alkalosis. Any reduction in urea cycle activity further increases bicarbonate and ammonia levels, worsening both alkalosis and hyperammonaemia.

The neurotoxic effects of ammonia include influencing brain function by impairing amino acid metabolism and energy use within the brain. It is also believed to affect astrocyte cells. These maintain electrolyte homoeostasis, provide neurotransmitter precursors and nutrients to the neurons and have a role in detoxification. An accumulation of neurotoxins, such as ammonia, can cause changes to the astrocytes as the neurotoxins gain access to the brain and influence regulation of the blood–brain barrier permeability. In acute liver failure (ALF) astrocytes appear to swell, contributing to cerebral oedema, whereas in chronic liver failure alongside the swelling, changes in the cell composition also appear to occur (Butterworth, 1999) similar to those seen in Alzheimer's disease. The swelling of astrocytes secondary to hyperammonaemia stimulates an increase in the synthesis of neurosteroids (Haussinger et al., 2000) which are believed to bind to GABA receptor complexes.

The gamma-amino butyric acid theory

GABA is an important inhibitory neurotransmitter that prevents excessive neurostimulation (Park and Navapurkar, 1994). It is produced in the gastrointestinal tract from glutamate and binds to the GABA receptor complex within the brain, which also has binding sites for benzodiazepines and barbiturates. Any binding with this site opens a chloride channel; the resulting changes in chloride levels stimulate neuroinhibition. These chloride channels are similarly influenced by hyperammonaemia (Jalan and Hayes, 1997; Haussinger et al., 2002; Sherlock and Dooley, 2002).

Although accumulation of GABA may contribute to encephalopathy, the role of the GABA receptor complex suggests endogenous benzodiazepines may also be implicated. Studies into the efficacy of flumazenil, a benzodiazepine receptor antagonist, reinforce this supposition, however study findings are at variance (Sherlock and Dooley, 2002).

False neurotransmitter theory

The false neurotransmitter theory suggests substances, such as phenylethanolamine, tyramine and octopamine, are generated by bacterial action in the colon. These are believed to inhibit cerebral neurotransmission by replacing the true transmitter, for example, resulting in reduced dopamine production. Changes to precursors of neurotransmitters may also be implicated, as levels of aromatic amino acids are increased in liver failure and branched-chain amino acids levels are decreased. The significance of these two groups of amino acids is they compete for uptake by the brain and create an imbalance in the permeability of the blood–brain barrier, predisposing to a vasogenic cause of cerebral oedema. The presence of aromatic amino acids is also thought to promote synthesis of the inhibitory transmitter, serotonin.

Other factors

Inflammation and sepsis has also been implicated as a contributory factor in the development and severity of encephalopathy (Rolando et al., 2000) exerting an influence on any of the proposed theories. Clearly, there are many overlaps between these theories reinforcing the supposition that they act synergistically to produce cerebral intoxication as a consequence of metabolic derangement.

These pathophysiological changes result in increased blood–brain barrier permeability and astrocyte swelling, raising the potential for cerebral oedema secondary to encephalopathy in the patient with ALF. Cerebral oedema is a complication which causes an increase in volume and pressure within the cranium with the potential for cerebral herniation or coning resulting in brainstem death.

Classification of hepatic encephalopathy

Hepatic encephalopathy has been defined into three types by a working party at a landmark conference (Ferenci et al., 2002):

■ *Encephalopathy associated with acute liver failure.* This is associated with cerebral oedema and raised intracranial pressure. It can develop rapidly in patients with acute liver failure and may lead to brainstem herniation and death (Knawy, 2004)

■ *Encephalopathy associated with portosystemic bypass and no intrinsic hepato-cellular disease.* Portosystemic shunts are generally associated with cirrhosis in liver failure, but may also occur without liver disease, such as following portocaval shunt surgery. This can be severe and intractable (Krige and Beckingham, 2001)

■ *Encephalopathy associated with cirrhosis and portal hypertension or porto-systemic shunts*

This was further subdivided by Ferenci et al. (2002):

■ Episodic encephalopathy which fluctuates in severity. It may be precipitated by recognised precipitating factors, or may occur spontaneously. Recurrent encephalopathy is defined as where more than two episodes of episodic encephalopathy occur in 1 year

■ Persistent encephalopathy where cognitive deficits have a negative impact on social and occupational functioning. This may be mild and only recognised by psychometric or neurophysiological testing, or severe according to the degree of autonomy (Blei and Cordoba, 2001). Patients with persistent encephalopathy may be treatment dependent where symptoms rapidly increase if there is any discontinuation in treatment (Ferenci et al., 2002)

■ Minimal encephalopathy is diagnosed in 30–80% of patients with liver cirrhosis (Knawy, 2004). This is demonstrated by psychometric tests and is significant as it will affect the patient's ability to be able to work and function normally at home

Quantifying the degree of hepatic encephalopathy can be difficult as diagnosis can be subjective. The West Haven grading system is commonly used and is based on changes in consciousness, intellectual function and behaviour (Table 6.2). Patients can be assessed for changes in their mental state using this or similar tools. Interpretation of the grades can, however, be subjective. In severe hepatic encephalopathy the use of the Glasgow coma score in addition to the grading system may help to quantify neurological impairment (Ferenci et al., 2002).

Diagnosis and investigations

Diagnosis of encephalopathy is made by clinical examination including a history of liver disease. There are no specific diagnostic investigations, although certain tests may be required to exclude any other cause. The neurological assessment and investigations that may be required are summarised in Table 6.3.

Laboratory results may show hepatic dysfunction, such as abnormal liver function tests and a raised PT/INR. Measurement of ammonia levels may be carried

Table 6.2 West Haven criteria for semiquantative grading of mental state. Reproduced from Ferenci P, Lockwood A, Mullen K, Tarter R, Weissenborn K, Blei AT (2002) Hepatic encephalopathy: definition, nomenclature, diagnosis, and quantification. Final report of the working party at the 11th World Congresses of Gastroenterology, Vienna 1998. *Hepatology* **35**:716–721 with permission from John Wiley and Sons.

Grade of hepatic encephalopathy	Clinical signs and symptoms
Grade 1	Trivial lack of awareness Euphoria or anxiety Shortened attention span Impaired performance of addition
Grade 2	Lethargy or apathy Minimal disorientation for time or place Subtle personality change Inappropriate behaviour Impaired performance of subtraction
Grade 3	Somnolence to semi-stupor, but responsive to verbal stimuli Confusion Gross disorientation
Grade 4	Coma (unresponsive to verbal or noxious stimulation)

Table 6.3 Summary of neurological assessment and investigations in hepatic encephalopathy.

Neurological examination	
Mental function	Orientation to time, place and person Changes in sleep–wake cycle (daytime sleeping with nocturnal waking) Cognitive changes apparent by decreasing ability to care for themselves West Haven criteria (Ferenci et al., 2002) and Glasgow coma score
Motor function	Cranial nerve function usually normal, although dysarthria where the patient has difficulty with speech may be present Evidence of increased tone and possibly tremors A 'flapping' tremor (asterexis) may be present when the patient's arms are outstretched by rapid flexion–extension movements at the metacarpophalangeal and wrist joints (Sherlock and Dooley, 2002)
Sensory function	Sensory changes are unusual and therefore other diagnoses should be considered if present

Investigations	
CT scan	Can confirm the absence of a space-occupying lesion such as tumour or bleed May show mild cerebral atrophy, generally in patients with alcohol-related cirrhosis In ALF may confirm presence of cerebral oedema, but is not routinely used
Lumbar puncture	May be required to rule out infection such as encephalitis
Electroencephalogram (EEG)	Changes may be present in encephalopathy of grade 2 or above. This is not conclusive evidence however as changes not specific to hepatic encephalopathy

Table 6.4 Risk factors for developing hepatic encephalopathy.

Level of risk	Risk factor
Low risk	Chronic hepatic failure but stable
Medium risk	Decompensated hepatic failure: ■ Sepsis ■ Recent gastrointestinal bleed ■ Renal failure
High risk	Acute liver failure, e.g. acetaminophen (paracetamol) overdose

out when making the initial diagnosis, although continued readings are not considered to be of any value in chronic liver disease patients (Blei and Cordoba, 2001). However, in ALF arterial ammonia levels >150 µmol/L have been associated with intracranial hypertension, so are useful in identifying patients who are at risk of cerebral complications (Clemmesen et al., 1999).

In advanced chronic liver disease encephalopathy is generally caused by precipitating events, such as a recent gastrointestinal bleed or sepsis (Table 6.4). Evidence of these precipitating factors should be specifically sought during examination and investigation to help with diagnosis.

Early signs of encephalopathy may include changes in personality and behaviour that may be subtle. As the encephalopathy progresses there may be an increase in apathy and inability to concentrate. These discrete changes in a patient's condition require the medical and nursing teams to be particularly observant and use of the encephalopathy grading system to help monitor changes.

Treatment and management of hepatic encephalopathy

The management of encephalopathy secondary to both acute and chronic liver failure involves the treatment and prevention of its precipitants and reduction of circulating ammonia levels. There are specific additional considerations concerning ALF which are discussed separately.

Treatment and prevention of precipitants

Sepsis

Rising ammonia levels in the blood resulting from increased tissue catabolism in sepsis may worsen encephalopathy. Patients with chronic ascites in liver disease are at risk of developing spontaneous bacterial peritonitis, the management of which is discussed in Chapter 5.

Reducing risk factors for infection through good infection control practice is essential. Dellinger et al. (2004) describe guidelines for the management of severe sepsis and septic shock. These guidelines, although not produced specifically for this group of patients, describe the same principles that are required. A full septic screen should be undertaken as soon as infection is suspected and should include an ascitic tap. Empirical antibiotic therapy may be started once cultures have been taken and should be reviewed regularly with microbiology advice. Preserving the integrity of the gut wall to decrease the risk of gut bacterial translocation can also help reduce sepsis (Buckley and MacFie, 1997) and this can be achieved by maintaining enteral feeding in mechanically ventilated patients.

Constipation

Constipation will increase the production and absorption of ammonia from the gut, and must therefore be avoided. Current treatment of encephalopathy assumes ammonia is mainly produced by colonic bacteria in the gut, so bowel cleansing could theoretically help reduce encephalopathy by reducing ammonia levels. The evidence to support this is limited; however the use of lactulose to treat and prevent encephalopathy is common practice (Shawcross and Jalan, 2005). Dosages of lactulose should be adjusted so that the patient has two to four semi-soft stools a day (Blei and Cordoba, 2001). This will require careful monitoring as excessive diarrhoea could worsen electrolyte imbalance. Phosphate enemas may be used for patients unable to tolerate oral lactulose although staff must be aware of the risk of rectal injuries and hyperphosphataemia (Davies, 2004).

Gastrointestinal bleeding

The presence of blood in the upper gastrointestinal tract can increase the absorption of ammonia and nitrogen from the gut which is thought to contribute to hepatic encephalopathy (Knawy, 2004). Treatment and prevention of upper gastrointestinal bleeding are important, as is ensuring adequate clearance of blood from the gut, with the use of lactulose and/or with phosphate enemas.

Renal failure

Renal impairment is another risk factor for encephalopathy, probably due to decreased clearance of nitrogenous substances including ammonia and urea. Common causes are sepsis, dehydration and hepatorenal syndrome. Treatment of the cause of renal impairment and renal replacement therapy when appropriate are important management strategies.

Fluid and electrolyte disturbances

Cirrhotic patients may become hypokalaemic as a result of losing potassium through vomiting, diarrhoea and through poor dietary intake. Hypokalaemia will be accompanied by extracellular alkalosis which it is thought contributes to renal synthesis and release of ammonia (Conn, 1994). Hypokalaemia can be avoided with intravenous or oral supplements when indicated. Potassium and sodium depletion may occur with diuretics and the diuresis may reduce hepatic blood flow which is also thought to contribute to encephalopathy. Diuretics should therefore be used with extreme care in those with liver failure.

Avoidance of sedatives

Some analgesics, barbiturates and other sedatives can induce encephalopathy (Krige and Beckingham, 2001). Managing patients with hepatic encephalopathy can be challenging as they may become confused and agitated, however unnecessary sedation should be avoided as it will exacerbate their neurological impairment. The use of appropriate benzodiazepine regimes for alcohol withdrawal syndrome is discussed in Chapter 7.

Ammonia reduction

Nutrition
There has been some debate about methods for reducing ammonia through dietary protein restriction. However, Cordoba et al. (2004) demonstrated that ensuring patients receive enough dietary protein could help reduce hepatic encephalopathy; therefore protein restriction is not advocated. Nutritional recommendations compiled by the European Society for Clinical Nutrition and Metabolism (ESPEN) suggest this may be achieved by providing supplements by both oral and enteral tube feeding (Plauth et al., 2006). When nutritional requirements are not met, nitrogenous products from muscle breakdown for gluconeogenesis may exacerbate hepatic encephalopathy. Meeting the patients' nutritional requirements can be particularly challenging, and are discussed further in Chapter 14.

Pharmacological and other treatments
There are various other tested treatments for hepatic encephalopathy which may be used whilst debate into their effectiveness continues. These are included in the treatment summary shown in Table 6.5.

General care and ongoing assessment

When caring for a patient with liver disease it is important to include neurological assessment as part of their ongoing care to detect any change. Some patients may live with a degree of encephalopathy manifested with short-term memory loss or sleep disturbances. Others may rapidly deteriorate over a few hours, such as in acute liver failure. When caring for a patient with liver disease an awareness of the risk factors for encephalopathy can help to identify those at greatest risk. This will highlight those patients requiring particularly close monitoring.

Table 6.5 Treatment options in hepatic encephalopathy.

Treatment	Mode of action
Probiotics	Used in dietary management. Modifies gut flora, reducing ammonia
Lactulose	Reduces absorption of ammonia from the gut
L-ornithine-L-aspartate	Stimulates urea cycle resulting in loss of ammonia
Sodium benzoate	Promotes urinary excretion of ammonia
Levodopa and bromocriptine	Correction of defect in dopamine neurotransmission
Flumazanil	A benzodiazepine receptor antagonist which has shown some improvement in patients with hepatic encephalopathy
Branched-chain amino acid	Used to counterbalance the ratio deficit between branched-chain amino acid and aromatic amino acid
Molecular Adsorbents Recirculating System (MARS)®	Extracorporeal blood detoxification of toxins such as ammonia. Used as bridge to liver transplantation in fulminant liver failure
Zinc	As a cofactor of all five enzymatic reactions in the urea cycle. Improvements in hepatic encephalopathy are especially noted in malnutrition

Nursing these patients may be challenging as they may become confused and uncooperative. Sedation or analgesia could depress the patient's neurological state further, whereas sleep deprivation or steroids may induce confusion and behaviour disturbances. Close observation of electrolytes and blood glucose are required as abnormalities may lead to neurological impairment and require correction. Endotracheal intubation may be required if the patient either becomes unmanageable or if the airway is compromised.

Hepatic encephalopathy in acute liver failure

With acute liver failure the rate of onset and progression of encephalopathy can be varied and unpredictable. The onset of encephalopathy marks the presence of true acute liver failure, and is often a determining factor in deciding on the need for transplantation. The key to caring for these patients is identification of the cause of acute liver failure and appropriate treatment. Initially this includes close observation and assessment of the subtle changes in their conscious level. As the patients' level of consciousness and activity deteriorates, assessment of physiological dynamics becomes necessary. It is at this point that patients with acute liver failure should be transferred to a critical care setting.

Patients who are approaching grade 3–4 hepatic encephalopathy have an 80% risk of developing cerebral oedema (Bersten et al., 2003); of these 35% may die due to brainstem herniation (Bernal and Wendon, 2004). The management of these patients then becomes focused on maintaining the integrity of the brain and its normal physiological functioning. The overall aim is to minimise fluctuations in cerebral blood flow achieved by managing the patient's mechanical ventilation,

Table 6.6 Summary of key points from recommendations (O'Neal et al., 2006).

Frequent neurological assessment:
- Pupillary reaction
- Close observation for seizure activity
- Transient episodes of cardiovascular instability

Adequate sedation
Suction as clinically indicated
Mild permissive hypocapnia
Application of ventilator care bundle:
- 30 degrees head elevation
- DVT prophylaxis
- Stress ulcer prophylaxis

Haemodynamic monitoring
Antifungal and antibiotic prophylaxis
Induced hypothermia
Management of renal failure
Tight glucose control

haemodynamics, positioning and other interventions as shown in Table 6.6. Further management strategies are discussed in detail in Chapter 13.

Chapter summary

Liver failure associated with hepatic encephalopathy in cirrhosis is responsible for approximately 20% of deaths from this disease (Youssef and McCullough, 2004). The degree of encephalopathy will correlate with the severity of the liver disease. Patients and their families may need to be realistic about a life-threatening illness. Decisions about possible transplantation may need to be made, or how far to continue treating a patient with multi-organ failure. Other patients with minimal hepatic encephalopathy may need to adapt to living with a degree of neurological impairment.

Illustrative case study

Mr R was a 41-year-old married man with two children. He had presented to the hospital 7 months earlier when he was diagnosed with alcoholic liver disease and had since abstained. He was admitted to the hepatology ward for treatment of his ascites 2 weeks before transfer to the high dependency unit (HDU) when his general condition had deteriorated. His blood results on admission to the HDU are illustrated in Table 6.7.

Table 6.7 Blood results on admission to HDU.

Parameter	Normal range	On admission to HDU
Urea (mmol/L)	<7.5	34.4
Creatinine (μmol/L)	35–135	198
Albumin (g/L)	30–44	28
CRP (mg/L)	0–6	21
Haemoglobin (g)	13–18	8
Platelets (×10⁹/L)	150–450	99
WBC (×10⁹/L)	4–11	41.4
PT (seconds)	11–14	17.2
APTT (seconds)	22.5–34.5	39.3

A full assessment was undertaken on transfer to the HDU. He was found to have pulmonary oedema diagnosed by crackles heard on auscultation, although he was not dyspnoeic. He required 2 L/min of oxygen to maintain saturations greater than 95%. A recent history of anuria had been treated with albumin, and he had a central venous pressure reading of 18 mmHg. He had a pyrexia and had become increasingly hypotensive with a blood pressure of 90/40 mmHg and a tachycardia of 110 beats per minute. An increase in white cell count and inflammatory marker (CRP) was attributed to the presence of an infection. Blood tests confirmed that he had developed renal failure with a rising creatinine and urea.

On neurological assessment he was found to be orientated to time and place, but appeared to have limited insight into his condition as he was frequently asking to go home. He was sleeping for much of the time, but intermittently had episodes of restlessness and some agitation. He was assessed as having grade 1 hepatic encephalopathy.

The deterioration in Mr R's condition was attributed to an infection. This had led to increasing encephalopathy as well as deterioration in his renal function. Cultures were taken to ensure that he was receiving the most appropriate antibiotics. His encephalopathy was managed by ensuring he opened his bowels three to five times a day by giving him daily phosphate enemas and lactulose. It was decided to start haemofiltration to reduce his uraemia which could improve his neurological condition and also reduce oedema and enable nasogastric feeding.

During the first 24 hours in the HDU his condition continued to deteriorate as he developed a grade 2 encephalopathy, becoming increasingly drowsy. He had a Glasgow coma score of 12 at this time as he was unable to obey commands and was more confused. Over the next few days, however, the sepsis started to resolve and both his cardiovascular and neurological status improved. Ten days after transfer to the HDU he returned to the ward, having stopped antibiotics.

On the ward he made a good physical recovery. He continued to have occasional episodes of confusion but was thought to have a good understanding of his condition. A CT scan was carried out of his head which excluded any other cause of his confusion, showing atrophic changes, no focal parenchysmal abnormality or haemorrhage. It was hoped that he would recover sufficiently to be assessed for possible liver transplantation in the future.

References

Bernal W, Wendon J (2004) Liver transplantation in adults with acute liver failure. *Journal of Hepatology* **40**(2):192–197

Bersten AD, Soni N, Oh TE (2003) *Oh's Intensive Care Manual*, 5th edn. Butterworth Heinemann Ltd, Edinburgh

Blei AT, Cordoba J (2001) Hepatic encephalopathy *The American Journal of Gastroenterology* **96**:1968–1975

Buckley PM, MacFie J (1997) Enteral nutrition in critically ill patients: a review. *Care of the Critically Ill* **13**(1):7–10

Butterworth RF (1999) Hepatic encephalopathy. In: Siegel GJ, Agranoff BW, Fisher SK, Albers RW, Uhler MD (1999) *Basic Neurochemistry: Molecular, Cellular and Medical Aspects*, 6th edn. Lippincott Williams and Wilkins, Philadelphia

Clemmesen JO, Larsen FS, Kondrup J, Hansen BA, Ott P (1999) Cerebral herniation in patients with acute liver failure is correlated with arterial ammonia concentrations. *Hepatology* **29**(3):648–653

Conn HO (1994) Effects of high-normal and low-normal serum potassium levels on hepatic encephalopathy: facts, half facts or artefacts? *Hepatology* **20**(6):1637–1640

Cordoba J, Lopez-Hellin J, Planas M, Sabin P, Sanpedro F, Castro F, Esteban R, Guardia J (2004) Normal protein diet for episodic encephalopathy: results of a randomised study. *Journal of Hepatology* **41**(1):38–43

Davies C (2004) The use of phosphate enemas in the treatment of constipation. *Nursing Times* **100**(18):32–35

Dellinger RP, Carlet JM, Masur H, Gerlach H, Calandra T, Cohen J, Gea-Banacloche J, Keh D, Marshall JC, Parker MM, Ramsay G, Zimmerman J, Vincent JL, Levy MM (2004) Surviving sepsis: guidelines for management of severe sepsis and septic shock. *Critical Care Medicine* **32**(3):858–873

Faint V (2006) The pathophysiology of hepatic encephalopathy. *Nursing in Critical Care* **11**(2):69–74

Ferenci P, Lockwood A, Mullen K, Tarter R, Weissenborn K, Blei AT (2002) Hepatic encephalopathy: definition, nomenclature, diagnosis, and quantification. Final report of the working party at the 11th World Congresses of Gastroenterology, Vienna 1998. *Hepatology* **35**:716–721

Haussinger D, Kircheis G, Fischer R, Schliess F, Vom Dahl S (2000) Hepatic encephalopathy in chronic liver disease: a clinical manifestation of astrocyte swelling and low grade cerebral edema? *Journal of Hepatology* **32**:1035–1038

Haussinger D, Schleiss F, Kircheis G (2002) Pathogenesis of hepatic encephalopathy. *Journal of Gastroenterology and Hepatology* **17**(Suppl 3):S256–S259

Jalan R, Hayes P (1997) Hepatic encephalopathy and ascites. *Lancet* **350**:1309–1315

Knawy BA (2004) Encephalopathy. In: Knawy BA, Shiffman ML, Wiesner RH (eds) *Hepatology: a Practical Approach*. Elsevier, Amsterdam, pp. 381–387

Krige JE, Beckingham IJ (2001) ABC of diseases of liver, pancreas and biliary system: portal hypertension – 2. Ascites, encephalopathy, and other conditions. *British Medical Journal* **322**:416–418

Nicolao F, Efrati C, Masini A, Merli M, Attili AF, Riggio O (2003) Role of determination of partial pressure of ammonia in cirrhotic patients with and without hepatic encephalopathy. *Journal of Hepatology* **38**:441–446

O'Neal H, Olds J, Webster N (2006) Managing patients with acute liver failure: developing a tool for practitioners. *Nursing in Critical Care* **11**(2):63–68

Park G, Navapurkar V (1994) Sedation in critically ill patients. *Care of the Critically Ill* **10**(1):5–9

Plauth M, Cabre E, Riggio O, Assis-Camilo M, Pirlich M, Kondrup J, Ferenci P, Hom E, vom Dahl S, Muller MJ, Notle W (2006) ESPEN guidelines on enteral nutrition: liver disease. *Clinical Nutrition* **25**(2):285–294

Rolando N, Wade J, Davalos M, Wendon J, Phillpott-Howard J, Williams R (2000) The systemic inflammatory response syndrome in acute liver failure. *Hepatology* **32**(4):734–739

Shawcross D, Jalan R (2005) Dispelling myths in the treatment of encephalopathy. *Lancet* **365**:431–434

Sherlock S and Dooley J (2002) *Diseases of the Liver and Biliary System*, 11th edn. Blackwell Publishing, Oxford

Voigt M, Conn H (1995) Hepatic encephalopathy. In: Kirsch R, Robson S, Trey C (eds) *Diagnosis and Management of Liver Disease*. Chapman and Hall Medical, London

Yousseff W, McCullough AJ (2004) Nutrition in liver disease. In: Knawy BA, Shiffman ML, Wiesner RH (eds) *Hepatology: a Practical Approach*. Elsevier, Amsterdam

Yurdaydin C (2003). Blood ammonia determination in cirrhosis: still confusing after all these years? *Hepatology* **38**(5):1307–1310

Alcohol-related liver disease

Kerry Webb

Introduction

Alcoholic liver disease (ALD) is the commonest cause of liver cirrhosis in the Western world (Stewart and Day, 2003). It is suggested that across all district general hospitals within the UK, 80% of cases of liver cirrhosis are alcohol related (O'Grady, 2002).

Incidence

Previously known as Laennec's disease, ALD has also been referred to as alcohol-induced cirrhosis and alcohol-related liver disease. In some ways ALD is an unhelpful term as it implies that developing the disease is as a consequence of being an *alcoholic*. There is no question that the relative risk of developing the disease increases with overall alcohol consumption (Gutjahr et al., 2001), however only around 20–30% of heavy drinkers will go on to develop the disease, and due to individual risk factors many of these patients will have been categorised as hazardous or harmful drinkers, whilst many alcohol-dependent patients (*alcoholics*) will avoid cirrhosis altogether (Lieber, 1993).

There have been attempts to quantify the total amount and length of alcohol consumption required to precipitate onset of the disease (Table 7.1). One report

Table 7.1 Relative risk of liver disease by gender and level of alcohol consumption. Adapted from Gutjar et al. (2001). Definition of drinking categories based on average volume of alcohol consumed. Category 1: for females 0–19.99 g pure alcohol daily; for males 0–39.99 g pure alcohol daily. Category 2: for females 20–39.99 g pure alcohol daily; for males 40–59.99 g pure alcohol daily. Category 3: for females 40 g of pure alcohol and above; for males 60 g pure alcohol and above. For comparison: a 75 cl bottle of wine contains about 70 g of pure alcohol. (ICD = international classification of diseases, the WHO disease classification process. The current version is version 10 of the manual, hence ICD-10)

			Females			Males		
Disease	ICD-9 4-digit	ICD-10 4-Digit	Drinking cat. 1	Drinking cat. 2	Drinking cat. 3	Drinking cat. 1	Drinking cat. 2	Drinking cat. 3
Liver cancer	155	C22	1.45	3.03	3.6	1.45	3.03	3.6
Liver cirrhosis	5.71	K70, K74	1.30	9.50	13.00	1.30	9.05	13.00

suggests that regular consumption of 80 g (10 units) of alcohol per day for men, and 60 g (7.5 units) for women over a period of 10–12 years is required, however it is clear that many people drink greater quantities over a longer period of time with no apparent liver disease (Grant et al., 1988). A Canadian study into the disease also provided evidence that up to 65% of diagnoses of non-alcohol-related liver disease were indeed attributable to alcohol (Ramstedt, 2003). Where alcohol consumption appears to be modest it is important to both exclude other aetiologies but also to attempt to corroborate the alcohol history through family members and medical notes (Paton, 1989).

While management of clinical symptoms of ALD has improved steadily over the years it is important to acknowledge that ongoing alcohol consumption is the single most significant contributor to increased morbidity and mortality, and conversely, abstinence from alcohol is the most beneficial intervention (Tilg and Day, 2007).

Metabolism of alcohol

Ethanol is the preferred fuel for the liver, displacing other substrates when present. It has been suggested that it is the process of metabolism, rather than the ethanol itself which leads to toxicity (Haber et al., 2003). About 10% of consumed alcohol is eliminated unchanged through the lungs and urine, whilst the other 90% is metabolised by the liver (NIAAA, 1997).

Metabolism can be described as the body converting ingested substances into other compounds. Toxicity can be increased or decreased by the metabolic process depending on the substance. Until all alcohol has been metabolised it is dispersed through various tissues and organs of the body remaining a potentially harmful toxin, with tissue concentrations similar to levels found in the blood (NIAAA, 1997).

Metabolism of ethanol (alcohol) involves a number of stages, the first one being oxidation. During this process alcohol dehydrogenase (ADH) – a mitochondrial liver enzyme – catalyses the conversion of ethanol to acetaldehyde. Acetaldehyde is highly reactive and thought to play a central role in hepatic damage (Haber et al., 2003). Other enzymes then convert acetaldehyde to acetate (acetic acid) before ultimately it is metabolised to carbon dioxide and water. It has also been found that hepatic enzyme metabolism differs between occasional drinkers and regular heavy drinkers. In the latter group there is additional induction of the cytochrome P450 enzyme system which further affects metabolism. Polymorphism in ethanol-metabolising enzymes has been suggested as an explanation for varying susceptibility of drinkers to ALD (Frenzer et al., 2002).

Pathophysiology

The role of ethanol is central to the pathogenesis of ALD, as is acetaldehyde and oxidative stress, as outlined above. Inflammation is the hallmark of alcoholic hepatitis and is characterised by the intrahepatic infiltration of neutrophils or mononuclear cells and by altered local and systemic expression of inflammatory cytokines (Haber et al., 2003). Cytokines with inflammatory effects, such as tumour necrosis factor beta (TNFß), interleukin (IL)-1 and IL-6, are presumed to play a significant role in the development of alcohol-related damage to the liver (O'Grady, 2002).

The development of fibrosis, or the *hepatic scar*, appears to come from the activation of the hepatic stellate cells (HSCs). When activated they appear to become myofibrinoblast-like, which results in both fibrinogenesis and cell proliferation (Friedman et al., 1993). In experimental studies, HSCs are directly stimulated by acetaldehyde. There is some evidence that HSC-induced fibrogenesis may be reversible (Iredale et al., 1998).

Clinical features

ALD is progressive and is best thought of on a continuum. It is widely thought to take upwards of 10 years of regular and excessive alcohol use before the disease manifests, and in some patients it can be much longer (Sheron, 2000; Carey, 2004). Whilst there can be clear markers for an ALD diagnosis, it is also worth noting that many clinical signs can be equivocal in identifying the aetiology. Liver biopsy can be a useful tool in establishing the diagnosis, however it is not always useful and there is a tendency to avoid routine liver biopsies in certain circumstances (Grant and Neuberger, 1999). This is discussed further in Chapter 2. It is important to screen and carefully assess alcohol use and to take a corroborative history to aid in the conclusion of a primary or secondary alcohol-related aetiology.

Stewart and Day (2003) describe a spectrum or staging of the disease process commonly beginning with steatosis (fatty liver), through steatohepatitis, fibrosis and finally cirrhosis. The three stages of ALD are described below, however, whilst this is useful for descriptive purposes, it must be remembered that in actuality they overlap and cannot truly be separated.

Steatosis (fatty liver)

Fatty liver is said to occur in around 90% of heavy drinkers at some point during their drinking career. It occurs when prolonged and excessive drinking causes an accumulation of abnormal amounts of fat within the cytoplasm of swollen hepatocytes (Sheron, 2000). At this stage the process is completely reversible upon abstinence or reduction to modest alcohol consumption. There are usually no observable clinical signs though there may be evidence of hepatomegaly on abdominal palpation. Fatty liver may occur in the absence of alcohol due to other causes such as obesity; the incidence of fatty liver in obese heavy drinkers is higher still.

Acute alcoholic steatohepatitis

Initial onset of acute alcoholic hepatitis may go unnoticed with the patient remaining clinically well. With gradual onset of the condition clinical signs will begin to appear. These commonly include loss of appetite, nausea, fatigue and a general feeling of being unwell. There may be low level spikes in temperature which should be monitored. As the condition progresses the symptoms become more aggressive with increasing nausea and usually with jaundice. Other symptoms in severe cases may include loss of muscle mass and ascites. Though by this stage the patient may well have been admitted to hospital and stopped drinking, their condition is likely to deteriorate over the following few weeks. Mortality in severe alcoholic hepatitis is high. This condition is further described later in this chapter.

Cirrhosis

When alcohol-related inflammation (alcoholic hepatitis) continues, fibrogenesis is triggered. Grant et al. (1988) suggest that approximately 40% of patients with severe hepatic fibrosis will develop cirrhosis within 5 years. Elsewhere, Galambos (1972) suggests that 38% of patients with alcoholic hepatitis, who continue to drink, will develop cirrhosis within 18 months. The pathophysiology of cirrhosis is described in Chapter 1.

Prognosis

In a clinically compensated cirrhotic patient, the 5-year survival rate is around 90% with abstinence, reducing to 70% if alcohol consumption continues (Tome and Lucey, 2004). However, once a patient develops decompensated cirrhosis, 5-year survival with ongoing alcohol consumption reduces to around 30% (Alexander et al., 1971).

Alcoholic hepatitis

Alcoholic hepatitis may be considered the most dramatic manifestation of ALD. Mortality rates in acute alcoholic hepatitis have been recorded as 40–50% at 1 month (Maddrey et al., 1978), and as high as 60% at 6 weeks (Edwards et al., 1997; Sargent, 2005), so the disease presents a significant medical and nursing challenge. According to Sheron (2000), death usually occurs as a result of liver failure, often associated with renal failure (hepatorenal syndrome), from uncontrolled sepsis or secondary to a variceal haemorrhage. Overall, however, mortality rates in alcoholic hepatitis are 15% (Philippe, 2007).

Pathogenesis

There is clear evidence of the multi-factorial processes involved in alcoholic hepatitis (Hill and Kugelmas, 1998). All hepatic cellular components, namely hepatocytes, Kupffer, stellate and endothelial cells, are involved at some stage in the pathogenesis of alcohol-induced liver injury (Sougioultzis et al., 2005). Haber et al. (2003) report that metabolism of ethanol to toxic metabolites, Kupffer cell stimulation by endotoxin, and nutritional impairment lead to hepatic injury, inflammation and fibrosis. However the mechanisms triggering the acute onset in a minority of alcoholic hepatitis patients are unknown (Ceccanti et al., 2006). Alcohol is directly associated with impaired hepatic regeneration.

Epidemiology

Alcoholic hepatitis has been estimated to occur in around 40% of chronic drinkers at some time (Hislop et al., 1983). However, because mild episodes of alcohol-induced liver inflammation (hepatitis) are commonly subclinical, a diagnosis may not always be made, or mild and non-specific symptoms may be attributed to other physical problems (Edwards et al., 1997; Ceccanti et al., 2006). Indeed complaints of nausea, abdominal discomfort and loss of appetite may be mistakenly considered a result of alcohol withdrawal and in the short term may appear improved in the alcohol-dependent drinker after they consume alcohol. In such mild cases the management of the hepatitis will usually occur in an outpatient setting whilst attention should be given to motivating the patient into engaging with alcohol treatment services (Tilg and Day, 2007).

In severe cases of acute alcoholic hepatitis the diagnosis of acute hepatitis is usually clear, though in order to clarify an alcohol aetiology it is again important to assess and establish an accurate alcohol history (O'Beirne et al., 2000).

Table 7.2 Clinical symptoms of alcoholic liver disease.

Clinical features of alcoholic hepatitis
Acute abdominal pain (upper outer quadrant)
Nausea
Malaise
Loss of appetite
Fever
Jaundice
Hepatomegaly

Symptoms related to portal hypertension may also be observed
Ascites
Variceal haemorrhaging
Hepatic encephalopathy

Clinical features

There is a cohort of clinical symptoms associated with alcoholic hepatitis (Table 7.2) and a patient may present with a combination or all of the symptoms.

Pathological features

Confirmation of a differential diagnosis requires a liver biopsy, however according to Talley et al. (1988), this is often not performed as it is unlikely to alter either diagnosis or therapy. O'Beirne et al. (2000) suggest that with a good history and consistent blood and radiological investigations, there should be sufficient data for establishing diagnosis. Other aetiologies may be excluded with a liver biopsy, however a percutaneous biopsy carries a risk of haemorrhaging in the presence of alcohol-induced severe thrombocytopenia (Ceccanti et al., 2006), whilst transjugular biopsy is a more specialist procedure that is not always available (Sargent, 2005).

Confirmatory features of a liver biopsy are likely to include:

- Neutrophil infiltration (usually)
- Enlargement of hepatocytes
- Mallory's hyaline (commonly)
- Pericellular fibrosis
- Infiltration of polymorphonuclear leucocytes
- Liver cell necrosis
- Steatosis

According to Bode (1999), there is usually a direct correlation between the frequency and intensity of the symptoms, and the severity of the histological features.

It is worth noting that some patients appear to decompensate upon alcohol detoxification. Whether the process of withdrawal triggers a paradoxical onset of alcoholic hepatitis is unclear, as the clinical condition of a patient with alcoholic hepatitis will continue to deteriorate for the first 2–3 weeks (Sheron, 2000).

Although it is not possible to predict the onset of alcoholic hepatitis there has been progress in charting its prognosis upon diagnosis. Biochemical and haematological features of alcoholic hepatitis are outlined in Table 7.3. Daily monitoring of liver function tests, coagulopathy and renal function is advocated until demonstration of sustained improvement (Sargent, 2005).

Assessment of prognosis

Much has been done in an attempt to predict outcome and improve treatment in alcoholic hepatitis.

Maddrey's discriminant function (DF) is a formula with good correlation and predictive value for 30-day mortality. It has been prospectively confirmed and appears to be the most clinically helpful for therapeutic decisions when severity of illness determines treatment.

$$DF = \text{prothrombin time prolongation} \times 4.6 + \text{serum bilirubin (mg/dL)}/17$$

A DF $\geq$32 signifies a poor prognosis, with a 3-month mortality rate of 55% (O'Beirne, 2000; Sargent, 2005). The prognostic value of this formula has other factors that correlate with poor prognosis. These include older age, impaired renal function, encephalopathy and a rise in the white blood cell count in the first 2 weeks of hospitalisation (Philippe, 2007).

Another validated scoring system for assessing outcome in alcoholic hepatitis is the Glasgow Alcoholic Hepatitis Score (GAHS) in which a GAHS $\geq$9 is predictive of a poor prognosis. This recent tool was the product of a UK-based multi-centre trial based on 241 patients across eight UK hospitals (Forrest et al., 2005). The biochemical markers and scoring criteria are shown in Table 7.4.

Management and treatment

At all stages of ALD it remains the case that abstinence from alcohol is the single most useful goal (Tome and Lucey, 2004; Sargent, 2005; Sougioultzis et al., 2005; Tilg and Day, 2007).

In the case of mild AH there is little indication for medical and nursing intervention (Carey, 2004). However, given the seriousness of an acute and severe alcoholic hepatitis, coupled with the high risk of mortality, hospital admission will be required and consideration of transfer to a specialist unit where possible (Moore, 2001).

If admission to hospital is not required, then referral for treatment of the harmful alcohol use is paramount. Where a patient is admitted, then assessment for alcohol

Table 7.3 Biochemical and haematological features of alcoholic hepatitis (AH). Adapted from Sargent (2005).

	Normal value	Changes seen in AH	Additional information
Bilirubin	<17 µmol/L	High	(50–1000 µmol/L)
Albumin	36–54 g/L	Low	Indicative of a decreased hepatic synthetic function
Alkaline phosphatase	35–115 U/L	Slightly elevated	Levels are normally mild
Aspartane aminotransferase (AST)	7–40 U/L	<200 U/L	In most patients there is moderated elevation of AST. An AST:ALT ratio of 2:1 is almost universal in AH
Alanine aminotransferase (ALT)	3–30 U/L	<200 U/L	ALT normal or mildly elevated
Gamma-glutamyl transpeptidase (GGT)	2–65 U/L	Elevated	An elevated level does not distinguish between AH and excessive alcohol use
Potassium	3.5–5.0 mmol/L	Low	Owing to low dietary protein intake, diarrhoea and secondary hyperaldosteronism
Sodium	135–146 mmol/L	Low	Hyponatraemia common in AH. Caused by excess body water because of the inability of these patients to adjust the amount of water excreted in the urine to that taken in
Urea	2.5–6.7 mmol/L	Low	Normally low unless hepatorenal syndrome present
Creatinine	60–100 µmol/L	Variable	High creatinine could be indicative of hepatorenal syndrome
Prothrombin time	12–16 seconds	Often prolonged	Over 5 seconds more than control. Important indicator of hepatic function
Mean corpuscular volume (MCV)	80–96 fL	High	Owing to alcohol effect on bone marrow
Leucocytosis	4–10 × 10^9/L	High often 12–20 × 10^9/L	Owing to neutrophil chemokine release in the liver
Ferritin	Male 20–260 µg/L Female 24–70 µg/L	High >1000 µg/litre	As an acute phase protein, ferritin is markedly elevated in AH, even in the absence of haemochromatosis. Levels fall over several months following cessation of alcohol
Serum immunoglobulin A concentration (IgA)	0.8–4 g/L	Increased	Increased levels are thought to be related to local stimulation of the secretory immune system. Levels do not necessarily fall following alcohol cessation

Table 7.4 Glasgow Alcohol Hepatitis Score (Forrest et al., 2005).

Score	1	2	3
Age	<50	≥50	–
WCC (×10⁹/L)	<15	≥15	–
Urea (mmol/L)	<5	≥5	–
PT ratio	<1.5	1.5–2.0	>2.0
Bilirubin (μmol/L)	<125	125–250	>250

withdrawal management, brief interventions and onward referral to alcohol services post discharge should form part of the treatment plan, as described elsewhere in this chapter (Carey, 2004; Sargent, 2005).

Management of decompensation

In severe alcoholic hepatitis there is a risk of hepatic decompensation which may give rise to any or one of the following:

- Ascites
- Variceal bleeding
- Hepatic encephalopathy
- Hepatorenal syndrome (HRS)

Management of these is described elsewhere in this book; however specific points to take into account include careful use, if any, of diuretics for management of ascites, due to the risk of precipitating HRS.

Nutrition

Nutrition is often neglected in those drinking alcohol to excessive levels. In particular, protein calorie malnutrition is a problem which can have a direct and untoward effect upon prognosis, and studies looking at nutritional supplementation in alcoholic hepatitis have shown promise (Mendenhall et al., 1984; Stewart and Day, 2003). See Chapter 14 for a comprehensive review on nutrition.

Antibiotic therapy

Prophylactic antibiotics and antifungals should be given due to the increased risk of bacterial translocation and fungal infection (e.g. ciprofloxacin 250 mg q12h and fluconazole 100 mg daily). Blood, urine and ascitic cultures should be taken before treatment with antibiotics or antifungals is started (O'Beirne et al., 2000). Due to the frequency of infection and its related morbidity and mortality (Moore, 2001), monitoring of the patient's temperature and prompt reporting are paramount (Sargent, 2005).

Corticosteroids

Use of this group of drugs has been extensive, and numerous studies have evaluated their use and benefit (Maddrey et al., 1978; Tilg and Day, 2007). There remains concern and controversy about the use of such drugs in this cohort; however, the tendency appears toward treating patients with severe alcoholic hepatitis (Maddrey's DF ≥32). Steroids are aimed at suppressing or 'switching off' the florid inflammatory response observed in liver biopsies from patients with severe AH. Two potential side effects of medium–high-dose steroids are poor wound healing and increased susceptibility to infection (Stewart and Day, 2003), with absolute contraindications to corticosteroid therapy including ongoing uncontrolled infection and uncontrollable variceal bleeding (Sheron, 2000).

Antioxidants

Heavy drinkers are deficient of various antioxidant elements and vitamins. In addition, Stewart and Day (2003) go on to describe the process by which oxidative stress has been implicated as a key mechanism in alcohol-mediated hepatotoxicity. These findings have led to clinical trials of the use of antioxidants including vitamins A–E, selenium and N-acetylcysteine in severe alcoholic hepatitis. Such trials, with and without concomitant use of corticosteroids, have been unconvincing and appear to show no survival benefits to patients with severe alcoholic hepatitis (Tilg and Day, 2007).

Pentoxifylline

Animal studies have demonstrated that TNFα plays a significiant role in disease pathogenesis (Yin et al., 1999). Pentoxifylline is a drug commonly used in peripheral vascular disease, however it is believed to be a TNF inhibitor due to its anticytokine effect (Carey, 2004) and exerts an antifibrinogenic action (Windmeier and Gressner, 1997). Akriviadis et al. (2000) demonstrated a reduction in mortality of 40% when using pentoxifylline rather than a placebo to treat severe alcoholic hepatitis.

Other pharmacotherapies

There have been numerous studies and clinical trials looking at other potential treatments including propylthiouracil, colchicine and phosphatidylcholine, with modest results. These have been described in greater detail elsewhere (Haber et al., 2003; Tilg and Day, 2007).

Liver transplantation

Orthotopic liver transplantation is now widely accepted as a treatment for end-stage liver disease (Prince and Hudson, 2002). Despite transplantation for ALD being a mainstream practice, transplantation for acute alcoholic hepatitis remains an exception rather than the rule. There are two main reasons for this. Firstly, ALD will often stabilise with a period of abstinence, negating the need for transplantation, and secondly, it is important to minimise the likelihood of a return to harmful alcohol use post transplant. Whilst evidence suggests that the length of pretransplant sobriety does not predict post-transplant abstinence (Tang et al., 1998), it remains controversial and emotive to transplant those actively drinking at the time of transplantation, notwithstanding the difficulty in engaging in any meaningful therapeutic relapse prevention work or risk assessment. To this end, the Liver Advisory Group (LAG) guidelines currently advise against transplantation for alcoholic hepatitis (Bathgate, 2006).

Nursing considerations

In the case of ALD nursing interventions are likely to be varied and influenced by the degree of pathology. It is possible that patients will feel embarrassed upon admission, particularly if they are aware that they have been consuming excessive alcohol which they attribute to their reason for presentation. It is unnecessary and unhelpful for a patient to feel awkward or guilty and this is likely to render them defensive or hostile regarding further discussion of their pattern of drinking (Millward, 2000). It is acknowledged that nurses are unlikely to set out to instil a sense of embarrassment or guilt within the patient, and any problem is likely to stem from the nurse's own lack of knowledge, training and confidence around addressing and managing alcohol-related issues (Brown et al., 1997; Owens et al., 2000).

As well as addressing alcohol screening, educational and attitudinal issues, there is a role in physical and psychological management of the alcohol-withdrawal syndrome (AWS). Management of AWS is described later in this chapter though it is important to be familiar with the local withdrawal regimen or protocol as well as the impact that support and reassurance can play in reducing symptom severity (Hawker, 1994). Whilst there is good indication for an alcohol-liaison specialist in the general hospital (Pirmohamed et al., 2000), complementary to – or in the absence of – this service, nursing staff should give consideration to the wealth of evidence supporting the use of brief interventions (Chick et al., 1985; Elvy et al., 1998). A brief intervention can be defined as a series of short interventions and low-intensity *opportunistic* engagements with a person who is a hazardous or harmful drinker. Whilst there is less certainty about the effect of such interventions in the alcohol-dependent group, their relatively cheap cost and short duration mean that they can be carried out by people who are not alcohol specialists, and hospital clinicians such as nursing staff are in an ideal position to implement this.

With regard to physical issues, a comprehensive list of physical assessment factors, history taking and its relation to nursing interventions is described by

Thomas (1999). The nurse must be aware that there is no specific management plan for a patient with alcoholic liver disease. Existing on a continuum means that the nurse needs to take into account which, if any, specific clinical signs and symptoms are present and work with medical staff to manage these accordingly. As reported above, patients may present asymptomatically or with mild and vague symptoms which are non-specific. Nevertheless, a nurse with a clear understanding of the spectrum of the disease will monitor the clinical situation accordingly and identify potential decompensation at an earlier stage.

Working with other members of the multi-disciplinary team and involving them accordingly is vital. In particular, key working relationships will include the dietician, pharmacist and alcohol specialist. Nursing considerations of management of clinical manifestations such as ascites, hepatic encephalopathy and oesophageal varices are described elsewhere; however it is worth mentioning that each of these can elicit its own concerns and anxieties, both for the patient and the relative, and therefore an ability to convey knowledge and reassurance in these conditions is paramount.

Alcohol-withdrawal therapies and protocols

For the vast majority of people stopping alcohol will not present a problem (Whitfield, 1980). However, once people begin to consume excessive amounts on a daily basis for more than a few weeks, and without periods of reduction or abstinence, then abrupt cessation of alcohol can precipitate the onset of alcohol-withdrawal syndrome (AWS). The clinician must appreciate that it is not possible to predict with absolute certainty what quantity of alcohol, consumed over what specific period, will engender an AWS response in any particular individual. Suggestions of daily use, with weekly consumption of more than 100 units of alcohol per week triggering an AWS are common, but reports of a withdrawal phenomenon with as little as 50 units per week have been described (Cooper, 1994).

Alcohol works as a central nervous system (CNS) depressant, by inhibition of the neurotransmission pathways (Fadda and Rosetti, 1998). Prolonged action over time causes compensation in the brain known as neuroadaption. Whilst the individual's drinking pattern remains stable this will not present with direct difficulties; however abrupt cessation of alcohol consumption, such as following admission to hospital, can cause a rebound process of neuroexcitation. In alcohol withdrawal, dopamine and N-methyl-D-aspartate (NMDA) levels are increased and GABA is decreased (Glue and Nutt, 1990). This sudden stimulation of the CNS manifests in physical and psychological symptoms of overexcitation which can range from minimal discomfiture to severe disturbance and, in the case of severe delirium tremens, occasionally death.

The initial onset of AWS commonly occurs within around 4 hours of the last drink. Early symptoms are usually mild but progress over the first 6–24 hours.

Table 7.5 Typical autonomic withdrawal symptoms in alcohol withdrawal.

Sweating
Nausea
Retching
Anxiety
Tachycardia (>100 bpm)
Hyper-reflexia
Tremor (characteristically in the hands but may spread to head and trunk in severe cases)
Vomiting
Insomnia
Agitation
Hypertension
Fever (37–38°C)

Hall and Zador (1997) describe the withdrawal process as commonly dividing into the following three stages.

■ *Autonomic hyperactivity*. These are the most likely symptoms experienced in alcohol withdrawal, usually peaking within 24–48 hours. Common symptoms are contained within Table 7.5

■ *Neuronal excitation*. Seizures are not uncommon in sudden withdrawal from alcohol. They are often called alcohol withdrawal fits and are usually of time-limited duration. According to O'Brien (1996), they are likely to occur 12–48 hours after the last drink, though clinically it is safer to monitor for fits for a number of days and the nursing care plan should take into account risk factors such as a patient wishing to leave the ward or take an unsupervised bath. Recent studies have suggested evidence of a 'kindling effect', whereby previous episodes of alcohol withdrawal significantly increase the risk of fits in subsequent withdrawals (Becker, 1996; Gonzalez et al., 2001)

■ *Delirium tremens (DTs)*. Prompt recognition of the risk of alcohol withdrawal and treatment with benzodiazepines will usually prevent DTs which, untreated, has a mortality rate of 20% (Hall and Zador, 1997). Onset of symptoms is commonly 48–72 hours after the last alcohol, though onset can be delayed for as long as 14 days (Victor, 1970). In 80% of cases the syndrome will resolve within 72 hours (Victor and Adams, 1953). Whilst the incidence of DTs is a less common manifestation of the alcohol withdrawal syndrome, it is certainly to be avoided. The effect on the patient is profound with abject fear being a key feature. It has often been described by patients as being awake but stuck in a nightmare. They may well have more pronounced autonomic symptoms (sweating profusely) during this stage but DTs must also be considered in the absence of such symptoms. The patient may have some disorientation in the three spheres (time, place and person), often only evident upon careful questioning. DTs are more likely to occur in patients over the age of 30 and with a long history of heavy alcohol use (Pristach et al., 1983). A past history of DTs is a significant predictor of further episodes upon sudden alcohol cessation. There is also a link between withdrawal symptom expectation and symptom severity (Hawker, 1994), and as such attention should be given to good withdrawal management as well as empathic reassurance and supportive nursing interventions

Alcoholic hallucinosis

Alcoholic hallucinosis is an acute mental syndrome characterised by vivid auditory hallucinations which occur shortly after the cessation or reduction of drinking. The differential diagnosis of acute alcoholic hallucinosis includes DTs, paranoid psychosis, borderline transient psychotic episode or other substance-related disorder (Jones, 2002). Alcohol withdrawal hallucinations can occur independently of DTs (Holloway et al., 1984) and as such are not predictive of them. It can be difficult to distinguish between alcoholic hallucinosis and hallucinations which occur secondary to a delirium, though the former are associated with a limited number of autonomic symptoms (Jones, 2002). Past research has suggested this syndrome occurs in around 25% of patients admitted to hospital with a history of at least 10 years' heavy drinking (Victor, 1966), though, whilst alcoholic hallucinosis remains a frequent occurrence on medical wards, improved identification and medication regimen may have reduced this figure somewhat. The hallucinations are predominantly visual, though auditory hallucinations do occur. Few cases ever progress to development of a schizophrenic illness (Glass, 1989a,b). Common phenomena include seeing bugs crawling on the floor or seeing faces in the bedside curtains. Hearing buzzes and clicks is common. Voices can be heard and tend to be overly critical or accusatory in content. Tactile (sensorial) hallucinations (formication hallucinosis) are also common with sensations such as spiders crawling over the skin (Holloway et al., 1984; Turner et al., 1989).

Alcohol-withdrawal management guidelines

Recognition and assessment

In order to manage alcohol withdrawal safely it is important to anticipate and undertake interventions at the earliest opportunity. Alcohol withdrawal may be a presenting feature or occur as an unexplained development in a patient who has recently been admitted for other reasons and consequently deprived of alcohol. It is useful to consider the merits of an alcohol screening tool to administer to all newly admitted patients. Examples of these include the Alcohol Use Disorders Identification Test (AUDIT) (Babor et al., 2001), the Fast Alcohol Screening Tool (FAST) (Hodgson et al., 2002) and the Paddington Alcohol Test (PAT) (Patton et al., 2004). It is also good practice for alcohol intake to be assessed as part of the admission process, including amount consumed, frequency and time of last drink (Paton, 1989). Where there is suggestion of an inaccurate history, then a corroborative history should be taken from relatives, the GP and past medical notes. If past admissions have resulted in alcohol-withdrawal symptoms then there should be a low threshold for introducing a medication regimen to manage this. A blood alcohol level can also be used to confirm suspicion of recent alcohol use, though this is ideally done with the consent of the patient. Withdrawal medication should not be withheld until a negative blood or breath alcohol level is obtained, as significant withdrawal symptoms are likely to have manifested long before this time in the alcohol-dependent patient.

Acute management of alcohol-withdrawal syndrome

Mild symptoms can generally be managed with reassurance and general support. A well lit, cool environment with sympathy and reassurance from nursing staff or relatives is ideal for the confused patient (Hawker, 1994; CRAG Working Group, 1998). Attention should be paid to optimising nutrition and fluid levels.

Risk factors for progression to severe withdrawal include (Raistrick, 2001):

- High alcohol intake (>15 units/day)
- Previous history of severe withdrawal, seizures or DTs
- Concomitant use of other psychotropic drugs
- Poor physical health
- High levels of anxiety or other psychiatric disorders
- Electrolyte disturbance
- Fever or sweating
- Insomnia
- Tachycardia

The greater the number of these symptoms, the greater the need for inpatient medical supervision to reduce the risk of seizures or DTs. In more severe cases, medication can reduce symptoms and reduce the risk of the patient developing convulsions or delirium tremens (Mayo-Smith, 1997; Williams and McBride, 1998).

Alcohol-withdrawal medication

There have been several studies and meta-analyses examining pharmacological management of alcohol withdrawal (Mayo-Smith, 1997; Williams and McBride, 1998). Overall consensus appears to favour the use of a medium to long-acting benzodiazepine such as chlordiazepoxide as the first-line treatment of choice for alcohol-withdrawal management. The benefits of the benzodiazepine group include cross-tolerance with alcohol, a long duration of action, anxiolytic properties and anticonvulsant effects (Chick, 1996; Hall and Zador, 1997; Mayo-Smith, 1997). While all benzodiazepines appear equally efficacious in withdrawal management, they do have individual benefits and drawbacks (Hall and Zador, 1997; Mayo-Smith, 1997).

The guiding principle for a withdrawal regimen is to start with a high dose (to replace the high alcohol intake) and gradually reduce over the following days

Table 7.6   Typical withdrawal regimen using chlordiazepoxide or oxazepam.

	Morning	Midday	Evening	Night	Total daily dose
Day 1	30 mg	30 mg	30 mg	30 mg	120 mg
Day 2	30 mg	20 mg	20 mg	30 mg	100 mg
Day 3	20 mg	20 mg	20 mg	20 mg	80 mg
Day 4	20 mg	10 mg	10 mg	20 mg	60 mg
Day 5	10 mg	10 mg	10 mg	10 mg	40 mg
Day 6	10 mg	10 mg	0	10 mg	30 mg
Day 7	10 mg	0	0	10 mg	20 mg

(Table 7.6). Ideally doses should remain regular (i.e. four times daily) until the latter stages to minimise the risk of breakthrough symptoms and the nocte dose should be loaded to cover for the extended period between doses. It should be remembered that all patients will respond individually to a withdrawal regimen, though, in general, the greater the alcohol consumption the greater the dose of medication. Those patients who are frail or elderly may well require a lower cumulative dose. Patients should always be monitored for benzodiazepine toxicity and it is good practice to have ready access to a benzodiazepine antagonist, i.e. flumazenil.

Chlordiazepoxide
This is commonly the first line drug of choice for alcohol-withdrawal management as outlined above. Table 7.6 provides a recommended withdrawal scale.

Diazepam
This is often used as an *alternative* to chlordiazepoxide. It has a longer half-life, and is therefore more prone to accumulation and toxicity. A similar reducing regime should be used as in Table 7.6, but remembering that 5 mg diazepam is equivalent to approximately 10–15 mg chlordiazepoxide.

Oxazepam and lorazepam
There may be situations where it may be appropriate to consider an *alternative* to the above. Oxazepam and lorazepam do not produce active metabolites and are inactivated and eliminated by simple glucoronidation (Chick, 1996). One of these drugs may therefore be used as an alternative to chlordiazepoxide, in a liver unit for example, where there are clinical signs or a history of *significant* liver function impairment. Although the benefits are a much shorter half-life and being less prone to accumulation and toxicity (McBride, 2002), nurses should be aware that this increases the risk of breakthrough withdrawal symptoms occurring between drug rounds. Use of a withdrawal measurement scale can be an invaluable tool (see below).

An oxazepam regime has the benefit of following the same dosage and pattern as chlordiazepoxide (see Table 7.6); 1 mg lorazepam equates to approximately 10 mg diazepam or 30 mg chlordiazepoxide.

Caution in benzodiazepine use

Benzodiazepines can cause respiratory depression as well as sedation. The use of such drugs should be carefully considered and monitored in certain clinical situations such as a suspected or recent head injury where neurological symptoms may be masked. In such instances a head CT scan should be considered and the situation balanced with the need to manage significant alcohol withdrawal effectively. Again, oxazepam may be more appropriate due to its shorter half-life.

It is important to note that benzodiazepines have a high incidence of abuse and concomitant use with alcohol can prove fatal. The provision of benzodiazepines for withdrawal management as a take home prescription (TTO) is therefore usually contraindicated unless with specialist advice or community follow-up. Extra caution should also be taken if a patient is suspected of ongoing alcohol consumption whilst undergoing inpatient care.

Severe withdrawal

Previously significant alcohol-withdrawal problems predict the likelihood of a difficult withdrawal programme (Gonzalez et al., 2001). The more severe the withdrawal syndrome the more significant the risk of complications including:

- Wernicke's encephalopathy
- Alcoholic hallucinosis
- Depression
- Suicidal ideation

Management of delirium tremens

Initial management of the severely confused or agitated patient requires the administration of adequate sedative doses of benzodiazepines (intravenously if necessary). The object of treatment is to make the patient calm and sedated but easily roused.

- For patients able to take oral medication, higher and more frequent doses of chlordiazepoxide may be necessary
- For patients requiring parenteral treatment, intravenous diazepam may be useful. Intramuscular diazepam should be avoided, but rectal diazepam may be useful where there is difficulty establishing venous access (CRAG Working Group, 1998)
- For patients with liver failure, intravenous lorazepam is an alternative and may be given intramuscularly
- Chlormethiazole is not recommended (Duncan and Taylor, 1996)

- Severe psychotic symptoms may be managed by the addition of haloperidol, although adequate treatment with benzodiazepines should be the priority
- Close monitoring of fluid balance is important. Urea and electrolytes (including magnesium) should be regularly checked (CRAG Working Group, 1998)

Nurses should be aware that the British National Formulary (BNF) recommends the use of long-acting benzodiazepines for the management of alcohol withdrawal. In clinical practice there may be a requirement to use an alternative (e.g. lorazepam in liver failure, or a combination of intravenous diazepam and haloperidol at doses exceeding the BNF recommended limits). In such cases it is advised to enlist the advice of a liaison psychiatrist or substance misuse specialist. It is also good practice to ensure that there are suitable local clinical management guidelines in place.

Wernicke's encephalopathy

Wernicke's encephalopathy (WE) is not to be confused with hepatic encephalopathy. It is a syndrome most commonly, though not exclusively, precipitated by abrupt cessation of alcohol withdrawal. Inappropriately managed this carries a mortality rate of over 15% (Victor et al., 1989; Sechi and Serra, 2007), and results in permanent brain damage (Korsakoff's psychosis) in 85% of survivors (Victor et al., 1989; Sechi and Serra, 2007).

WE presents as a consequence of thiamine (vitamin B_1) deficiency. Thiamine pyrophosphate (the biologically active form of thiamine) is an essential coenzyme in a number of biochemical brain pathways (Sechi and Serra, 2007). As thiamine deficiency develops, enzymes and systems dependent upon thiamine begin to function less well, ultimately leading to cell death (Thomson et al., 2002).

The classical triad of signs of WE (acute confusion, ataxia and ophthalmoplegia) occur in only around 10% of patients (Harper et al., 1986). Therefore the triad cannot be used as the basis of diagnosis and a high index of suspicion is needed. The presence of only one of the following signs should be sufficient to assign a diagnosis and commence treatment (Cook, 2000):

- Acute confusion
- Decreased consciousness level including unconsciousness or coma
- Memory disturbance
- Ataxia/unsteadiness
- Ophthalmoplegia
- Nystagmus
- Unexplained hypotension with hypothermia

Treatment of WE is by replacement of thiamine and is considered a medical emergency (Sechi and Serra, 2007). In a recent Cochrane review, Day et al. (2004) reported insufficient evidence from randomised control trials to guide clinicians in the dose, frequency, route or duration of thiamine treatment for prophylaxis against or treatment of WE. Nevertheless, there is clearly supported advice for both prophylactic and treatment regimen (Harper et al., 1986; Victor et al., 1989; Chick, 1996; Cook, 2000).

Treatment

Give Pabrinex® IV High Potency (HP) two ampoule pairs (four ampoules in total) three times daily for 2–3 days, followed by Pabrinex® IV HP one ampoule pair (two ampoules in total) daily for 3–5 days. Pabrinex® should be continued until improvement of the clinical symptoms stops. Use of oral supplementation will then be useful (thiamine 100 mg q12h + vitamin B Co Strong ii q24h).

Pabrinex® IV HP should be given by infusion over 30 minutes, following dilution of ampoule pairs in 100 ml normal saline (Sechi and Serra, 2007).

Prophylaxis

Increased demands on the already depleted B vitamin stores raise the risk of precipitating WE. Therefore any patient undergoing alcohol withdrawal should be treated prophylactically. This includes any patient admitted for another reason and subsequently found to require detoxification, as well as those with a known history of alcohol dependence and any of the following:

- Intercurrent illness
- DTs
- Alcohol-related seizures
- Head injury
- Poor diet, signs of malnutrition or significant weight loss
- Recent diarrhoea or vomiting
- Drinking >20 units of alcohol per day
- Peripheral neuropathy

Give Pabrinex® IV HP one ampoule pair daily for 3–5 days, followed by oral supplementation (thiamine 100 mg q12h + vitamin B Co Strong q24h). Intravenous dextrose should not be given before Pabrinex® due to the risk of precipitating WE. This is because glucose metabolism utilises thiamine and therefore may deplete reserves.

Alcohol-withdrawal scales

It is good practice to employ an objective screening scale to monitor symptom severity in alcohol withdrawal. One such tool is the Clinical Institute Withdrawal Assessment for Alcohol – Revised (CIWA-R) which allows clinicians to objectively score a patient's alcohol-withdrawal symptoms, thus guiding administration of the reducing scale of the benzodiazepine medication. The frequency of when CIWA-R should be utilised depends upon individual clinical experience, however, if a patient is in the early stages of withdrawal it is recommended that this is used every 90 minutes.

The tool will enable the clinician to decipher whether the patient requires additional PRN medication. It is recommended that if the patient scores >10 then the patient should receive supplementary PRN chlordiazepoxide (or equivalent). If the patient scores <10 then no PRN medication should be given. However, the regular prescribed medication should be given at all times unless the patient becomes overly sedated (Sullivan et al., 1989).

Chapter summary

Alcohol-related liver injury remains the most serious consequence of alcohol abuse and is a frequent cause of liver cirrhosis in the Western world, resulting in substantial mortality and morbidity. This chapter has highlighted the variety of spectrums of disease presentation and clinical management. However, a thread throughout the chapter highlights the importance of addressing the underlying drinking behaviour and encouraging treatment engagement.

Illustrative case study

A 32-year-old man is admitted to the ward with symptoms of nausea and abdominal pain in the right upper quadrant. He complains of having no energy and feeling generally unwell. He has no appetite. His temperature is generally within normal range but there are occasional moderate spikes. The medical examination reveals evidence of jaundice, hepatomegaly and probable mild ascites. There is some mild jaundice.

The patient is asked about excess alcohol and states that he has stopped drinking and was a social drinker previously. With a provisional diagnosis of acute hepatitis the alcohol history is revisited and the patient's wife is also solicited. It transpires that the patient did indeed stop drinking 2 days ago, however prior to that was drinking 5 pints of normal strength (4.1%) beer every evening after work in the pub, and 8 pints on a Friday, Saturday and Sunday (88 units per week).

The following day the jaundice worsens and the patient's temperature begins to soar. He becomes tachycardic and is sweating. He is unable to eat and though there is no sign of a liver flap, his hands are moderately tremulous.

Blood results show an elevated AST (120 U/L), with an AST:ALT ratio of 2:1. Bilirubin has risen to over 350 µmol/L. Albumin is 29 g/L, GGT is 256 U/L and sodium is 115 mmol/L. MCV is 100.4 fL. PT is 17 seconds (vitamin K corrected).

There is no sign of sepsis and no sign of bleeding. The presumed diagnosis at this point is acute alcoholic hepatitis and concomitant acute alcohol-withdrawal syndrome.

Treatment includes a reducing scale of oxazepam (monitored using the CIWA-R withdrawal scale), a prophylactic Pabrinex® regimen, ciprofloxacin 250 mg q12h and fluconazole 100 mg q24h.

There is some debate medically about whether to perform a liver biopsy, however as a transjugular biopsy is an option in this unit this is undertaken. It confirms marked inflammation suggestive of alcoholic hepatitis.

Maddrey's (modified) discriminant function (mDF) is 44. There is no obvious sepsis or bleeding. Renal function is reasonable. As a consequence the medical team cautiously instigate corticosteroid therapy (prednisolone 30 mg/day) for 4 weeks, though reviewed daily.

In the initial 7 days the clinical picture deteriorates and then stabilises. During this time nutritional advice is sought from the dietician and comprehensive enteral feeding is established. By the beginning of week 3 the clinical symptoms are improving.

In week 5 the patient appears symptom free. During the latter stages of the admission the nursing and medical staff have had opportunity to advise and educate the patient on the correlation between the alcohol use and liver disease. Prior to discharge the patient is seen by the alcohol liaison specialist who explores the patient's goals regarding alcohol use post transplant. Advice from the medical team is for ongoing abstinence and the focus of alcohol interventions is to work with the patient, and family where possible, on a menu of options to enable change to be sustained upon discharge home. The patient also accepts referral to the local community alcohol team for ongoing supportive counselling. Consistent advice from all members of the treatment team regarding alcohol use (or abstinence from) help to reduce the likelihood of the patient selectively adopting more liberal advice, such as 'one drink won't hurt'.

References

Akriviadis E, Botla R, Briggs W, Han S, Reynolds T, Shakil O (2000) Pentoxifylline improves short-term survival in severe acute alcoholic hepatitis: a double-blind, placebo-controlled trial. *Gastroenterology* **119**:1637–1648

Alexander JF, Lichner MW, Galambos JT (1971) Natural history of alcoholic hepatitis: the long term prognosis. *American Journal of Gastroenterology* **56**:515–525

Ali A, Hassiotis A (2006) Alcohol misuse: diagnosis and management. *British Journal of Hospital Medicine* **67**(10):M182–185

Babor T, Higgins-Biddle J, Saunders J, Monteiro M (2001) *AUDIT: The Alcohol Use Disorders Identification Test, Guidelines For Use In Primary Care*, 2nd edn. World Health Organization, Geneva

Bathgate AJ (2006) Recommendations for alcohol-related liver disease. *Lancet* 367:2045–2046

Becker H (1996) The alcohol withdrawal 'kindling' phenomenon: clinical and experimental findings. *Alcoholism, Clinical and Experimental Research* 20(8):121A–124A

Bode J (1999) Alcoholic liver disease. In: Bianchi Porro G, Cremer M, Krejs G, Ramadori G, Madsen J (eds) *Gastroenterology and Hepatology*. McGraw-Hill, Maidenhead

Brown C, Pirmohamed M, Park BK (1997) Nurses' confidence in caring for patients with alcohol-related problems. *Professional Nurse* 13(2):83–86

Carey W (2004) Alcohol-induced liver disease. In: Al Knawy B, Shiffman M, Wiesner R (eds) *Hepatology: A Practical Approach*. Elsevier, London

Ceccanti M, Attili A, Balducci G, Attilia F, Giacomelli S, Rotondo C, Sasso G, Xirouchakis E, Attilia M (2006) Acute alcoholic hepatitis. *Journal of Clinical Gastroenterology* 40(9):833–841

Chick J (1996) Medication in the treatment of alcohol dependence. *Advances in Psychiatric Treatment* 2:249–257

Chick J, Lloyd G, Crombie E (1985) Counselling problem drinkers on medical wards: a controlled study. *British Medical Journal (Clinical Research Edition)* 290:965–967

Cook CCH (2000) Prevention and treatment of Wernicke-Korsakoff syndrome. *Alcohol & Alcoholism* 35(Suppl. 1):19–20

Cooper D (1994) *Alcohol Home Detoxification and Assessment*. Radcliffe Medical Press, Oxford

CRAG Working Group on Mental Illness (1998) *The Management of Alcohol Withdrawal and Delirium Tremens*. The Scottish Executive, Edinburgh

Day E, Bentham P, Callaghan R, Kuruvilla T, George S (2004) Thiamine for Wernicke-Korsakoff syndrome in people at risk from alcohol abuse. *Cochrane Database of Systematic Reviews*, Issue 1. Art. No.: CD004033. DOI: 10.1002/14651858.CD004033.pub2

Duncan D, Taylor D (1996) Chlormethiazole or chlordiazepoxide in alcohol detoxification. *Psychiatric Bulletin* 20:599–601

Edwards G, Marshall EJ, Cook CH (1997) Physical complications of excessive drinking. In: Edwards G, Marshall EJ, Cook CH (eds) *The Treatment of Drinking Problems: A Guide for the Helping Professions*, 3rd edn. Cambridge University Press, Cambridge

Elvy GA, Wells JE, Baird KA (1998) Attempted referral as intervention for problem drinking in the general hospital. *British Journal of Addiction* 83(1):83–89

Fadda F, Rosetti ZL (1998) Chronic ethanol consumption: from neuroadaption to neurodegeneration. *Progress in Neurobiology* 54(4):385–431

Forrest EH, Evans CD, Stewart S, Phillips M, Oo YH, MvAvoy NC, Fisher NC, Singhal S, Brind A, Haydon G, O'Grady J, Day CP, Hayes PC, Murray LS, Morris AJ (2005) Analysis of factors predictive of mortality in alcoholic hepatitis and derivation and validation of the Glasgow alcoholic hepatitis score. *Gut* 54(18):1174–1179

Frenzer A, Butler WJ, Norton ID, Wilson JS, Apte MV, Pirola RC, Ryan P, Roberts-Thompson IC (2002) Polymorphism in alcohol-metabolizing enzymes, glutathione *S*-transferases and apolipoprotein E and susceptibility to alcohol-induced cirrhosis and chronic pancreatitis. *Journal of Gastroenterology and Hepatology* 17(1):177–182

Friedman S, Wei S, Blaner S (1993) Retinol release by activated rat hepatic lipocytes: regulation by Kuppfer cell-conditioned medium and PDGF. *American Journal of Physiology* 264:G247–252

Galambos JT (1972) Alcoholic hepatitis: its therapy and prognosis. *Progress in Liver Diseases* 4:567–588

Glass I (1989a) Alcoholic hallucinosis: a psychiatric enigma – 1. The development of an idea. *The British Journal of Addiction* 84:29–41

Glass I (1989b) Alcoholic hallucinosis: a psychiatric enigma – 2. Follow-up studies. *The British Journal of Addiction* 84:151–164

Glue P, Nutt D (1990) Overexcitement and disinhibition. Dynamic neurotransmitter interactions in alcohol withdrawal. *British Journal of Psychiatry* 157:491–499

Gonzalez LP, Veatch LM, Ticku MK, Becker HC (2001) Alcohol withdrawal kindling: mechanisms and implications for treatment. *Alcoholism: Clinical & Experimental Research* 25(5 Suppl):197S–201S

Grant A, Neuberger J (1999) Guidelines on the use of liver biopsy in clinical practice. *Gut* 45(Suppl 4):1V1–1V11

Grant BF, Dufour MC, Hartford TC (1988) Epidemiology of alcoholic liver disease. *Seminars in Liver Disease* 8(1):12–25

Gutjahr E, Gmel G, Rehm J (2001) Relation between average alcohol consumption and disease: an overview. *European Addiction Research* 7(3):117–127

Haber P, Warner R, Seth D, Gorrell M, McCaughan G (2003) Pathogenesis and management of alcoholic hepatitis. *Journal of Gastroenterology and Hepatology* 18:1332–1344

Hall W, Zador D (1997) The alcohol withdrawal syndrome. *Lancet* 349:1897–1900

Harper, CG, Giles M, Finlay-Jones, R (1986) Clinical signs in the Wernicke-Korsakoff complex: a retrospective analysis of 131 cases diagnosed at necropsy. *Journal of Neurology, Neurosurgery, and Psychiatry* 49(4):341–345

Hawker R (1994) Alcohol withdrawal: a physical or psychological syndrome? *New Directions in the Study of Alcohol* 19:29–43

Hill DB, Kugelmas M (1998) Alcoholic liver disease: treatment strategies for the potentially reversible stages. *Postgraduate Medicine* 103(4):261–264, 267–268, 273–275

Hislop WS, Bouchier IA, Allan JG, Brunt PW, Eastwood M, Finlayson ND, James O, Russell RI, Watkinson G (1983) Alcoholic liver disease in Scotland and North-Eastern England. *Quarterly Journal of Medicine* 52:232–243

Hodgson R, Alwyn T, John B, Thom B, Smith A (2002) The FAST alcohol screening test. *Alcohol and Alcoholism* 37(1):61–66

Holloway H, Hales P, Watanabe H (1984) Recognition and treatment of acute alcohol withdrawal syndromes. *The Psychiatric Clinics of North America* 7:729–743

Iredale JP, Benyon RE, Pickering J, McCullen M, Northrop M, Pawley S, Hovell C, Arthur MJ (1998) Mechanisms of spontaneous resolution of rat liver fibrosis. Hepatic stellate cell apoptosis and reduced hepatic expression of metalloproteinase inhibitors. *Journal of Clinical Investigation* 102(3):538–549

Jones P (2002) Alcohol addiction: a psychobiological approach. *Behavioural Medicine*. Associates Comprehensive Modern Mental Health Services. http://www.bma-wellness.com/papers/EtOH_Psychobiology.html (accessed 17/05/07)

Lieber CS (1993) Aetiology and pathogenesis of alcoholic liver disease. *Clinical Gastroenterology* 7:581–608

Maddrey WC, Boitnott JK, Bedine MS, Weber FL, Mezey E, White R (1978) Corticosteroid therapy of alcoholic hepatitis. *Gastroenterology* 75:193–199

Madhotra R, Gilmore I (2003) Recent developments in the treatment of alcoholic hepatitis. *Quarterly Journal of Medicine* 96:391–400

Mayo-Smith M (1997) Pharmacological treatment of alcohol withdrawal: a meta-analysis and evidence-based practice guideline. American Society of Addiction Medicine Working Group on pharmacological management of alcohol withdrawal. *Journal of the American Medical Association* 278:144–151

McBride A (2002) Medical approaches and prescribing: alcohol. In: Petersen T, McBride A (eds) *Working with Substance Misusers: A Guide to Theory and Practice*. Routledge, London

Mendenhall CL, Anderson S, Weesner RE, Goldberg SJ, Crolic KA (1984) Protein-calorie malnutrition associated with alcoholic hepatitis. Veterans Administrative Cooperative Study Group on Alcoholic Hepatitis. *American Journal of Medicine* 76(2):211–222

Millward L (2000) Attitudes towards alcoholics: staff-patient relationships in the acute hospital setting. Unpublished PhD Thesis, University of London

Moore K (2001) Management of alcoholic hepatitis. *Clinical Medicine* 1(4):281–284

National Institute on Alcohol Abuse and Alcoholism (NIAAA) (1997) Alcohol metabolism. *Alcohol Alert* No. 35; PH 371

O'Beirne J, Patch D, Holt S, Hamilton M, Burroughs A (2000) Alcoholic hepatitis – the case for intensive management. *Postgraduate Medical Journal* 76:504–507

O'Brien CP (1996) Drug addiction and drug abuse. In: *Goodman and Gilman's The Pharmacological Basis of Therapeutics*, 9th edn. McGraw-Hill, New York

O'Grady J (2002) Liver and biliary tract disease. In: Souhami R and Moxham J (eds) *Textbook of Medicine*, 4th edn. Churchill Livingstone, Edinburgh

Owens L, Gilmore I, Pirmohamed M (2000) General practice nurses' knowledge of alcohol use and misuse: a questionnaire survey. *Alcohol and Alcoholism* 35:259–262

Paton A (1989) Alcohol misuse and the hospital doctor. *British Journal of Hospital Medicine* **42**(5):394–398

Patton R, Hilton C, Crawford M, Touquet R (2004) The Paddington Alcohol Test: a short report. *Alcohol and Alcoholism* **39**(3):266–268

Philippe, L (2007) Acute alcoholic hepatitis. http://www.hepatitis.org/hepatalcool_angl.htm

Pirmohamed M, Brown C, Owens L, Luke C, Gilmore I, Breckenridge A, Park B (2000) The burden of alcohol misuse on an inner city general hospital. *Quarterly Journal of Medicine* **93**(5):291–295

Prince MI, Hudson M (2002) Liver transplantation for chronic liver disease: advances and controversies in an era of organ shortages. *Postgraduate Medicine Journal* **78**(917):135–141

Pristach CA, Smith CM, Whitney RP (1983) Alcohol withdrawal syndromes – prediction from detailed medical and drinking histories. *Drug and Alcohol Dependence* **11**(2):177–199

Raistrick D (2001) Alcohol withdrawal and detoxification. In: Heather N, Peters TJ, Stockwell T (eds) *International Handbook of Alcohol Dependence and Problems*. John Wiley & Sons, Chichester

Ramstedt M (2003) Alcohol consumption and liver cirrhosis mortality with and without mention of alcohol: the case of Canada. *Addiction* **98**:1267–1276

Sargent S (2005) The aetiology, management and complications of alcoholic hepatitis. *British Journal of Nursing* **14**(10):556–562

Sechi G, Serra A (2007) Wernicke's encephalopathy: new clinical settings and recent advances in diagnosis and management. *The Lancet Neurology* **6**(5):442–455

Sheron N (2000) Alcoholic liver disease. In: O'Grady J, Lake J, Howdle P (eds) *Comprehensive Clinical Hepatology*. Harcourt, London

Sougioultzis S, Dalakas E, Hayes P, Plevris JN (2005) Alcoholic hepatitis: from pathogenesis to treatment. *Current Medical Research and Opinion* **21**(9):1337–1346

Stewart SF, Day CP (2003) The management of alcoholic liver disease. *Journal of Hepatology* **38**(suppl 1):S2–S13

Sullivan JT, Sylora K, Schneiderman J, Naranjo CA, Sellers EM (1989) Assessment of alcohol withdrawal: the revised clinical institute withdrawal assessment for alcohol scale (CIWA-Ar). *British Journal of Addiction* **84**(11):1353–1357

Talley NJ, Roth A, Woods J, Hench V (1988) Diagnostic value of liver biopsy in alcoholic liver disease. *Journal of Clinical Gastroenterology* **10**:647–650

Tang H, Boulton R, Gunson B, Hubscher S, Neuberger J (1998) Patterns of alcohol consumption after liver transplantation. *Gut* **43**(1):140–145

Thomas D (1999) Management of persons with problems of the hepatic system. In: Phipps W, Sands J, Marek J (eds) *Medical–Surgical Nursing: Concepts and Clinical Practice*, 6th edn. Mosby, Missouri

Thomson AD, Cook CC, Touquet R, Henry JA (2002) The Royal College of Physicians' report on alcohol: guidelines for managing Wernicke's encephalopathy in the accident and emergency department. *Alcohol and Alcoholism* **37**(6):513–521

Tilg H, Day C (2007) Management strategies in alcoholic liver disease. *Nature Clinical Practice Gastroenterology Hepatology* **4**(1):24–34

Tome S, Lucey M (2004) Current management of alcoholic liver sisease. *Alimentary Pharmacology and Therapy* **19**(7):707–714

Turner RC, Lichstein PR, Peden JG, Busher JT, Waivers LE (1989) Alcohol withdrawal syndromes: a review of pathophysiology, clinical presentation and treatment. *Journal of General Internal Medicine* **4**:432–444

Victor M (1966) The treatment of alcoholic intoxication and the withdrawal syndrome. *Psychosomatic Medicine* **28**:636–650

Victor M (1970) The alcohol withdrawal syndrome. *Postgraduate Medicine* **47**(6):68–72

Victor M, Adams RD (1953) Effect of alcohol on the nervous system. *Research Publications – Association for Research in Nervous and Mental Disease* **32**:526–533

Victor M, Adams RD, Collins GH (1989) *The Wernicke–Korsakoff Syndrome and Related Neurological Disorders Due to Alcoholism and Malnutrition.* FA Davis Company, Philadelphia

Whitfield CL (1980) Non-drug treatment of alcohol withdrawal. *Current Psychiatric Therapies* **19**:101–109

Williams D, McBride AJ (1998) The drug treatment of alcohol withdrawal symptoms: a systematic review. *Alcohol & Alcoholism* **33**(2):103–115

Windmeier C, Gressner A (1997) Pharmacological aspects of pentoxifylline with emphasis on its inhibitory actions on hepatic fibrogenesis. *General Pharmacology* **29**(2):181–196

Yin M, Wheeler MD, Kono H, Bradford B, Gallucci R, Luste M, Thurman R (1999) Essential role of tumour necrosis factor alpha in alcohol-induced liver injury in mice. *Gastroenterology* **117**(4):942–952

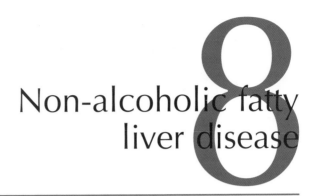

Non-alcoholic fatty liver disease

Antonis Nikolopoulos and Jude A. Oben

Introduction

Non-alcoholic fatty liver disease (NAFLD), a liver disease predominantly caused by obesity, is now the leading cause of chronic liver dysfunction in developed countries. In some patients it may progress to cirrhosis. The pathogenesis implicates insulin resistance and increased oxidant stress with subsequent activation of collagen-making cells in the liver. There is at present no single diagnostic test for NAFLD. The treatment similarly is largely experimental presently but emerging therapies include metformin, glitazones, vitamin E, angiotensin-receptor blockers and alpha-antagonists.

Definition

The first people to describe NAFLD as a clinical entity were Ludwig et al. (1980). NAFLD is now accepted as the most common cause of chronic disease in developed countries (Falck-Ytter et al., 2001). It is a spectrum of chronic liver disease that is histologically similar to alcoholic fatty liver disease but occurs in an individual who drinks little or no alcohol. The definition of little or no alcohol has changed over the years but presently the United States National Institutes of Health, Non-Alcoholic Fatty Liver Disease Clinical Research Network accepts an alcohol

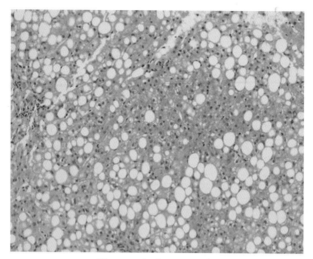

Macrovesicular steatosis.

Figure 8.1   Macrovesicular steatosis. For a colour version of this figure, please see Plate 7 in the colour plate section.

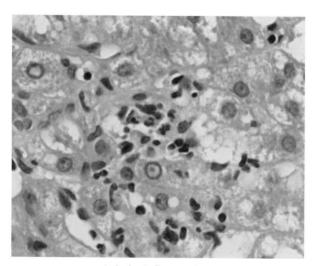

Lobular inflammation
(acute or chronic).

Figure 8.2   Lobular inflammation. For a colour version of this figure, please see Plate 8 in the colour plate section.

consumption of less than 140 g (17.5 units) per week for men and less than 70 g (8.75 units) per week for women, as being compatible with the diagnosis.

At one end of the spectrum of NAFLD is hepatosteatosis (fatty liver), which may progress to fat with inflammation (steatohepatitis or non-alcoholic steato-hepatitis, NASH) (Figures 8.1, 8.2, Plates 7, 8); this may progress to fibrosis and in some patients to cirrhosis and hepatocellular carcinoma (Powell et al., 1990; Bugianesi et al., 2002). It is important to note that by the time patients with NAFLD reach cirrhosis, there is most often a decrease in the degree of steatosis (Powell et al., 1990).

Regarding the nomenclature, NASH and NAFLD therefore are not synonymous terms. NASH is the more severe stage of NAFLD, just as myocardial infarction is the more severe stage of ischaemic heart disease. It is also now accepted that NAFLD is the underlying diagnosis in the majority of cases previously designated as cryptogenic cirrhosis (Bugianesi et al., 2002).

Disease prevalence

The population prevalence of NAFLD has been estimated at 7–35%, depending on whether an elevation of alanine transaminase, ultrasound appearances or magnetic resonance spectroscopy (MRS) appearances are used (Bellentani et al., 2000; Clark et al., 2003; Ruhl and Everhart, 2003; Bedogni et al., 2005; Szczepaniak et al., 2005) with the MRS series probably most accurate. Estimates of the more severe stage NASH are at about 2.5% (Underwood Ground, 1984; Wanless and Lentz, 1990; Yu and Keeffe, 2002). Even with the estimates of NASH at 2.5%, it is more common than chronic hepatitis C, chronic hepatitis B, alcoholic liver disease and the metabolic liver diseases.

Risk factors

NAFLD is primarily associated with the (dys)metabolic syndrome comprising of features including obesity, type 2 diabetes, insulin resistance, hypertension and dyslipidaemia (Marchesini et al., 2001, 2003; Bugianesi et al., 2005). NAFLD may, however, also occur in lean individuals (Underwood Ground, 1984; Wanless and Lentz, 1990; Pratt and Kaplan, 2000). The increasing rates of obesity in developed and developing countries (Mokdad et al., 2001, 2003) make NAFLD the most common cause of chronic liver disease in developed countries and predicts that the prevalence of NAFLD will increase. In keeping with this predicted increase in the prevalence of NAFLD, the projected numbers of patients being transplanted for NAFLD is expected to exceed those being transplanted for chronic hepatitis C within the next decade, if current rates of obesity continue (Michael, 2004).

Natural history of NAFLD

The natural history of NAFLD is imprecisely known but probably the best study so far to document the natural history is the recent study from two Scandinavian hospitals, with a mean follow-up period of some 14 years (Ekstedt et al., 2006). In essence, this study involved patients with biopsy-proven NAFLD. They were divided into those with steatosis (hepatosteatosis) alone and those with steatosis and inflammation (steatohepatitis). The findings may be summarised as showing that hepatosteatosis progresses but with a low risk of cirrhosis, but that NASH progresses more aggressively, because about 20% of the patients with NASH at inception of the study progressed to cirrhosis over the follow-up period.

Conversely, although none of the hepatosteatosis group progressed to cirrhosis, there was, however, some progression to a more severe stage of fibrosis in about half of the patients. The inference then is that whilst hepatosteatosis may not progress to cirrhosis in the medium term, a proportion of patients will probably progress to cirrhosis in the longer term (Ekstedt et al., 2006). The survival of patients with NASH in this study was also reduced compared to the general population (Ekstedt et al., 2006) as was that of unstaged NAFLD patients in an earlier study (Adams et al., 2005; Ekstedt et al., 2006).

The risk of cardiovascular disease is, not unsurprisingly, increased in NAFLD (Villanova et al., 2005) and is the leading cause of death in these patients (Adams et al., 2005). This is not to denigrate the importance of liver-related mortality in NAFLD because in the Adams et al. study, liver disease was the third leading cause of death in patients with NAFLD compared to 13th in the general population (Adams et al., 2005). The risk of hepatocellular carcinoma has also been demonstrated convincingly to be increased in a very large prospective cohort study involving almost 1 million patients with probable NAFLD in association with type 2 diabetes with other causes of chronic liver diseases excluded (El-Serag et al., 2004).

Clinical features

Most patients with NAFLD are asymptomatic in the early stages. Symptoms when they occur include right upper quadrant discomfort and fatigue. On examination there may be hepatomegaly and right upper quadrant tenderness which, given the phenotype of the typical patient with NAFLD, may be mistaken for gallstone disease (McCullough, 2002). Palmar erythema, jaundice, spider naevi, gynaecomastia, ascites or splenomegaly may be present if cirrhosis develops.

Diagnosis

There is at present no single diagnostic test that reliably detects NAFLD. The diagnosis therefore remains largely one of exclusion in obese, insulin-resistant, dyslipidaemic individuals with abnormal liver function tests, who deny and have had corroboration of absence of excessive alcohol consumption, have negative imaging for focal liver lesions and negative serology for hepatitis A, B and C, normal autoimmune profile, ferritin and transferrin saturation, copper and caeruloplasmin.

Most patients with NAFLD have abnormal liver function tests but abnormalities such as elevated serum transaminases and GGT lack sensitivity and specificity not only for NAFLD but for any liver disease. The ALT is usually elevated but may be normal in the presence of radiological evidence of hepatosteatosis (Browning et al., 2004) and may even normalise with progressive disease. The AST:ALT ratio is usually less than 1, as compared to alcohol-induced liver disease where it is usually greater than 1. In NAFLD a reversal of the AST:ALT ratio, so that it is greater than 1, implies an advanced fibrotic stage.

The ALP and GGT are usually increased some two- to three-fold in >50% of cases. Serum bilirubin and albumin are usually normal unless the patient is cirrhotic. The ferritin, if increased in the presence of normal iron indices, is reflective of a low level inflammatory state that exists in obesity and NAFLD, and the increased ferritin here is an acute phase reactant (Powell et al., 1990; Bacon et al., 1994; Brunt, 2001). Anti-nuclear antibodies and anti-smooth muscle antibodies may be abnormal in up to 25% of patients with NAFLD and their presence augers more severe injury and inflammation (Adams et al., 2004)

Imaging as a diagnostic tool in NAFLD

Of the present imaging modalities ultrasound scanning is the most cost effective and detects steatosis with a sensitivity of 66–100%, although this is reduced if the fat content is less than 33% (Caturelli et al., 1992; Saadeh et al., 2002). CT has about the same sensitivity and specificity as ultrasound scanning but is more expensive (Saadeh et al., 2002). MRI is of the same utility as CT and ultrasound scanning, but it is in any case impractical as a screening tool because of its expense. MRS is the most sensitive technique and is able to detect fat at around 5%, unlike the other modalities where maximal detection occurs after about 33% (Szczepaniak et al., 2005). It is worth stressing that none of the imaging modalities can distinguish between the various stages of NAFLD, i.e. they cannot indicate whether fat alone is present or whether the fat is present with inflammation (Saadeh et al., 2002); this information is of clear prognostic importance.

The role of liver biopsy in diagnosing NAFLD

A liver biopsy is considered by many to be mandatory to both confirm the diagnosis and stage the disease. The utility of the liver biopsy is underscored by a recent paper by Skelley et al. (2001) which showed that in a group of 354 patients being investigated for abnormal liver function tests in the presence of negative liver serology, some 34% had a revised diagnosis after the liver biopsy. Liver biopsy is not, however, without its limitations. First of all, a needle biopsy sample usually represents around 1/50 000 of the total mass of the liver (Bravo et al., 2001). In addition it has been shown that the histological lesions of NASH are unevenly distributed throughout the liver parenchyma. Therefore the inherent sampling error of a liver biopsy can result in potential misdiagnosis or staging inaccuracies (Ratziu et al., 2005).

Liver biopsy, moreover, is an invasive test with potential risk of complications as described in Chapter 2 (Bravo et al., 2001). A few hours' admission for observation of the patient is also needed following a liver biopsy. Another test that has recently been validated for assessing liver fibrosis in patients with chronic liver disease, especially chronic hepatitis C, is transient elastography (FibroScan). FibroScan is a non-invasive test that measures liver stiffness but it is less sensitive in obese patients (Kettaneh et al., 2007).

Histology of NAFLD

The histological features of NAFLD on haemotoxylin and eosin staining include macrovesicular steatosis, an acute or chronic inflammatory cell infiltrate, Mallory's hyaline and, on connective tissue staining, pericellular fibrosis (Figures 8.1–8.3, Plates 7–9). These features are also found in alcohol-induced liver disease and this

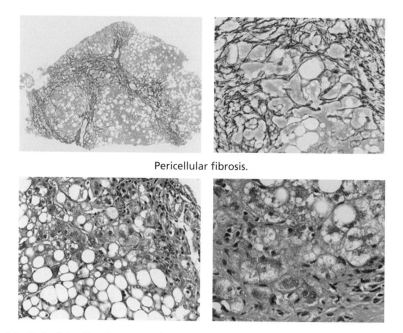

Pericellular fibrosis.

Figure 8.3 Pericellular fibrosis. For a colour version of this figure, please see Plate 9 in the colour plate section.

underlies the importance of corroborating the patient's alcohol history. Recently a scoring system has been devised by Brunt and colleagues to aid the scoring of liver biopsies in NAFLD (Brunt, 2005, 2007; Kleiner et al., 2005).

Pathogenesis

The pathogenesis of NAFLD remains poorly understood. It is known, however, that insulin resistance, in association with obesity, is a key mechanism leading to hepatic steatosis. Resistance to insulin is presently thought to enhance peripheral lipolysis and delivery of free fatty acids to the liver. This insulin resistance has been referred to as the first hit in the pathogenesis of NAFLD (Day and James, 1998).

High circulating insulin, secondary to insulin resistance, also results in defective fatty acid oxidation in the hepatic mitochondria, reduced export of triglycerides and increased de novo synthesis of triglycerides within the liver, all resulting in intracytoplasmic accumulation of triglycerides (Harrison and Di Bisceglie, 2003). As a consequence there is enhanced lipid peroxidation and activation of profibrogenic and proinflammatory cytokine pathways with TNFα and adiponectin being key players (Tilg and Diehl, 2000; Hui et al., 2004; Kamada et al., 2007a). The role of lipid peroxidation in NASH has been suggested by studies showing its presence in both animal models of non-alcoholic fatty liver and humans with steatosis of different aetiologies (Letteron et al., 1996). The second hit, therefore, is the increased oxidant stress secondary to increased lipid peroxidation and the increase in profibrogenic and proinflammatory cytokines (Day and James, 1998). The pathogenic role of triglycerides has been questioned recently because of data showing that hepatocyte accumulation of triglycerides may actually be a protective mechanism to reduce the toxicity from free fatty acids delivered from the periphery to the liver (Yamaguchi et al., 2007).

Nielsen et al. (2004) have suggested that free fatty acids might also directly mediate inflammation in NAFLD. They have shown that central obesity, which has been linked to an increased risk of NASH, is associated with an increased lipolysis of visceral adipose tissue and an increased hepatic supply of free fatty acids. Furthermore a recent study using stable isotope methodology has demonstrated that almost two thirds of fat in the liver of patients with NAFLD is derived from circulatory free fatty acids as opposed to dietary sources or de novo lipogenesis (Donnelly et al., 2005).

Hepatic iron, anti-oxidant deficiencies and intestinal bacteria have all been implicated as potential oxidative stressors with recent studies showing that HFE gene mutations or increased hepatic iron are associated with enhanced liver injury in NAFLD (George et al., 1998; Nelson et al., 2007). It is still not clear why some patients develop hepatosteatosis and do not progress for years without any complications whereas others go on to develop inflammation, fibrosis and eventually liver cirrhosis.

Obesity-related hepatic steatosis has also been shown to be associated with an increased production of inflammatory cytokines by hepatocytes. Recent studies in rodents have shown conclusively that hepatic steatosis is associated with a state of chronic inflammation with an increase in TNFα and a reduction in the anti-inflammatory adipokine, adiponectin (Cai et al., 2005). In this regard, experimental animals with induced NASH, lacking adiponectin, are more likely than controls to develop hepatocellular carcinoma (Kamada et al., 2007b) This chronic inflammation state is often, as above, reflected in an elevated ferritin as an acute phase reactant.

Ingestion of a wide variety of therapeutic drugs may also lead to hepatic steatosis. Amiodarone, antiviral agents (zidovudin and interferon), non-steroidal anti-inflammatory drugs, tetracycline and sodium valporate have all been implicated. Accumulation of fat results predominantly from the inhibition of the mitochondrial beta-oxidation of fatty acids by a variety of mechanisms (Fromenty and Pessayre, 1995). Drugs like amiodarone not only cause steatosis but also provide a mechanism for increased oxidative stress and are capable of inducing steatohepatitis-like lesions.

From the findings of a NASH model of genetically obese ob/ob mice, it has been suggested that gut bacterial flora might be implicated in the development of fatty liver, as the endogenous ethanol production by the intestinal flora is significantly increased (Cope et al., 2000). In patients, Nair et al. (2001) found a positive correlation between breath ethanol concentrations and obesity in a small group of individuals who denied recent consumption of alcoholic beverages.

As regards the development of fibrosis, it is probable that obesity-related activation of the sympathetic nervous system (SNS) directly or indirectly via raised leptin levels may hasten the fibrosis because the absence of SNS, either through genetic or pharmacological manipulation or reduced angiotensin-1 signalling, markedly abrogates the extent of fibrosis in animal models of NASH (Oben et al., 2003b, 2004; Hirose et al., 2007).

Disease management

There is at present no proven therapy for NAFLD. As a significant proportion of patients with NAFLD are obese, have type 2 diabetes or are dyslipidaemic, i.e. have features of the metabolic syndrome, initial therapy is aimed at reducing the drivers for the disease – namely obesity and insulin resistance. Initial therapy would therefore include an alteration of lifestyle, dietary advice with support from a nutritionist and increased exercise. In this regard, bariatric surgery has been shown in recent series to improve histological features of NAFLD (Clark et al., 2005; Klein et al., 2006). Exercise similarly improves the biochemical and histological parameters in NAFLD (Ueno et al., 1997), partially through enhancing insulin sensitivity. Too rapid or extreme weight loss in a short space of time has been associated with accelerated progression of the disease in some patients with NAFLD (Capron et al., 1982). Ideally, controlled weight loss should be the result of a planned structured approach by a dedicated bariatric service that comprises lipidologists, dieticians, psychologists/psychiatrists and hepatologists.

Pharmacotherapy may also be used to aid weight loss. Available drugs are orlistat, sirbutramine and, most recently, rimonabant. There is some evidence from small series studies that orlistat and sirbutramine may be of benefit in NAFLD (Clark, 2006). Trials of the cannabinoid receptor blocker, rimonabant, in NAFLD are planned.

Besides lifestyle modifications and pharmacotherapy to reduce weight and enhance insulin sensitivity, agents such as metformin which directly enhance insulin sensitivity have also been used. Metformin decreases circulating glucose levels primarily by decreasing hepatic gluconeogenesis and glycogenolysis and moderately increasing skeletal muscle glucose uptake. In animal models it has been found to reverse fatty liver in obese, leptin-deficient ob/ob mice (Lin et al., 2000). Metformin has also been shown to prevent lipid-induced insulin resistance in animal models (Cleasby et al., 2004). Nair et al. (2004) have also shown that metformin treatment transiently normalised markers of hepatic inflammation and the degree of hepaosteatosis in a small study in patients with NAFLD.

Thiazolidinediones (TZDs), like troglitazone, have also been used as a treatment of NAFLD. Cadwell et al. (2001) reported that treatment with troglitazone significantly improved liver enzyme abnormalities and somewhat improved hepatic histology in a small series of patients with NAFLD. It should be mentioned though that troglitazone has been withdrawn as a first-line therapy for type 2 diabetes because of rare but potentially lethal hepatotoxicity. A recent placebo-controlled trial of another TZD, pioglitazone, in NAFLD showed that it improved liver function tests, hepatic fat content and insulin sensitivity in subjects with NASH. It did not, however, improve fibrosis (Belfort et al., 2006). Cholesterol-lowering agents such as 3-hydroxy-coenzyme A reductase inhibitors, atorvastatin, have also been shown in a small group of patients with NAFLD to have beneficial effects (Gomez-Dominguez et al., 2006). Statins appear to be safe in NAFLD and the present consensus would favour their use in patients with NAFLD and dyslipidaemia. This stance on their safety in NAFLD is supported by data from the large Dallas heart study (Browning, 2006).

Pilot studies with the anti-oxidant vitamin E have demonstrated improved histological parameters in NAFLD (Sanyal et al., 2004). Cytoprotective agents like ursodeoxycholic acid (UDCA) have also been evaluated. Lindor et al. (2004) studied the effects of 13 and 15 mg/kg/day dose of UDCA for 2 years in 126 patients with biopsy-proven NASH and found that although safe and well tolerated it was no better than placebo. The study, however, may have been under-powered (Clark and Brancati, 2004; Lindor et al., 2004). Other emerging treatments of NAFLD include probiotics, through their alteration of gut flora and reduction of TNFα (Solga and Diehl, 2003), angiotensin-1 receptor blockers (Yokohama et al., 2004; Hirose et al., 2007) and alpha-adrenoceptor antagonists which reduce liver injury, enhance liver regeneration and also reduce the fibrogenesis in animal models of NASH, the more severe stage of NAFLD (Oben et al., 2003a, 2004).

Chapter summary

NAFLD is a spectrum of chronic liver disease ranging from hepatosteatosis through steatosis with inflammation to fibrosis, cirrhosis and hepatocellular carcinoma. It is presently the most common cause of chronic liver disease in developed countries. Its increase is secondary to the increasing rates of obesity and type 2 diabetes. Insulin resistance seems to be the key pathogenic requirement with increased oxidant stress and proinflammatory cytokines also clearly involved. There is no accepted single diagnostic test for NAFLD. It remains a diagnosis of exclusion which, in some patients, requires a liver biopsy to reliably diagnose and stage the disease.

There is currently no approved treatment for NAFLD. Treatments strategies usually start with lifestyle modifications and may include pharmacotherapy to aid weight loss or enhance insulin sensitivity. Bariatric surgery in morbidly obese patients with NAFLD appears effective. Therapeutic trials are planned for drugs such as rimonabant, adrenoceptor antagonists and angiotensin-1 receptor blockers which show promise in experimental studies.

Illustrative case study

Mr ZK, a 77-year-old, lean man, was a retired tailor. He had been a type 2 diabetic for several years but had of late lost weight at the insistence of his family. He presented acutely with melaena. He had no previous upper gastrointestinal complaints and no history of non-steroidal use. He did not drink alcohol immoderately and certainly on corroboration from his family drank at most 1 unit per month. He was previously fit and well.

On initial examination, he was cardiovascularly stable and had no overt stigmata of chronic liver disease. Investigations revealed a slightly low haemoglobin, low platelets, a low albumin and a prolonged INR (1.6). An urgent endoscopy showed portal hypertensive gastropathy and small oesophageal varices not amenable to band ligation. A liver disease aetiology database was unrevealing. A subsequent abdominal ultrasound scan showed a small shrunken liver with a coarse echo pattern, suggestive of cirrhosis. A liver biopsy showed severe macrovesicular steatosis, an inflammatory cell infiltrate, marked pericellular fibrosis and incomplete cirrhosis. The features were consistent with alcoholic liver disease or NAFLD. Given the corroborated alcohol history the diagnosis was NAFLD with developing cirrhosis.

References

Adams LA, Lindor KD, Angula P (2004) The prevalence of autoantibodies and autoimmune hepatitis in patients with nonalcoholic fatty liver disease. *The American Journal of Gastroenterology* **99**:1316–1320

Adams LA, Lymp JF, St Sauver J, Sanderson SO, Lindor KD, Feldstein A, Angulo P (2005) The natural history of nonalcoholic fatty liver disease: a population-based cohort study. *Gastroenterology* **129**:113–121

Bacon BR, Farahvash MJ, Janney CG, Neuschwander-Tetri BA (1994) Nonalcoholic steatohepatitis: an expanded clinical entity. *Gastroenterology* **107**:1103–1109

Bedogni G, Miglioli L, Masutti F, Tiribelli C, Marchesini G, Bellentani S (2005) Prevalence of and risk factors for nonalcoholic fatty liver disease: the Dionysos nutrition and liver study. *Hepatology* **42**:44–52

Belfort R, Harrison SA, Brown K, Darland C, Finch J, Hardies J, Balas B, Gastaldelli A, Tio F, Pulcini J, Berria R, Ma JZ, Dwivedi S, Havranek R, Fincke C, Defronzo R, Bannayan GA, Schenker S, Cusi K (2006) A placebo-controlled trial of pioglitazone in subjects with nonalcoholic steatohepatitis. *New England Journal of Medicine* **355**:2297–2307

Bellentani S, Saccoccio G, Masutti F, Croce LS, Brandi G, Sasso F, Cristanni G, Tiribelli C (2000) Prevalence of and risk factors for hepatic steatosis in Northern Italy. *Annals of Internal Medicine* **132**:112–117

Bravo AA, Sheth SG, Chopra S (2001) Liver biopsy. *New England Journal of Medicine* **344**:495–500

Browning JD (2006) Statins and hepatic steatosis: perspectives from the Dallas Heart Study. *Hepatology* **44**:466–471

Browning JD, Szczepaniak LS, Dobbins R, Nuremberg P, Horton JD, Cohen JC, Grundy SM, Hobbs HH (2004) Prevalence of hepatic steatosis in an urban population in the United States: impact of ethnicity. *Hepatology* **40**:1387–1395

Brunt EM (2001) Nonalcoholic steatohepatitis: definition and pathology. *Seminars in Liver Disease* **21**:3–16

Brunt EM (2005) Nonalcoholic steatohepatitis: pathologic features and differential diagnosis. *Seminars in Diagnosis and Pathology* **22**:330–338

Brunt EM (2007) Pathology of fatty liver disease. *Modern Pathology* **20**(Suppl 1): S40–48

Bugianesi E, Gastaldelli A, Vanni E, Gambino R, Cassader M, Baldi S, Ponti V, Pagano G, Ferrannini E, Rizzetto M (2005) Insulin resistance in non-diabetic patients with non-alcoholic fatty liver disease: sites and mechanisms. *Diabetologia* **48**:634–642

Bugianesi E, Leone N, Vanni E, Marchesini G, Brunello F, Carucci P, Musso A, De Paolis P, Capussotti L, Salizzoni M, Rizzetto M (2002) Expanding the natural history of nonalcoholic steatohepatitis: from cryptogenic cirrhosis to hepatocellular carcinoma. *Gastroenterology* **123**:134–140

Cai D, Yuan M, Frantz DF, Melendez PA, Hansen L, Lee J, Shoelson SE (2005) Local and systemic insulin resistance resulting from hepatic activation of IKK-beta and NF-kappaB. *Nature Medicine* **11**:183–190

Cadwell SH, Hespenheide EE, Redick JA, Iezzoni JC, Battle EH, Sheppard BL (2001) A pilot study of a thiazolidinedione, troglitazone, in nonalcoholic steato-hepatitis. *American Journal of Gastroenterology* **96**:519–525

Capron JP, Delmarre J, Dupas JL, Braillon A, Degott C, Quenum C (1982) Fasting in obesity: another cause of liver injury with alcoholic hyaline? *Digestive Disease Science* **27**:265–268

Caturelli E, Squillante MM, Andriulli A, Cedrone A, Cellerion C, Pompili M, Manoja ER, Rapaccini GL (1992) Hypoechoic lesions in the 'bright liver': a reliable indicator of fatty change. A prospective study. *Journal of Gastroenterology and Hepatology* **7**:469–472

Clark JM (2006) Weight loss as a treatment for nonalcoholic fatty liver disease. *Journal of Clinical Gastroenterology* **40**:S39–43

Clark JM, Alkhuraishi ARA, Solga SF, Alli P, Diehl AM, Magnuson TH (2005) Roux-en-Y gastric bypass improves liver histology in patients with non-alcoholic fatty liver disease. *Obesity Research* **13**:1180–1186

Clark JM, Brancati FL (2004) Negative trials in nonalcoholic steatohepatitis: why they happen and what they teach us. *Hepatology* **39**:602–603

Clark J, Brancati DL, Diehl AM (2003) The prevalence and etiology of elevated aminotransferase levels in the United States. *American Journal of Gastroenterology* **98**:960–967

Cleasby ME, Dzamko N, Hegarty BD, Cooney GJ, Kraege EW, Ye JM (2004) Metformin prevents the development of acute lipid-induced insulin resistance in the rat through altered hepatic signaling mechanisms. *Diabetes* **53**:3258–3266

Cope K, Risby T, Diehl AM (2000) Increased gastrointestinal ethanol production in obese mice: implications for fatty liver disease pathogenesis. *Gastroenterology* **119**:1340–1347

Day CP, James OF (1998) Steatohepatitis: a tale of two 'hits'? *Gastroenterology* **114**:842–845

Donnelly KL, Smith CI, Schwarzenberg SJ, Jessurun J, Boldt MD, Parks EJ (2005) Sources of fatty acids stored in liver and secreted via lipoproteins in patients with nonalcoholic fatty liver disease. *Journal of Clinical Investigation* **115**: 1343–1351

Ekstedt M, Franzen LE, Mathiesen UL, Thorelius L, Holmqvist M, Bodemar G, Kechagiag S (2006) Long-term follow-up of patients with NAFLD and elevated liver enzymes. *Hepatology* **44**:865–873

El-Serag HB, Tran T, Everhart JE (2004) Diabetes increases the risk of chronic liver disease and hepatocellular carcinoma. *Gastroenterology* **126**:460–468

Falck-Ytter Y, Younossi ZM, Marchesini G, McCullough AJ (2001) Clinical features and natural history of nonalcoholic steatosis syndromes. *Seminars in Liver Disease* **21**:17–26

Fromenty B, Pessayre D (1995) Inhibition of mitochondrial beta-oxidation as a mechanism of hepatotoxicity. *Pharmacology and Therapeutics* **67**:101–154

George DK, Goldwurm S, MacDonald GA, Cowley LL, Walker NI, Ward PJ, Jazwinska EC, Powell LW (1998) Increased hepatic iron concentration in non-alcoholic steatohepatitis is associated with increased fibrosis. *Gastroenterology* **114**:311–318

Gomez-Dominguez E, Gisbert JP, Moreno-Montegudo JA, Garcia-Buey L, Moreno-Otero RO (2006) A pilot study of atorvastatin treatment in dyslipemid, non-alcoholic fatty liver patients. *Alimentary Pharmacology & Therapeutics* **23**:1643–1647

Harrison SA, Di Bisceglie (2003) Advances in the understanding and treatment of nonalcoholic fatty liver disease. *Drugs* **63**:2379–2394

Hirose A, Ono M, Saibara T, Nozaki Y, Masuda K, Yoshioka AA, Takahashi M, Akisawa N, Iwasaki S, Oben JA, Onishi S (2007) Angiotensin II type 1 receptor blocker inhibits fibrosis in rat nonalcoholic steatohepatitis. *Hepatology* **45**: 1375–1381

Hui JM, Hodge A, Farrell GC, Kench JG, Kriketos A, George J (2004) Beyond insulin resistance in NASH: TNF-alpha or adiponectin? *Hepatology* **40**:46–54

Kamada Y, Matsumoto H, Tamura S, Fukushima J, Kiso S, Fukui K, Igura T, Maeda N, Kihara S, Funahashi T, Matsuzawa Y, Shimomura I, Hayashi N (2007a) Hypoadiponectinemia accelerates hepatic tumor formation in a non-alcoholic steatohepatitis mouse model. *Journal of Hepatology* **47**:556–564

Kamada Y, Matsumoto H, Tamura S, Fukushima J, Kiso S, Fukui K, Igura T, Maeda N, Kihara S, Funahashi T, Matsuzawa Y, Shimomura I, Hayashi N (2007b) Hypoadiponectinemia accelerates hepatic tumor formation in a non-alcoholic steatohepatitis mouse model. *Journal of Hepatology* **47**:556–564

Kettaneh A, Marcellini P, Douvin C, Poupon R, Ziol M, Beaugrand M, De Ledinghen V (2007) Features associated with success rate and performance of FibroScan measurements for the diagnosis of cirrhosis in HCV patients: a prospective study of 935 patients. *Journal of Hepatology* **46**:628–634

Klein S, Mittendorfer B, Eagon JC, Patterson B, Grant L, Feirt N, Seki E, Brenner D, Korenblat K, McCrea J (2006) Gastric bypass surgery improves metabolic and hepatic abnormalities associated with nonalcoholic fatty liver disease. *Gastroenterology* **130**:1564–1572

Kleiner DE, Brunt EM, Van Natta M, Behling C, Contos MJ, Cummings OW, Ferrell LD, Liu YC, Torbenson MS, Unalp-Arida A, Yeh M, McCullough AJ, Sanyal AJ (2005) Design and validation of a histological scoring system for nonalcoholic fatty liver disease. *Hepatology* **41**:1313–1321

Letteron P, Fromenty B, Terris B, Degott C, Pessayre D (1996) Acute and chronic hepatic steatosis lead to in vivo lipid peroxidation in mice. *Journal of Hepatology* **24**:200–208

Lin HZ, Yang SQ, Kujhada F, Ronnet G, Kiehl AM (2000) Metformin reverses nonalcoholic fatty liver disease in obese leptin-deficient mice. *Nature Medicine* **6**:998–1003

Lindor KD, Kowdley KV, Heathcoate EJ, Harrison ME, Jorgensen R, Angulo P, Lymp JF, Burgart L, Colin P (2004) Ursodeoxycholic acid for treatment of non-alcoholic steatohepatitis: results of a randomized trial. *Hepatology* **39**:770–778

Ludwig J, Viggiano TR, Mcgill DB, Oh BJ (1980) Nonalcoholic steatohepatitis: Mayo Clinic experiences with a hitherto unnamed disease. *Mayo Clinic Proceedings* **55**:434–438

Marchesini G, Brizi M, Bianchi G, Tomassetti S, Bugianesi E, Lenzi M, McCullough AJ, Natale S, Forlani G, Melchionda N (2001) Nonalcoholic fatty liver disease: a feature of the metabolic syndrome. *Diabetes* **50**:1844–1850

Marchesini G, Bugianesi E, Forlani G, Cerrelli F, Lenzi M, Manini R, Natale S, Vanni E, Villanova N, Melchionda N, Rizzetto M (2003) Nonalcoholic fatty liver, steatohepatitis, and the metabolic syndrome. *Hepatology* **37**:917–923

McCullough AJ (2002) Update on nonalcoholic fatty liver disease. *Journal of Clinical Gastroenterology* **34**:255–262

Michael C (2004) Nonalcoholic fatty liver disease: a review of current understanding and future impact. *Clinical Gastroenterology and Hepatology* **2**(12):1048–1058

Mokdad AH, Ford ES, Bowman BA, Dietz WH, Vinicor F, Bales VS, Marks JS (2003) Prevalence of obesity, diabetes, and obesity-related health risk factors, 2001. *Journal of the American Medical Association* **289**:76–79

Mokdad AH, Ford ES, Bowman BA, Nelson DE, Engelgau MM, Vinicor F, Marks JS (2001) The continuing increase of diabetes in the US. *Diabetes Care* **24**:412

Nair S, Cope K, Risby TH, Diehl AM (2001) Obesity and female gender increase breath ethanol concentration: potential implications for the pathogenesis of non-alcoholic steatohepatitis. *American Journal of Gastroenterology* **96**:1200–1204

Nair S, Diehl AM, Wiseman M, Farr GH Jr, Perrillo RP (2004) Metformin in the treatment of non-alcoholic steatohepatitis: a pilot open label trial. *Alimentary Pharmacology & Therapeutics* **20**:23–28

Nelson JE, Bhattacharya R, Lindor KD, Chalasani N, Raaka S, Heathcote EJ, Miskovsky E, Shaffer E, Rulyak SJ, Kowdley KV (2007) HFE C282Y mutations are associated with advanced hepatic fibrosis in Caucasians with nonalcoholic steatohepatitis. *Hepatology* **46**:723–729

Nielsen S, Guo Z, Johnson CM, Hensrud DD, Jensen MD (2004) Splanchnic lipolysis in human obesity. *Journal of Clinical Investigation* **113**:1582–1588

Oben JA, Roskams T, Yang S, Lin H, Sinelli N, Li Z, Torbenson M, Huang J, Guarino P, Kafrouni M, Diehl AM (2003a) Sympathetic nervous system inhibition increases hepatic progenitors and reduces liver injury. *Hepatology* **38**:664–673

Oben JA, Roskams T, Yang S, Lin H, Sinelli N, Li Z, Torbenson M, Thomas SA, Diehl AM (2003b) Norepinephrine induces hepatic fibrogenesis in leptin deficient ob/ob mice. *Biochemical and Biophysical Research Communications* **308**:284–292

Oben JA, Roskams T, Yang S, Lin H, Sinelli N, Torbenson M, Smedh U, Moran TH, Li Z, Huang J, Thomas SA, Diehl AM (2004) Hepatic fibrogenesis requires sympathetic neurotransmitters. *Gut* **53**:438–445

Powell EE, Cooksley WG, Hanson R, Searle J, Halliday JW, Powell LW (1990) The natural history of nonalcoholic steatohepatitis: a follow-up study of forty-two patients for up to 21 years. *Hepatology* **11**:74–80

Pratt DS, Kaplan MM (2000) Evaluation of abnormal liver-enzyme results in asymptomatic patients. *New England Journal of Medicine* **342**:1266–1271

Ratziu V, Charlotte F, Heurtier A, Gombert S, Giral P, Bruckert E, Grimaldi A, Capron F, Poynard T (2005) Sampling variability of liver biopsy in nonalcoholic fatty liver disease. *Gastroenterology* **128**:1898–1906

Ruhl CE, Everhart JE (2003) Determinants of the association of overweight with elevated serum alanine aminotransferase activity in the United States. *Gastroenterology* **124**:71–79

Saadeh S, Younossi ZM, Remer EM, Gramlich T, Ong JP, Hurley M, Mullen KD, Cooper JN, Sheridan MJ (2002) The utility of radiological imaging in nonalcoholic fatty liver disease. *Gastroenterology* **123**:745–750

Sanyal AJ, Mofrad PS, Contos MJ, Sargeant C, Luketic VA, Sterling RK, Stravitz RT, Shiffman ML, Clore J, Mills AS (2004) A pilot study of vitamin E versus vitamin E and pioglitazone for the treatment of nonalcoholic steatohepatitis. *Clinical Gastroenterology and Hepatology* **2**:1107–1115

Skelly MM, James PD, Ryder SD (2001) Findings on liver biopsy to investigate abnormal liver function tests in the absence of diagnostic serology. *Journal of Hepatology* **35**:195–199

Solga SF, Diehl AM (2003) Non-alcoholic fatty liver disease: lumen-liver interactions and possible role for probiotics. *Journal of Hepatology* **38**:681–687

Szczepaniak LS, Nurenberg P, Leonard D, Browning JD, Reingold JS, Grundy S, Hobbs HH, Dobbins RL (2005) Magnetic resonance spectroscopy to measure hepatic triglyceride content: prevalence of hepatic steatosis in the general population. *American Journal of Physiology. Endocrinology and Metabolism* **288**: E462–468

Tilg H, Diehl AM (2000) Cytokines in alcoholic and nonalcoholic steatohepatitis. *New England Journal of Medicine* **343**:1467–1476

Ueno T, Sugawara H, Sujaku K, Hashimoto O, Tsuji R, Tamaki S, Torimura T, Inuzuka S, Sata M, Tanikawa K (1997) Therapeutic effects of restricted diet and exercise in obese patients with fatty liver. *Journal of Hepatology* **27**:103–107

Underwood Ground K (1984) Prevalence of fatty liver in healthy male adults accidentally killed. *Aviation, Space, and Environmental Medicine* **55**:59–61

Villanova N, Moscatiello S, Ramilli S, Bugianesi S, Magalotti D, Vanni E, Zoli M, Marchesini G (2005) Endothelial dysfunction and cardiovascular risk profile in nonalcoholic fatty liver disease. *Hepatology* **42**:473–480

Wanless IR, Lentz JS (1990) Fatty liver hepatitis (steatohepatitis) and obesity: an autopsy study with analysis of risk factors. *Hepatology* **12**:1106–1110

Yamaguchi K, Yang L, McCall S, Huang J, Yu XX, Pandey SK, Bhanot S, Monia BP, Li YX, Diehl AM (2007) Inhibiting triglyceride synthesis improves hepatic steatosis but exacerbates liver damage and fibrosis in obese mice with nonalcoholic steatohepatitis. *Hepatology* **45**:1366–1374

Yokohama S, Yoneda M, Haneda M, Okamato S, Okada M, Aso K, Hasegawa T, Tokusashi Y, Miyokawa N, Nakamura K (2004) Therapeutic efficacy of an angiotensin II receptor antagonist in patients with nonalcoholic steatohepatitis. *Hepatology* 40:1222–1225

Yu AS, Keefe EB (2002) Nonalcoholic fatty liver disease. *Reviews in Gastroenterological Disorders* 2:11–19

Viral hepatitis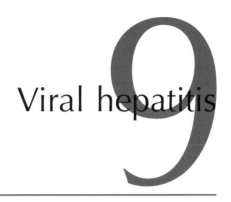

Tracey Dudley

Introduction

Hepatitis, or inflammation of the liver, has many causes. These include toxins, such as alcohol, some medicines, autoimmune and genetic conditions, and viral infection.

Viral hepatitis is a major cause of morbidity and mortality worldwide, causing both acute and chronic illness. The spectrum of disease is broad, ranging from asymptomatic, self-limiting infection to chronic hepatitis, acute liver failure (ALF), or liver cirrhosis. Also, hepatitis virus infection is the most common cause of liver cancer. By far the greatest burden of disease is caused by chronic viral hepatitis, and specifically hepatitis B virus (HBV) and hepatitis C virus (HCV) infection.

Viruses hijack the cellular machinery of the host organism to reproduce, or replicate. Often, the virus itself is not directly cytopathic. Liver damage is a consequence of the immune response to infection which destroys infected hepatocytes. Blood tests show raised ALT and AST levels indicative of liver damage. Following acute infection and eradication of the virus, inflammation resolves and healthy liver tissue regenerates. In chronic infection, ongoing inflammation leads to the development of scar tissue, or fibrosis, in the liver. Eventually, interlinking areas of fibrosis replace healthy liver tissue leading to cirrhosis.

Chronic HBV and HCV infections contribute significantly to the development of liver cirrhosis and liver cancer, both leading causes of death worldwide. Co-infection with human immunodeficiency virus (HIV) accelerates the progression of liver disease in patients with hepatitis infection.

The chapter will discuss both acute and chronic viral hepatitis, and co-infection with HIV.

Hepatitis A virus

Epidemiology

The hepatitis A virus (HAV) is a ribonucleic acid (RNA) virus of the picornaviridae family. HAV is the commonest cause of acute viral hepatitis worldwide. It produces an acute and self-limiting illness. As a water- and food-borne disease, it is most commonly transmitted via the faecal–oral route as a consequence of poor standards of sanitation and hygiene. Although relatively uncommon in the UK, HAV is endemic in Africa, Asia, Central and South America (WHO, 2000a). In endemic areas, HAV infection occurs in childhood, and is usually an asymptomatic disease. By early adulthood, the majority of the population will be immune (WHO, 2000a).

HAV is extremely infectious. It is present, in high titres, in the stools of infected individuals before symptoms are apparent, and it can be detected for some weeks after the onset of jaundice. HAV is a resilient virus that can survive in the environment for a period of time. Contaminated water supplies, inadequate waste disposal and poor personal hygiene are responsible for the transmission of disease. Shellfish from infected waters are a common source of infection. Identified risk factors include:

- Contact with an infected person
- Overseas travel
- Living or working in residential care/correctional settings
- Injecting and non-injecting drug use
- Oral–anal sex (WHO, 2000a)

Diagnosis

Acute HAV infection is confirmed by the presence of anti-HAV IgM antibodies in serum. Anti-HAV IgG will be detectable approximately 3 weeks after the onset of jaundice. Over time, anti-HAV IgM titres decline to undetectable levels. IgG antibodies persist. The presence of anti-HAV IgG, without anti-HAV IgM, confirms previous exposure and immunity to infection (Thimme et al., 2005).

Clinical features

The virus has no direct cytopathic effect. Hepatitis is the result of the destruction of infected hepatocytes by the immune response (Thimme et al., 2005; Naomov, 2007).

The incubation period of HAV infection is between 10 and 50 days (WHO 2000a). Adult-acquired infection is often symptomatic. Jaundice is a frequent feature, accompanied by pale stools and dark urine. A prodromal syndrome can be identified, with symptoms including fever, fatigue, anorexia, nausea, vomiting and abdominal pain (Thimme et al., 2005). Most individuals recover with complete resolution of symptoms within 6 months. There is no chronic form of the disease and infection confers life-long immunity. Severe hepatitis is more likely with advancing age, and in patients with pre-existing chronic liver disease (WHO 2000a; Thimme et al. 2005). HAV infection may lead to the development of ALF (<1%) from which approximately 50% of patients will recover spontaneously (Taylor et al., 2006). For some, liver transplantation may be the only option. Patients with ALF should be managed in a specialist liver unit where timely assessment of the need for transplantation can be made.

Atypical forms of HAV infection have also been reported. These are *cholestatic hepatitis* and *relapsing hepatitis*. Cholestatic hepatitis is characterised by a prolonged period of jaundice (2–8 months) with pruritis, fatigue, weight loss and loose stools. Relapsing hepatitis typically has a biphasic pattern of jaundice with apparent recovery followed by relapse. Both cholestatic and relapsing patterns of HAV infection are followed by spontaneous recovery (Thimme et al., 2005).

Treatment

Treatment is not usually required in HAV infection. Management involves supportive care, encouraging rest, fluids and good nutrition. As in all acute hepatic illnesses, alcohol should be avoided. A short course of corticosteroids may be helpful in cholestatic HAV. Hospitalisation is uncommon but may be necessary if patients become dehydrated, or in the presence of severe hepatitis (Thimme et al., 2005).

Prevention and health promotion

Effective vaccines are available. Passive protection with anti-HAV immunoglobulins has now largely been replaced by active immunisation. However, immunoglobulins may be given as post-exposure prophylaxis to prevent the development, or reduce the severity, of HAV infection. Vaccination is advised for all high-risk groups.

Travellers to endemic areas are advised to:

- Drink bottled water, and avoid ice not made from bottled water
- Avoid uncooked/unpeeled fruit and vegetables, and know how these foods have been washed and prepared
- Avoid uncooked shellfish

Hepatitis E virus

Epidemiology

Although uncommon in the UK, hepatitis E virus (HEV) is endemic in many developing countries of the world, including parts of Asia, the Middle East, north and west Africa and parts of central America (WHO, 2007a). The majority of HEV infection in endemic areas is found in the 15–34-year age group. It is a water-borne infection, transmitted via the faecal–oral route. In areas of high prevalence, HEV occurs in sporadic outbreaks or as epidemics. The latter is particularly likely after heavy rains, when inadequate sanitation systems are unable to cope with flooding. In developed countries, HEV infection may be associated with travel to endemic areas. However, more recently, sporadic indigenous HEV infection has been identified, often in an older population (Dalton et al., 2007).

HEV is an RNA virus (WHO, 2007a). Unlike other hepatitides, it is thought that liver damage may result from a combination of a cytopathic effect and the immune response (Thimme et al., 2005).

Diagnosis

The diagnosis is usually made by the presence of anti-HEV IgM. Unlike HAV infection, immunity to HEV is not life-long. Antibody titres decline after acute infection, and individuals remain susceptible to re-infection.

Clinical features

The mean incubation period is 40 days and infection is usually asymptomatic. A prodromal phase with fever and malaise can sometimes be identified. The commonest sign is jaundice. Other symptoms include anorexia, arthralgia, abdominal pain, diarrhoea, vomiting and urticaria (Thimme et al., 2005; WHO, 2007a). HEV does not lead to chronic disease. However, a more aggressive pattern of disease may be seen during pregnancy, occasionally causing ALF (Khuroo and Kamili, 2003). HEV infection of patients with chronic liver disease may be associated with significant mortality.

HEV is found in the stools of infected individuals, but unlike HAV infection the risk of person-to-person transmission is low. This is possibly because the amount of virus shed in stools is lower than in HAV, and the period of viral shedding is relatively short (Thimme et al., 2005). Thus, humans are unlikely to be the source of continuing infection, and there is evidence to suggest that animals, particularly pigs, may be reservoirs of virus in both endemic (Shukla et al., 2007) and non-endemic (Dalton et al., 2007) areas.

Treatment

Treatment for HEV is rarely required, and management is aimed at symptom relief. Patients with ALF will require management in specialist liver units.

Prevention and health promotion

A vaccine for HEV infection is not available, though some are being evaluated in clinical trials.

Measures to prevent the spread of infection include the provision of safe drinking water, good personal hygiene and sanitary disposal of waste.

Advice to travellers is similar to that given for the prevention of HAV infection.

Hepatitis B virus

Epidemiology

Hepatitis B is a major public health problem. Worldwide, approximately 350 million people have chronic HBV infection, and 1 million people die each year from cirrhosis, liver failure or hepatocellular carcinoma (HCC) as a consequence (Lavanchy, 2004). Global rates of prevalence vary from less than 1% to as high as 20% (WHO, 2004) (Figure 9.1).

HBV is highly infectious, transmitted by the blood and body fluids of an infected person. In areas of high prevalence, HBV is most commonly passed from mother to baby at the time of birth (vertical transmission). Vertical transmission and transmission between children are responsible for the majority of chronic infection in areas of intermediate prevalence. Infected blood products and contaminated medical equipment are also sources of infection. In parts of the world where infection occurs sporadically, HBV is usually acquired sexually, or as a result of injecting drug use (Hahne et al., 2004; Lavanchy, 2004).

Diagnosis

HBV is a deoxyribonucleic acid (DNA) virus of the hepadnaviridae family. It is comprised of a nucleocapsid core protein known as the hepatitis B core antigen (HBcAg), enclosed by a surface lipoprotein comprising hepatitis B surface antigen (HBsAg). HBsAg is produced in excess and circulates in the blood of an infected individual. Another protein, closely resembling the HBcAg, can also be detected in the blood of some patients with HBV infection. This is called the hepatitis B e

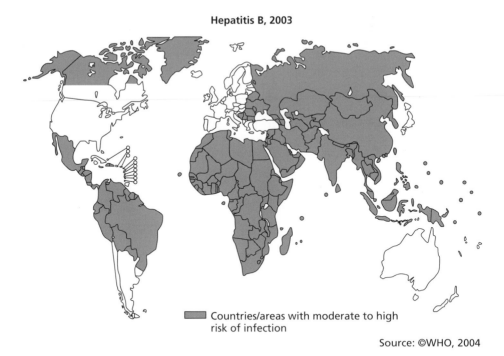

Hepatitis B, 2003

Countries/areas with moderate to high
risk of infection

Source: ©WHO, 2004

Figure 9.1 Geographical prevalence of HBV. Used with permission from International Travel and Health, 2007 with permission from WHO.

antigen (HBeAg). The presence of the HBeAg is associated with high rates of viral replication. The amount of virus is best measured by quantitation of the HBV genome, HBV DNA. The results of this test are typically reported as virus copies per millilitre of blood (copies/mL).

In response to infection, antibodies to each of the antigens are produced (anti-HBs, anti-HBc and anti-HBe). HBsAg, HBeAg and HBV DNA can be detected within 6 weeks of infection. Antibodies to HBcAg (anti-HBc) appear approximately 8 weeks after infection. Table 9.1 illustrates some common serology results with their interpretation.

Clinical features

HBV causes acute or chronic infection. When infection is acquired in adulthood, it is likely to be self-limiting (Lok and McMahon, 2007). In contrast, 90% of those infected at birth will develop chronic HBV infection.

Acute HBV infection

The average incubation period of HBV infection is 75 days (WHO, 2004). Acute HBV infection may be asymptomatic. Symptoms, if present, include jaundice,

Table 9.1 HBV serology results.

Diagnosis	Antigen/antibody	Result
Chronic HBV infection	HBsAg	+
	AntiHBc IgM	−
	Total AntiHBc	+
	AntiHBs	−
Acute HBV infection	HBsAg	+
	AntiHBc IgM	+
	Total AntiHBc	+
	AntiHBs	−
Resolved HBV infection (immune)	HBsAg	−
	AntiHBc	+
	AntiHBs	+/−
Vaccinated (immune)	HBsAg	−
	AntiHBc	−
	AntiHBs	+

pruritis, fatigue, malaise and arthralgia. No specific treatment is required and the majority of adult-acquired infection resolves within 2 months of the onset of jaundice (Thomas, 2007). The disappearance of HBsAg and the appearance of antibodies to HBsAg (anti-HBs) is called HBsAg seroconversion and indicates resolution of infection. The individual is no longer infectious and most cases will have life-long immunity to HBV infection. Fulminant HBV infection is rare (<1%), and these patients will need to be transferred to a specialist liver unit. Transplantation may be indicated (Thimme et al., 2005; Thomas, 2007).

Chronic HBV infection

The persistence of HBsAg for 6 months indicates chronic HBV infection. HBV is not cytopathic. However, the immune response to infected hepatocytes causes inflammation which, over time, can lead to fibrosis and eventually to cirrhosis. Once chronic infection is established, it is rare for individuals to eradicate the virus (Lok and McMahon, 2007).

Most chronic infection is a consequence of infection by HBV at a young age. Under this circumstance, four phases of chronic infection may be observed:

- The immune tolerance phase
- The immune clearance phase
- An inactive carrier state
- Reactivation of replication (Yim and Lok, 2006)

The immune tolerance phase (HBeAg-positive)

Children and young adults most frequently demonstrate the immune tolerance phase of the disease. This phase is characterised by HBeAg positivity with high levels of HBV DNA (usually more than 1 million copies/mL). Serum ALT is often normal, indicating little or no immune response to the virus. The risk of liver damage during this phase is very low.

The immune clearance phase (HBeAg-positive)

During this phase, the immune system mounts a determined attack on infected hepatocytes. This is associated with disappearance from the blood of HBeAg and the appearance of antibodies to HBeAg (anti-HBe). This event is called HBeAg seroconversion and it is associated with reduced viral replication and a dramatic fall in HBV DNA levels (usually to less than 10 000 copies/mL). The process of HBeAg seroconversion is occasionally incomplete, producing bursts of increased inflammatory activity but without a sustained decline in HBV DNA levels. These are known as hepatitis 'flares' and are characterised by peaks in ALT levels. Successful HBeAg seroconversion occurs spontaneously at a rate of around 10% per year and the majority (approximately 90%) of individuals will have seroconverted by the age of 40 years (Chu and Liaw, 2007).

The inactive carrier state (HBeAg-negative)

The reduction in viral titres usually leads to a reduction in inflammatory activity. HBV DNA levels remain low, or undetectable, and ALT may be normal. For some patients, this phase will continue indefinitely. For others reactivation of replication can occur.

Reactivation of viral replication (HBeAg-negative)

HBeAg remains negative but viral replication increases. HBV DNA levels fluctuate, but frequently exceed 100 000 copies/mL. Viral replication is not as high as observed in HBeAg-positive hepatitis (see above), but a rising ALT is evidence of resumed inflammatory activity.

Complications of chronic HBV infection

In both eAg-positive and eAg-negative disease, persistently high levels of HBV DNA and inflammatory activity will result in the development of fibrosis. Many develop cirrhosis (Yim and Lok, 2006). In the cirrhotic patient, the risk for progression to liver failure is 3–5% per annum. HBV infection is also strongly associated with the development of HCC. In cirrhotic patients, HCC incidence is 2–3% per annum, but it can also occur in the absence of cirrhosis. It is estimated that 15–40% of people with HBV infection will develop cirrhosis, liver failure or HCC (Lok and McMahon, 2007). Common risk factors for the development of cirrhosis and HCC include male gender, persistent high levels of viral replication, alcohol consumption and co-infection with HCV, HDV or HIV (Yim and Lok, 2006).

Treatment

Treatment in HBV infection aims to suppress viral replication and to reduce inflammation. Treatment is required, in both HBeAg-positive and HBeAg-negative disease (when the level of virus is high), to prevent fibrosis progression and the development of cirrhosis. In the UK, two groups of drugs are currently licensed for the treatment of HBV infection. These are alfa interferons – interferon alfa-2b, interferon alfa-2a and pegylated interferon alfa-2a (PEG-IFN) – and nucleos(t)ide analogues (NAs) – lamivudine, adefovir, tenofovir and entecavir. Interferons augment the host immune response to HBV infection. NAs interrupt the process of viral replication. There are advantages and disadvantages to consider when deciding which drug to use.

The aim of treatment for patients with HBeAg-positivity is to induce HBeAg seroconversion. Clinical trials have shown that higher rates of HBeAg seroconversion are achieved by PEG-IFN in comparison with lamivudine (Marcellin et al., 2004). However, interferon therapy is expensive, has significant side effects and is probably unacceptable for prolonged treatment. Also, it is unsuitable for use in patients with advanced disease. NAs can be used for a longer duration, and HBeAg seroconversion rates may be improved by prolonged treatment. Patients usually report fewer side effects of NA therapy. However, prolonged NA therapy carries the risk of the development of drug-resistant virus. The rates for development of drug resistance vary quite considerably between the different NAs.

The decision to begin treatment for HBV infection depends upon several factors, including the amount of fibrosis, the degree of inflammatory activity, and also the predicted risk of future liver damage for an individual patient. For example, a 22-year-old HBeAg-positive female may have very high levels of HBV DNA, but she will usually have normal ALT, indicating immune tolerance and no inflammation. At this stage, the likelihood of liver damage is minimal. Also, she may undergo spontaneous HBeAg seroconversion before the development of liver damage. Observation, without treatment, seems appropriate for this type of patient. In contrast, for a 40-year-old HBeAg-positive male, with high levels of HBV DNA and a history of repeated flares of inflammatory activity, treatment is clearly required to suppress viral replication, to reduce inflammation and to prevent progression to cirrhosis. Current opinions are divided on the optimum management of HBV infection and it is not within the scope of this chapter to discuss the different treatment options in more detail. Comprehensive information is available in the guidelines of the American Association for the Study of Liver Diseases (Lok and McMahon, 2007), and in guidance from the National Institute for Health and Clinical Excellence (2006a).

It is important to remember that the course of HBV infection is unpredictable. Viral titres fluctuate, and there are no outward signs of damaging inflammatory activity. Once diagnosed, life-long monitoring will be required.

Prevention and health promotion

Hepatitis B is a preventable disease. Vaccination confers protection of >95% in babies, children and young adults. Three doses are required, and protection lasts for approximately 15 years, and may be life-long (WHO, 2004; Department of Health, 2006). A combination vaccine against HBV and HAV is also available (Department of Health, 2006). Many in the UK argue in favour of universal vaccination against HBV infection. However, current UK recommendations are for vaccination of high-risk groups (Department of Heath, 2006). These are:

- Injecting drug users
- Individuals with multiple sexual partners, particularly commercial sex workers
- Sexual partners of HBV-positive individuals
- Household contacts of HBV individuals
- Families adopting children from countries with high/intermediate prevalence of HBV infection
- Foster carers
- Individuals receiving regular transfusions of blood or blood products
- Patients with chronic liver disease
- Inmates of custodial institutions
- Travellers to areas of high/intermediate prevalence
- Individuals with occupational risk, e.g. health care workers, laboratory staff, staff working in residential homes for people with learning difficulties, prison staff
- Babies born to HBV-positive mothers

The risk of transmission from infected mother to baby is high, but can be prevented by an accelerated course of vaccination. Babies born to mothers with high levels of viral replication will be given, in addition to vaccination, protection with hepatitis B immunoglobulin. Breast-feeding is not contraindicated if the baby receives a full course of vaccination starting at birth (Department of Health, 2004).

The presence of the virus in blood and body fluids means that the risk of sexual transmission is high. Sexual partners should be vaccinated. Injecting drug users with HBV infection should not share injecting equipment. Cleaning with bleach does not guarantee destruction of the virus. Household items that may be contaminated with blood, particularly razors, nail scissors and toothbrushes, should not be shared.

Hepatitis D virus

Epidemiology

The hepatitis D virus (HDV), or delta virus, requires the HBsAg for survival. Therefore, it is only ever seen in patients who also suffer from HBV infection. An estimated 5% of HBV-infected individuals also have HDV infection. This equates to approximately 15 million carriers worldwide (Farci and Lai, 2005).

The prevalence of HDV infection is highest in South America, the South Pacific islands, western Africa, some parts of the Mediterranean, the Middle East and central Asia. In these areas, HDV may be acquired sexually or from close contact with other infected individuals. In northern Europe and North America where the prevalence is low, injecting drug use is the commonest route of transmission (Farci and Lai, 2005).

Diagnosis

HDV infection is confirmed by the presence of HDV RNA and HDV antibodies (anti-HDV). Hepatitis D virus antigen (HDVAg) is present in liver tissue, and can be detected in blood. HDV infection often suppresses replication of HBV DNA to low levels. Thus, the HDV is more responsible than the HBV for ongoing liver damage.

Clinical features

HDV infection can be acquired at the time of HBV infection (co-infection), or on top of existing HBV infection (super-infection). Both co-infection and super-infection can cause acute liver failure. In co-infection, the majority of individuals will have an acute, self-limiting infection. In contrast, most cases of super-infection present as an episode of acute hepatitis progressing to a chronic form of the disease. Like HBV infection, symptoms may include malaise, fatigue, anorexia and abdominal discomfort. However, the infection may be asymptomatic. HDV infection causes a rapidly accelerated progression of disease (Thomas, 2007). Seventy percent of individuals will develop cirrhosis, 15% within 1–2 years of infection. In addition, the risk of decompensated cirrhosis and hepatocellular carcinoma is higher than in HBV infection alone (Farci and Lai, 2005). Debate exists on whether liver damage is caused by a direct cytopathic effect or as a result of the host immune response.

Treatment

Interferon alfa is the only treatment that has been effective in the treatment of HDV infection. PEG-IFN appears to demonstrate more effective HDV RNA inhibition and ALT normalisation than conventional interferon, and also improved long-term outcome and survival (Farci, 2006).

Prevention and health promotion

Vaccination against HBV infection will protect against HDV infection. However, no vaccine is currently available for individuals with HBV infection to protect against super-infection (Farci and Lai, 2005).

Health promotion advice is as for HBV infection.

Hepatitis C virus

HCV infection is a major cause of liver disease, and is the leading indication for liver transplantation worldwide. Identified in 1989, HCV was originally named post-transfusion non-A non-B hepatitis. By the time the virus was identified, millions of people had already been infected, many of whom had advanced stages of liver disease.

Epidemiology

Current estimates suggest that around 180 million people worldwide, or 3% of the world's population, are carriers of HCV infection (WHO, 2000b). The highest disease prevalence is seen in Africa, central and south-eastern Asia and parts of South America (Figure 9.2). In Egypt, the country with the world's highest prevalence, as many as 60% of people in some parts are estimated to have HCV infection.

HCV is an RNA virus of the Flaviviridae family. Genetically, there is great variability in its structure. There are six main types of HCV, known as genotypes. These are identified by number, for example genotype 1, genotype 2, genotype 3

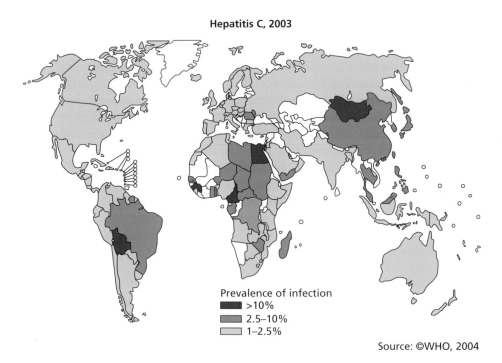

Hepatitis C, 2003

Prevalence of infection
- \>10%
- 2.5–10%
- 1–2.5%

Source: ©WHO, 2004

Figure 9.2   Geographical prevalence of HC virus. Used with permission from International Travel and Health, 2007 with permission from WHO.

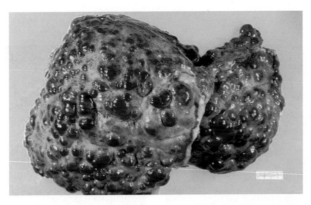

Plate 1 Photograph showing extensive liver cirrhosis. Used with permission from Bernard Portmann.

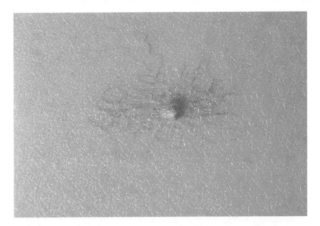

Plate 2 A spider naevus. The central arteriole resembles a spider's body and the radiating vessels the spider's legs. Reprinted with permission from eMedicine.com, 2007. Available at: http://www.emedicine.com/derm.topic293.htm.

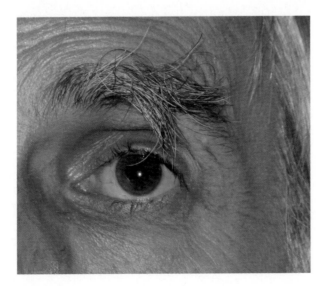

Plate 3 The jaundiced patient.

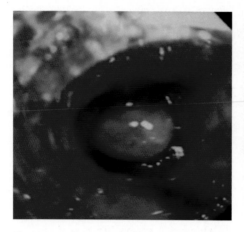

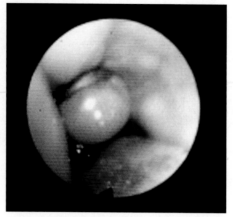

Plate 4 Endoscopic view of an oesophageal varix.

Plate 5 Band ligation on an oesophageal varix. Reproduced with permission from Krige JE, Beckingham IJ (2001) ABC of diseases of liver, pancreas, and biliary system. Portal hypertension – 1: varices. *British Medical Journal* **322**:348–351.

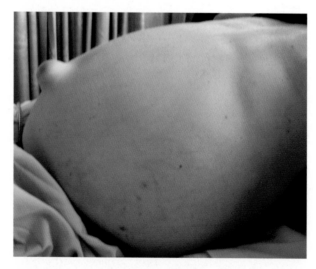

Plate 6 Patient with tense ascites with an umbilical hernia.

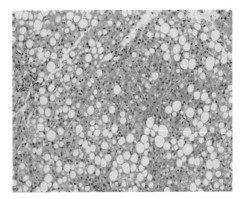

Macrovesicular steatosis.

Plate 7   Macrovesicular steatosis.

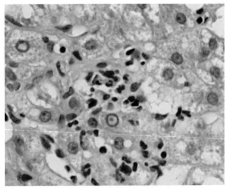

Lobular inflammation
(acute or chronic).

Plate 8   Lobular inflammation.

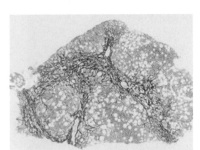

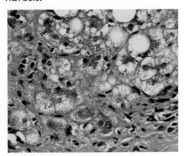

Pericellular fibrosis.

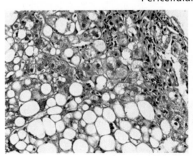

Plate 9   Pericellular fibrosis.

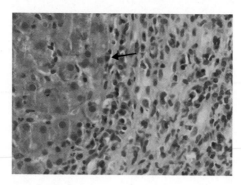

Plate 10 Photomicrograph of a liver biopsy specimen from a patient with autoimmune hepatitis, showing interface hepatitis with plasma cell infiltrate (arrowed). Photomicrograph provided by Dr Alberto Quaglia.

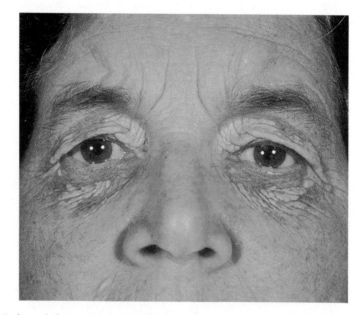

Plate 11 Both xanthelasma and pigmentation in a patient with primary biliary cirrhosis. Reproduced with permission from Sherlock S, Dooley J (2002) *Diseases of the Liver and Biliary System*, 11th edn. Blackwell Publishing.

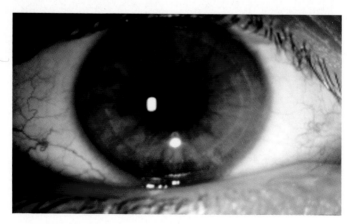

Plate 12 Kayser-Fleischer ring in a patient with Wilson's disease. Reproduced with permission from Ryder SD, Beckingham IJ (2001) ABC of diseases of liver, pancreas, and biliary system: Other causes of parenchymal liver disease. *British Medical Journal* **322**:290–292.

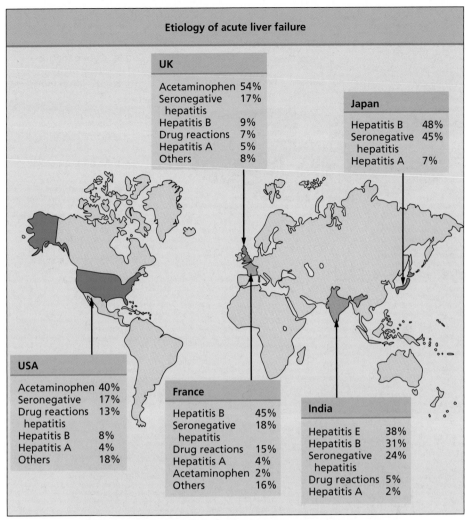

Etiology of acute liver failure

UK

Acetaminophen	54%
Seronegative hepatitis	17%
Hepatitis B	9%
Drug reactions	7%
Hepatitis A	5%
Others	8%

Japan

Hepatitis B	48%
Seronegative hepatitis	45%
Hepatitis A	7%

USA

Acetaminophen	40%
Seronegative	17%
Drug reactions hepatitis	13%
Hepatitis B	8%
Hepatitis A	4%
Others	18%

France

Hepatitis B	45%
Seronegative hepatitis	18%
Drug reactions	15%
Hepatitis A	4%
Acetaminophen	2%
Others	16%

India

Hepatitis E	38%
Hepatitis B	31%
Seronegative hepatitis	24%
Drug reactions	5%
Hepatitis A	2%

Plate 13 Worldwide aetiology of acute liver failure. Reproduced from Bacon et al. (2006) with permission from Elsevier.

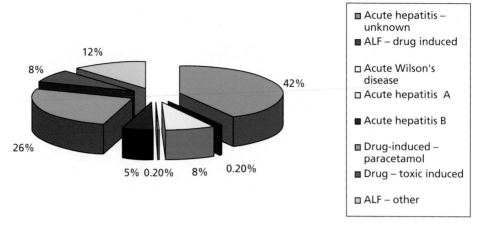

Legend:
- Acute hepatitis – unknown
- ALF – drug induced
- Acute Wilson's disease
- Acute hepatitis A
- Acute hepatitis B
- Drug-induced – paracetamol
- Drug – toxic induced
- ALF – other

12%
8%
42%
26%
5% 0.20% 8% 0.20%

Plate 14 UK aetiologies for ALF transplants 2001–2006 (UK Transplant, 2006).

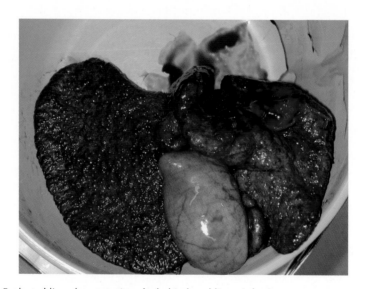

Plate 15 Explanted liver demonstrating alcohol-induced liver cirrhosis.

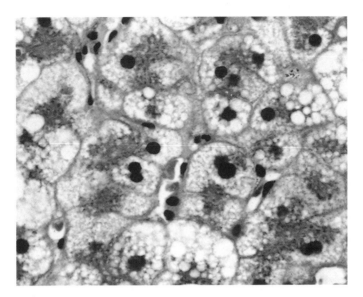

Plate 16 Liver biopsy demonstrating changes in acute fatty liver of pregnancy. Reproduced with permission from Sherlock S, Dooley J (2002) *Diseases of the Liver and Biliary System*, 11th edn, Blackwell Publishing.

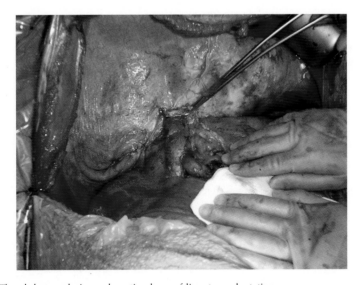

Plate 17 The abdomen during anhepatic phase of liver transplantation.

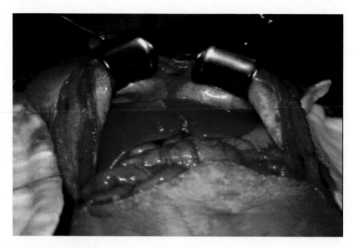

Plate 18 Abdomen following transplant with new liver in situ.

etc. Each genotype has further subtypes, of which there are over 100 in total: genotype 1a, genotype 3b etc (Forns and Sanchez-Tapias, 2005). Genotype does not determine the severity of disease, but some genotypes respond better to treatment than others.

HCV is a blood-borne infection. Globally, modes of transmission vary. In the developed world, the most common route of HCV transmission is injecting drug use. In England, the Health Protection Agency identified injecting drug use as the risk factor for HCV infection in 92% of reported infections between 1996 and 2005. Although the prevalence of HCV infection in the UK is low, the prevalence amongst the current injecting drug user population is estimated to be around 45% (HPA, 2006). Another risk factor is a history of receiving transfused blood, or blood products, before the introduction of screening for HCV infection. One group of individuals particularly affected by transfusion-associated infection are those with haemophilia and related clotting disorders, many of whom acquired HCV (and other blood-borne infections) from infected clotting factor concentrates. Transmission of HCV from infected mother to newborn is uncommon, but the risk increases when the mother has high levels of the virus, and if the mother also has HIV co-infection. Tattooing, acupuncture and body piercing using non-sterile equipment are also known to have transmitted the infection. Unlike HBV infection, the risk of sexual transmission, particularly in monogamous relationships, is low. However, multiple sexual partners, aggressive sexual activity and HIV co-infection are known to increase this risk (Terrault, 2002).

In the developing world, the spread of infection is more likely to be the result of unhygienic health care practices (Shepard et al., 2005). This includes the use of unscreened blood donations, and injections or other clinical procedures involving contaminated unsterilised medical equipment.

Diagnosis

Serological tests for HCV infection are more straightforward than those for HBV. Two tests are necessary. The first test looks for the presence of the antibody to HCV infection, commonly expressed as anti-HCV. The second test looks for the virus itself, or the HCV RNA. Most often, the virus RNA is detected and measured by a laboratory method called the polymerase chain reaction (PCR). Thus, infected patients are often called 'PCR-positive'. Antibodies to HCV will be detectable in the blood of any individual who has ever been in contact with the HCV virus. The presence of HCV RNA confirms that the individual is still infected. In individuals who clear the virus, HCV RNA will not be detectable, but anti-HCV will remain. Anti-HCV antibodies do not protect against re-infection, either with the same or a different genotype. The persistence of detectable HCV RNA after 6 months indicates the transition from acute to chronic HCV infection. Spontaneous subsequent clearance of the virus is unlikely.

Other serological investigations include HCV genotype and HCV viral titre. These tests are important when treatment is being considered.

Clinical features

Acute infection is most often asymptomatic. If present, symptoms are usually non-specific and the majority of individuals will not develop jaundice (Dusheiko, 2007). Indeed, it is not uncommon for the infection to remain undetected until the chronic phase of infection when abnormal liver function tests are found incidentally, or until features of advanced liver disease develop. HCV rarely causes acute liver failure.

The incubation period for HCV infection is 15–150 days (WHO, 2000b). Only a minority of infected individuals will clear the virus, with approximately 85% becoming chronic carriers of the disease (Shiffman, 2003).

A prolonged period of chronic infection may remain unsuspected and un-detected. Liver inflammation causes fibrosis leading to cirrhosis. Liver biopsy is the gold standard investigation for evaluating the extent of liver damage caused by HCV. It measures both inflammation and fibrosis stage (Ishak et al., 1995). The rate at which cirrhosis will develop is difficult to predict. In a large cross-sectional study of patients with HCV infection, the median time from infection to cirrhosis was 30 years (Poynard et al., 1997). However, for some individuals, fibrosis pro-gresses at a much faster rate, while others never develop advanced liver disease. Despite the variable disease trajectory, several factors are known to accelerate the rate of fibrosis progression. These factors are male gender, excessive alcohol intake, acquiring the virus at an older age (Poynard et al., 1997) and co-infection with HIV (Poynard et al., 2003).

When cirrhosis is complicated by the development of a liver cancer (1.4% per year), or liver failure (3.9% per year) (Fattovich et al., 1997), transplantation can be a life-saving option.

Treatment

Current treatment for chronic HCV infection uses a combination of PEG-IFN, given by weekly subcutaneous injection, and twice daily oral ribavirin. Treatment has been approved by the National Institute for Health and Clinical Excellence (NICE, 2004/2006b). Patients with genotypes 2 and 3 infection require 6 months of therapy. Twelve months of treatment is given for the more difficult to treat genotypes 1, 4, 5 or 6. Successful treatment is associated with serum HCV RNA negativity during treatment and for at least 6 months after treatment. If the virus remains undetectable for at least 6 months post-treatment, this is referred to as a sustained virological response (SVR). SVR indicates that the patient is cured of HCV infection. The published trials of PEG-IFN and ribavirin reported SVR rates of 42–52% for genotype 1 infection, and 77–88% for genotypes 2/3 infection (Manns et al., 2001; Fried et al., 2002).

HCV treatment is demanding, many patients will experience significant side effects (Table 9.2), and some will fail to complete the planned duration of therapy

Table 9.2 Side effects of HCV treatment (Fried, 2002).

Flu-like symptoms
Fatigue
Depression
Poor concentration
Anorexia and weight loss
Hair loss
Skin rashes
Neutropenia
Anaemia
Thrombocytopenia
Diabetes
Thyroid dysfunction

(Fried, 2002). Selecting the optimum time for treatment and taking an individual patient's circumstances into account make adherence with treatment more likely. Adherence is a key determinant of treatment success. When contemplating antiviral treatment for HCV, important factors to consider include the severity of liver disease, social circumstances, physical and psychological health, and the patient's readiness to undergo a 6- or 12-month course of treatment. Pre-treatment counselling must include information on the risks and benefits of antiviral therapy, possible side effects and their management and likely response rates. A psychological assessment may also be helpful. During treatment, close monitoring and support are required. Most patients attend clinic each week initially, and then at least monthly.

The optimum time for treatment is before extensive liver damage has occurred. At this stage, the chance of achieving a SVR is highest.

Very good response rates have been reported in patients with acute HCV infection. Acute HCV requires treatment with PEG-IFN monotherapy for 24 weeks, regardless of genotype (Santantonio et al., 2005).

As a result of the silent nature of HCV, many patients present with chronic hepatitis, and some with established cirrhosis. For cirrhotic patients with good synthetic function, viral eradication can reduce the risk of hepatic decompensation which is a compelling incentive for treatment. However, treatment after cirrhosis has developed is difficult and often poorly tolerated. Dose reductions are common and response rates are lower than in the non-cirrhotic population. Anaemia and thrombocytopenia are usually more profound, and with little hepatic reserve, there is a high risk of hepatic decompensation. Antiviral treatment is contraindicated in decompensated cirrhosis.

Extrahepatic manifestations of HCV infection

Several diseases have been associated with HCV infection, including:

- Cryoglobulinaemia
- Membranoproliferative glomerulonephritis
- Diabetes mellitus
- Lichen planus
- Sjögren's syndrome
- Non-Hodgkins lymphoma

Living with HCV infection

Many patients with HCV report symptoms such as fatigue, poor concentration, poor memory and depression. Certainly there is evidence that patients with HCV infection experience worse health-related quality of life (HRQoL) than the general population (von Wagner and Lee, 2006). This may be proportional to the severity of liver disease (Bonkovsky et al., 2007). Other factors leading to poor HRQoL have also been proposed including non-specific HCV-associated symptoms, living with a chronic health problem, the stigma of infectious disease, the risk to future health, uncertainty of response to treatment and the side effects of antiviral treatment (Heitkemper et al., 2001). Some studies report poor HRQoL in HCV-positive patients who are unaware of their diagnosis, or who believe that they have been cured of infection. This implies that the disease process itself, and not simply the psychological reaction to it, may be responsible for poor quality of life (Rodger et al., 1999; Bonkovsky et al., 2007). The impact of pre-morbid conditions, such as substance misuse and its known association with mental health problems, must also be considered. Finally, there is a growing evidence for direct HCV effects in extrahepatic sites, including the presence of the infection in the central nervous system (Laskus et al., 2005). This finding raises the possibility of poor HRQoL resulting from direct neurotoxicity. Defining the contributory factors to HRQoL in HCV infection remains an important topic for future investigation.

Prevention and health promotion

There is no vaccine available to protect against HCV infection. Health promotion initiatives focus on identifying and treating infected individuals, and preventing further spread of the disease.

Harm-reduction strategies are required for high-risk populations such as injecting drug users. This should include the provision of needle exchange programmes and information on safe injecting practices. HCV infection is not transmitted on household items, such as cutlery and crockery, where there is no blood-to-blood contact. However, items that may be contaminated with blood, particularly razors, nail scissors and toothbrushes, should not be shared.

Minimal alcohol consumption should be encouraged. Many patients abstain from alcohol after the diagnosis of HCV infection has been made, an attitude which should be supported. Dietary restrictions are not required and patients should be encouraged to eat a well balanced and nutritious diet.

The risk of sexual transmission is low but not zero. HCV, at low levels, has been found in body fluids other than blood, including genital secretions. In patients with HIV co-infection or who have other sexually transmitted diseases, the risk of HCV transmission is higher. In monogamous relationships, couples should be reassured. The sexual partner of the HCV-positive patient may wish to undergo testing for HCV. Most long-term monogamous couples choose not to change their sexual practices, including the use (or not) of contraception. That approach seems sensible. Barrier methods of contraception should be recommended for individuals with multiple sexual partners and/or those who participate in high-risk sexual activities (Terrault, 2002).

The risk of transmission of infection from HCV-infected mother to newborn is low, particularly in women with low levels of the virus. Breast-feeding is not thought to transmit infection as long there is no bleeding from the nipples, and the skin is not cracked. HIV co-infection increases the risk of mother-to-baby transmission (Roberts and Yeung, 2002).

Hepatitis and HIV co-infection

Epidemiology

HIV is a major cause of morbidity and mortality worldwide, affecting approximately 40 million individuals. The development of highly active anti-retroviral therapy (HAART) has improved the outcome of HIV infection significantly (Palella et al., 1998). However, where access to HAART is limited, progression to acquired immune deficiency syndrome (AIDS) remains an inevitable outcome (Joint United Nations Programme on HIV/AIDS (UNAIDS) and World Health Organisation, 2006). As a blood-borne virus, HIV shares common routes of transmission with HBV and HCV infection, and co-infection is common. An estimated 2–4 million HIV-positive individuals have HIV/HBV infection, and 4–5 million are co-infected with HCV (Alter, 2006). Individuals with the highest risk of HIV/HCV co-infection are injecting drug users and recipients of blood and blood products. Co-infection also increases the risk of perinatal (Alter, 2006) and sexual (Nelson et al., 2003) transmission of HCV.

HIV/HBV co-infection is usually a consequence of sexual transmission or due to injecting drug use (Alter, 2006). In the pre-HAART era, death in patients with HIV/hepatitis co-infection was frequently the result of an AIDS-related illness, and unrelated to the development of liver disease. However, HAART prevents the progression to AIDS. Thus, HIV/hepatitis co-infected patients may be expected to live long enough to develop cirrhosis and its complications.

Clinical features

Patients with HBV/HIV and HCV/HIV co-infection are at risk of developing more severe liver disease compared to those with mono-infection. This is principally because HIV alters the ability of the immune system to modulate HBV or HCV viral replication. Consequently, co-infection is characterised by high viral titres, a more rapid progression to cirrhosis and an increased risk of decompensated liver disease. The rate of development of liver damage is inversely correlated with the degree of immune suppression (as reflected by the CD4 count) (Graham et al., 2001). In addition, the risk of HAART-associated drug hepatotoxicity appears higher in patients with co-existent hepatitis infection.

The immunosuppression associated with HIV infection can prevent anti-HCV antibody production. Thus, false-negative tests for anti-HCV can be seen, and can confound the diagnostic process. Therefore, HIV-positive patients with risk factors for HCV and/or abnormal liver function tests should be tested for HCV RNA (even if the anti-HCV test is negative).

Treatment

HCV and HIV

In HCV/HIV co-infection, antiviral treatment presents unique challenges. Combination treatment with PEG-IFN and ribavirin for 12 months is recommended for all HCV genotypes. Published studies have reported lower response rates than observed for treatment of mono-infection, particularly in genotype 1 infection. Some studies also report higher treatment discontinuation rates. HIV drug interactions with ribavirin are possible, and didanosine (ddI), in particular, should be avoided if possible (Nelson et al., 2003).

Despite the challenges, eradication of HCV infection will prevent significant liver disease and should be considered for all HIV/HCV co-infected patients. Treatment is more effective and better tolerated before the development of advanced liver disease, and with well controlled HIV infection. The CD4 count is used as a guide to immune competence and it has been suggested that a level of at least 200×10^9 cells/L is required for successful HCV treatment. HCV treatment in patients with lower CD4 counts will be less effective and HAART therapy should take priority (Nelson et al., 2003).

HBV and HIV

Some antiviral treatments, for example lamivudine and tenofovir, are active against both HIV and HBV infection. This dual action makes them very useful in the co-infection setting. However, because of the high risk of HIV drug resistance, special consideration should be given to the stage of each disease, and the likely future requirement for treatment. When treatment is indicated for HBV alone, the guiding principle is to avoid drugs with anti-HIV activity.

Strategies for the treatment of HBV/HIV and HCV/HIV co-infection are evolving as new antiviral therapies emerge. Management of this complex group of patients requires expertise in the management of both HIV and hepatitis infections.

Chapter summary

Viral hepatitis is a major cause of morbidity and mortality worldwide, producing both acute and chronic illness. This chapter has examined the epidemiology, diagnosis, clinical features and treatment of viral hepatitis, in addition to health promotion advice and important measures to prevent the spread of infection.

By far the greatest burden of disease is caused by chronic viral hepatitis, and specifically hepatitis B virus (HBV) and hepatitis C virus (HCV) infection. HBV infection is a major public health problem. Worldwide, 1 million people die each year from cirrhosis, liver failure or HCC as a consequence of the disease. HCV infection is a major cause of liver disease, and is the leading indication for liver transplantation worldwide. As a blood-borne virus, HIV shares common routes of transmission with HBV and HCV infection, and co-infection is common, therefore consideration of the impact of HBV/HIV and HCV/HIV co-infection has additionally been explored.

Illustrative case study

Mr X is a 51-year-old accountant. He has not donated blood for many years, but attends a session organised at the company where he works. He later receives a letter from the Blood Transfusion Service to inform him that he may have HCV infection, and asking him to attend his GP. His GP informs him that he has HCV infection and refers him to a hepatologist for further management. He is fit and well with no significant past medical history. He is a non-smoker and drinks an occasional glass of wine at the weekend. Blood tests reveal abnormal liver function tests. His ALT is 83 U/L and his AST is 69 U/L. Bilirubin and ALP levels are within normal limits. Mr X admits that he injected drugs, on only a couple of occasions, at university many years previously.

Mr X is devastated by the diagnosis. His main concern is that he could have passed the virus on to his wife and three children. He is reassured that this is unlikely, but is advised that the family could be tested by the GP. Further investigations confirm genotype 1 infection. A liver biopsy shows fibrosis with minimal inflammation. Twelve months' treatment is planned. Mr X defers treatment for 9 months because he does not want to start until his 16-year-old son has completed his school exams. PEG-IFN and ribavirin are prescribed. Mr X completes the full course of treatment with acceptable side effects. His main problems are flu-like symptoms on the day of injection, tiredness, dry itchy skin and, during the final 2 months of treatment, some shortness of breath on exertion. His haemoglobin level falls from pretreatment 15.2 g/L to 11.3 g/L at conclusion of treatment. Mr X continues full-time employment during his treatment. At the end of treatment, his HCV titre is below the level of detection (PCR-negative). Six months after the end of treatment, the virus is still undetectable, confirming that his HCV infection is cured (he has had a SVR). His liver function is normal, and 2 years after the end of treatment, he is discharged from the hepatologist's care.

References

Alter MJ (2006) Epidemiology of viral hepatitis and HIV co-infection. *Journal of Hepatology* **44**(Suppl 1):S6–S9

Bonkovsky HL, Snow KK, Malet PF, Back-Madruga C, Fontana RJ, Sterling RK, Kulig CC, Di Bisceglie AM, Morgan TR, Dienstag JL, Ghany MG, Gretch DR, HALT-C Trial Group (2007) Health-related quality of life in patients with chronic hepatitis C and advanced fibrosis. *Journal of Hepatology* **46**:420–431

Chu C-M, Liaw Y-F (2007) Chronic hepatitis B virus infection acquired in childhood: special emphasis on prognostic and therapeutic implication of delayed HBeAg seroconversion. *Journal of Viral Hepatitis* **14**:147–152

Dalton HR, Thurairajah PH, Fellows HJ, Hussaini HS, Mitchell J, Bendall R, Banks M, Ijaz S, Teo CG, Levine DF (2007) Autochthonous hepatitis E in southwest England. *Journal of Viral Hepatitis* **14**:304–309

Department of Health (2004) Children in need and blood-borne viruses: HIV and hepatitis. http://www.dh.gov.uk/en/Publicationsandstatistics/Publications/PublicationsPolicyAndGuidance/DH_4093509 (accessed March 2007)

Department of Health (2006) Immunisation against infectious disease – 'The Green Book'. http://www.dh.gov.uk/en/Policyandguidance/Healthandsocialcaretopics/Greenbook/DH_4097254 (accessed March 2007)

Dusheiko G (2007) Hepatitis C. *Medicine* **35**(1):43–48

Farci P (2006) Treatment of chronic hepatitis D: new advances, old challenges. *Hepatology* **44**(3):536–539

Farci P, Lai ME (2005) Chronic viral hepatitis D. In: Weinstein WM, Hawkey CJ, Bosch J (eds) *Clinical Gastroenterology and Hepatology*. Elsevier Mosby, Philadelphia, pp. 609–612

Fattovich G, Giustina G, Degos F, Tremolada F, Diodati G, Almasio P, Nevens F, Solinas A, Mura D, Brouwer JT, Thomas H, Njapoum C, Casarin C, Bonetti P, Fuschi P, Basho J, Tocco A, Bhalla A, Galassini R, Noventa F, Schalm SW, Realdi G (1997) Morbidity and mortality in compensated cirrhosis type C: a retrospective follow-up study of 384 patients. *Gastroenterology* **112**(2):463–472

Forns X, Sanchez-Tapias JM (2005) Chronic viral hepatitis C. In: Weinstein WM, Hawkey CJ, Bosch J (eds) *Clinical Gastroenterology and Hepatology*. Elsevier Mosby, Philadelphia, pp. 601–607

Fried MW (2002) Side effects of therapy of hepatitis C and their management. *Hepatology* **36**(5 Suppl. 1):S237–S244

Fried MW, Shiffman ML, Reddy KR, Smith C, Marinos G, Gonçales FL Jr, Häussinger D, Diago M, Carosi G, Dhumeaux D, Craxi A, Lin A, Hoffman J,

Yu J (2002) Peginterferon alfa-2a plus ribavirin for chronic hepatitis C virus infection. *New England Journal of Medicine* 347:975–982

Graham CS, Baden LR, Yu E, Mrus JM, Carnie J, Heeren T, Koziel MJ (2001) Influence of human immunodeficiency virus infection on the course of hepatitis C infection: a meta-analysis. *Clinical Infectious Diseases* 33:562–569

Hahne S, Ramsay M, Balogun K, Edmunds WJ, Mortimer P (2004) Incidence and transmission of hepatitis B virus in England and Wales, 1995–2000: implications for immunisation policy. *Journal of Clinical Virology* 29:211–220

Health Protection Agency (2006) *Hepatitis C in England: an update 2006*. Health Protection Agency Centre for Infections, London

Heitkemper M, Jarrett M, Kurashige EM, Carithers R (2001) Chronic hepatitis C: implications for health-related quality of life. *Gastroenterology Nursing* 24(4):169–175

Ishak K, Baptista A, Bianchi L, Callea F, De Groote J, Gudat F, Denk H, Desmet V, Korb G, MacSween RN, et al. (1995) Histological grading and staging of chronic hepatitis. *Journal of Hepatology* 22:696–699

Joint United Nations Programme on HIV/AIDS (UNAIDS) and World Health Organisation (WHO). Aids epidemic update 2006. http://www.unaids.org/en/HIV_data/epi2006/default.asp (accessed May 2007)

Khuroo MS, Kamili S (2003) Aetiology, clinical course and outcome of sporadic acute viral hepatitis in pregnancy. *Journal of Viral Hepatitis* 10:61–69

Laskus T, Radkowski M, Adair DM, Wilkinson J, Scheck AC, Rakela J (2005) Emerging evidence of hepatitis C neuroinvasion. *AIDS* 19(Suppl. 3): S140–S144

Lavanchy D (2004) Hepatitis B virus epidemiology, disease burden, treatment, and current and emerging prevention and control measures. *Journal of Viral Hepatitis* 11:97–107

Lok AS-F, McMahon BJ (2007) Chronic hepatitis B. *Hepatology* 45(2):507–539

Manns MP, McHutchison JG, Gordon SC, Rustgi VK, Shiffman M, Reindollar R, Goodman ZD, Koury K, Ling M, Albrecht JK (2001) Peginterferon alfa-2b plus ribavirin compared with interferon alfa-2b plus ribavirin for initial treatment of chronic hepatitis C: a randomised trial. *The Lancet* 358:958–965

Marcellin P, Lau GK, Bonino F, Farci P, Hadziyannis S, Jin R, Lu ZM, Piratvisuth T, Germanidis G, Yurdaydin C, Diago M, Gurel S, Lai MY, Button P, Pluck N; Peginterferon Alfa-2a HBeAg-Negative Chronic Hepatitis B Study Group (2004) Peginterferon alfa-2a alone, lamivudine alone, and the two in combination in patients with HBeAg-negative chronic hepatitis B. *New England Journal of Medicine* 351(12):1206–217

Naomov NV (2007) Hepatitis A and E. *Medicine* 35(1):35–38

National Institute for Clinical Excellence (2004) Interferon alfa (pegylated and non-pegylated) and ribavirin for the treatment of chronic hepatitis C. http://www.nice.org.uk/TA075guidance (accessed February 2007)

National Institute for Health and Clinical Excellence (2006a) Adefovir Dipivoxil and peginterferon alfa-2a for the treatment of chronic hepatitis B. http://guidance.nice.org.uk/TA96 (accessed February 2007)

National Institute for Health and Clinical Excellence (2006b) Peginterferon alfa and ribavirin for the treatment of mild chronic hepatitis C. http://guidance.nice.org.uk/TA106 (accessed February 2007)

Nelson MR, Matthews G, Brook MG, Main J (2003) BHIVA guidelines: coinfection with HIV and chronic hepatitis C virus. *HIV Medicine* 4:52–62

Palella FJ Jr, Delaney KM, Moorman AC, Loveless MO, Fuhrer J, Satten GA, Aschman DJ, Holmberg SD (1998) Declining morbidity and mortality among patients with advanced human immunodeficiency virus infection. *New England Journal of Medicine* 338(13):853–860

Poynard T, Bedossa P, Opolon P (1997) Natural history of liver fibrosis progression in patients with chronic hepatitis C. *The Lancet* 349:825–832

Poynard T, Mathurin P, Lai CL, Guyader D, Poupon R, Tainturier MH, Myers RP, Muntenau M, Ratziu V, Manns M, Vogel A, Capron F, Chedid A, Bedossa P; PANFIBROSIS Group. (2003) A comparison of fibrosis progression in chronic liver diseases. *Journal of Hepatology* 38:257–265

Roberts EA, Yeung L (2002) Maternal-infant transmission of hepatitis C virus infection. *Hepatology* 36(5 Suppl 1):S106–S113

Rodger AJ, Jolley D, Thompson SC, Lanigan A, Crofts N (1999) The impact of diagnosis of hepatitis C virus on quality of life. *Hepatology* 30:1299–1301

Santantonio T, Fasano M, Sinisi E, Guastadisegni A, Casalino C, Mazzola M, Francavilla R, Pastore G (2005) Efficacy of a 24-week course of PEG-interferon alfa-2b monotherapy in patients with acute hepatitis C after failure of spontaneous clearance. *Journal of Hepatology* 42:329–333

Shepard CW, Finelli L, Alter MJ (2005) Global epidemiology of hepatitis C virus infection. *The Lancet Infectious Diseases* 5:558–567

Shiffman ML (2003) Natural history and risk factors for progression of hepatitis C virus disease and development of hepatocellular cancer before liver transplantation. *Liver Transplantation* 9(11 Suppl 3):S14–S20

Shukla P, Chauhan UK, Naik S, Anderson D, Aggarwal R (2007) Heptitis E infection among animals in northern India: an unlikely source of human disease. *Journal of Viral Hepatitis* 14:310–317

Taylor RM, Davern T, Munoz S, Han SH, McGuire B, Larson AM, Hynan L, Lee WM, Fontana RJ; US Acute Liver Failure Study Group (2006) Fulminant hepatitis A virus infection in the United States: incidence, prognosis and outcomes. *Hepatology* 44(6):1589–1597

Terrault NA (2002) Sexual activity as a risk factor for hepatitis C. *Hepatology* 36(5 Suppl 1):S99–S105

Thimme R, Spangenburg HC, Blum HE (2005) Acute viral hepatitis. In: Weinstein WM, Hawkey CJ, Bosch J (eds) *Clinical Gastroenterology and Hepatology.* Elsevier Mosby, Philadelphia, pp. 583–593

Thomas HC (2007) Hepatitis B and D. *Medicine* 35(1):39–42

von Wagner M, Lee J-H (2006) Impaired health-related quality of life in patients with chronic hepatitis C and persistently normal aminotransferase levels. *Journal of Viral Hepatitis* 13(12):828–834

World Health Organisation (2000a) Hepatitis A. http://www.who.int/csr/disease/hepatitis/HepatitisA_whocdscsredc2000_7.pdf (accessed May 2007)

World Health Organisation (2000b) Hepatitis C. http://www.who.int/mediacentre/factsheets/fs164/en/index.html (accessed March 2007)

World Health Organisation (2004) Position paper on hepatitis B. http://www.who.int/immunization/wer7928HepB_July04_position_paper.pdf (accessed March 2007)

World Health Organisation (2007a) Hepatitis E. http://www.who.int/vaccine_research/diseases/zoonotic/en/index2.html (accessed May 2007)

World Health Organisation (2007b) International Travel and Health. http://www.who.int/ith/en/ (accessed June 2007)

Yim HJ, Lok AS-F (2006) Natural history of chronic hepatitis B infection: what we knew in 1981 and what we know in 2005. *Hepatology* **43**(2 Suppl 1):S173–S181

10

Autoimmune hepatitis

Sarah Hughes and Michael Heneghan

Introduction

Autoimmune hepatitis (AIH) is a progressive condition of unknown aetiology resulting in unresolving hepatocellular inflammation. It can occur in both children and adults, and, as with most autoimmune conditions, is more common in women than in men. The diagnosis of AIH is based on recognised clinical and laboratory abnormalities, with abnormal levels of serum immunoglobulins and the presence of circulating autoantibodies, in conjunction with typical histological features. The natural history of the disease is characterised by fluctuating activity. The majority of cases which require treatment respond well. If left untreated, however, severe cases incur a high mortality. Ongoing liver injury can ultimately lead to the development of cirrhosis, and, with it, the complications of chronic liver disease.

Historical perspective

In 1950, Jan Waldenstrom described a distinct group of young women with raised gamma globulins and liver disease of silent onset to the German Society for Digestive and Metabolic Disorders. In the same year, a physician from New York, Kunkel, reported on a group of patients with similar features. It was recognised that these patients had a complex clinical syndrome including joint pain, acne, hirsutism, skin rashes, Cushingoid facies and absence of normal menstruation. In

1956 Ian Mackay, an Australian rheumatologist, coined the term lupoid hepatitis, and subsequently, the presence of anti-nuclear antibodies in serum was recognised as a determining feature of the condition (Reuben, 2003). Although years of research have expanded our knowledge of the pathogenesis, natural history, diagnostic criteria, complications and treatment of the condition, much remains poorly defined. After the application of many different labels, the term autoimmune hepatitis was accepted in 1992 by a panel of experts (Johnson and McFarlane, 1993).

Pathogenesis

It has been proposed that AIH occurs as a result of an environmental trigger in a genetically susceptible individual. This results in activation of the immune system against the liver, leading to ongoing inflammation and subsequent scar formation.

Potential triggers

Viruses

The environmental trigger causing immune activation in a susceptible individual is not known. Several viruses have been proposed, based on clinical observations and associations. These include measles virus, cytomegalovirus (CMV) and Epstein-Barr virus (EBV) as potential culprits, although the best evidence exists for some of the hepatitis viruses. There are numerous cases of autoimmune hepatitis occurring after acute hepatitis A virus infection and cases of an association between hepatitis C virus (HCV) infection and type-2 AIH have been described. It is difficult to prove that viruses are a trigger, since they may induce changes in the cellular immune system long before the autoimmune disease becomes manifest.

There are two suggested mechanisms by which viruses could trigger autoimmunity. The first is the phenomenon of molecular mimicry, in which there is a structural similarity between parts of the virus (viral epitopes) and components of the liver (liver antigens). This results in the activation of a clone of T-cells that cross-react to the virus, but also to self-liver antigens. The second is that the virus triggers the release of chemicals which activate a population of autoreactive T-cells that interfere with self-antigen processing and presentation.

Drugs

Various drugs have been reported as inducing liver damage which mimics AIH. These include oxyphenacetin, methyldopa, nitrofurantoin, diclofenac, interferon, minocycline and some of the statins. What is not clear is whether these drugs unmask or induce a true AIH or whether they cause a drug-induced hepatitis with autoimmune features.

Genetic susceptibilty

Studies have shown that a family of genes called human leucocyte antigen (HLA) genes, found within the major histocompatibility complex (MHC) on the short arm of chromosome 6, have a dominant role in the genetic predisposition to AIH. HLA molecules present antigens to the immune system. In type 1 AIH, characterised by circulating anti-nuclear antibodies (ANA), smooth muscle antibodies (SMA), anti-actin antibodies, atypical perinuclear anti-neutrophilic cytoplasmic antibody (pANCA), and antibodies to soluble liver and liver pancreas antigens (SLA/LP), there is an association with the HLA DR3 and HLA DR4 serotypes. Eighty to 85% of patients with type 1 AIH have the DR3 and/or DR4 serotype (Czaja et al., 1997).

Genotyping for HLA by PCR techniques shows that the principal susceptibility allele amongst white northern Europeans and Americans is HLA-DRB1*0301 (this correlates with the DR3 serotype) and the second highest frequency allele is HLA-DRB1*0401 (which correlates with the DR4 serotype). Each of these two alleles codes for a six amino acid motif, found in the antigen binding groove of the HLA DR molecule. In South Americans the allele HLA-DRB1*1301 has been found to occur with high frequency amongst those with autoimmune hepatitis, just as HLA-DRB1*0405 does in the Japanese population (where the DR3 association is rare). In children HLA-DRB1*03 and HLA-DRB1*13 are seen to occur with high frequency (Krawitt, 2006).

The importance of genes relates not just to susceptibility. The DR3 serotype has been seen to be associated with more severe forms of AIH, often in girls and young women. DR4 is associated more with adult onset, milder disease, with a better response to steroids and often with more extrahepatic manifestations.

In type 2 AIH, characterised by circulating antibodies against liver/kidney microsome type 1 (LKM-1) and liver cytosol 1 (LC-1), the HLA-DRB1*0701 allele may confer susceptibility, as may DQB1 alleles. Studies suggest that HLA-DR2 may be protective against type 2 AIH (Djilali-Saiah et al., 2004).

Other genetic susceptibility mechanisms, involving immune promoter genes outside the MHC, have also been studied, although their relevance is uncertain.

Clinical features

Presentation

The incidence of AIH is approximately 2 per 100 000 of the population in white northern Europeans. The prevalence is estimated at 17 per 100 000 in the same group, although it may be higher than this, as the condition can go unrecognised in the presence of chronic viral hepatitis which is very common. All ages are affected, particularly with type 1 AIH. Type 2 AIH occurs predominantly in children. Overall women are affected more frequently than men with a ratio of 4:1.

The ratio is higher than this in type 2 AIH, where women are predominantly affected. AIH is a global condition which has been reported in most ethnic groups (Czaja and Freese, 2002).

The mode of presentation of AIH is varied and 40% of patients present acutely. Many of these will have had subclinical disease for some time. A small number of patients have a fulminant (acute liver failure) presentation with the development of hepatic encephalopathy within 8 weeks of presentation. The majority of patients, however, present insidiously, some cases being picked up incidentally in the investigation of a patient with unexpected abnormal liver function tests. AIH may also present during pregnancy and the early postpartum period.

Regarding symptoms at presentation, many patients are asymptomatic and non-specific symptoms, such as lethargy, fatigue, anorexia, nausea, abdominal pain and pruritis, are often reported. Joint pain is a common complaint. Patients may also present with varying degrees of jaundice, which can be profound in severe cases. Less commonly, a patient's first presentation may be with symptoms related to decompensation of chronic liver disease, such as ascites, jaundice, confusion and gastrointestinal bleeding. There may also be symptoms related to the presence of other autoimmune conditions, such as thyroiditis, ulcerative colitis, type 1 diabetes mellitus, rheumatoid arthritis and coeliac disease. A history of these conditions should alert the physician to the possible presence of AIH in the relevant setting (Krawitt, 2006).

The physical examination of the patient will vary from normal to the presence of hepatomegaly, splenomegaly, jaundice and the peripheral stigmata of chronic liver disease, including palmar erythema, Duypuytren's contracture, spider naevi, gynaecomastia and caput medusae.

Laboratory abnormalities

The common laboratory abnormalities seen in autoimmune hepatitis are derangement of the liver function tests, elevation of serum globulins and the presence of significant concentrations of circulating autoantibodies. Liver function tests often show the serum aminotransferases, AST and ALT, to be the predominant abnormality, and these are usually raised more than the serum bilirubin and ALP. There are cases which present with a more cholestatic set of liver function tests, but this is unusual and requires exclusion of extrahepatic biliary obstruction, drug reactions, primary biliary cirrhosis, primary sclerosing cholangitis or a variant auto-immune syndrome in the first instance. There is usually a generalised elevation in serum globulins, but IgG levels are particularly raised, to 1.2–3 times the upper limit of normal.

The common circulating non-organ specific autoantibodies are anti-nuclear antibody (ANA), smooth muscle antibody (SMA) and anti-liver/kidney microsome type 1 (LKM-1). Anti-mitochondrial antibody, the hallmark of another auto-immune liver disease, primary biliary cirrhosis, is rarely, if ever, present. Further autoantibodies, such as anti-actin antibody, soluble liver antigen/liver-pancreas

(SLA/LP) antibodies, anti-neutrophil cytoplasmic antibody (ANCA) and anti-liver cytosol-1 (LC-1), can support a diagnosis of suspected autoimmune hepatitis if the conventional antibodies are negative. Studies have attempted to determine the role of these alternative antibodies in achieving a diagnosis of AIH, and also whether they are associated with particular clinical characteristics, such as response to treatment and prognosis (Czaja and Homburger, 2001).

Classification

A proposed system of classification for AIH is based on autoantibody patterns. This arose because of the observation that the clinical features of the disease and HLA serotypes vary depending on whether ANA and SMA or LKM-1 antibodies are positive. Type-1 AIH is characterised by ANA and SMA at titres equal to or greater than 1:80. Anti-actin antibodies are more specific for type 1 AIH. SLA/LP is actually the most specific antibody for type 1 disease, but is not sensitive, being present in only 10–30% of cases. In fact, SLA/LP-positive autoimmune hepatitis has been proposed as type-3 AIH, but patients have clinical and laboratory abnormalities indistinguishable from those seen in type-1 AIH (Czaja and Manns, 1995).

Type-2 AIH is characterised by anti-LKM-1 positivity. Anti-LC-1 may also be present, and usually occurs with LKM-1. Anti-LKM-1 has been seen to occur in patients with chronic hepatitis C, but its pathogenicity in this situation is debated. Table 10.1 summarises this classification and the differences in clinical features between the two main types of AIH. Based on the lack of distinct aetiological factors for each of the subclassifications, this system has not been endorsed by the

Table 10.1   Classification of autoimmune hepatitis.

Feature	Type 1 autoimmune hepatitis	Type 2 autoimmune hepatitis
Characteristic autoantibodies	ANA SMA Anti-actin antibody Anti-SLA/LP antibodies Atypical p-ANCA	Anti-LKM-1 antibody Anti-LC-1 antibody
Geographic variation	Worldwide	Worldwide; rare in North America
Age at presentation	Any age	Predominantly childhood and young adulthood
Sex of patients	Female in c. 75% of cases	Female in c. 95% of cases
Clinical severity	Broad range	Generally severe
Histopathological features at presentation	Broad range	Generally advanced
Treatment failure	Infrequent	Frequent
Relapse after drug withdrawal	Variable	Common
Need for long-term maintenance	Variable	Approximately 100%

International Autoimmune Hepatitis Group, but is still frequently referred to in clinical practice.

Diagnosis

As AIH is such a heterogeneous condition it can be difficult to achieve a firm diagnosis. The diagnosis requires the presence of characteristic features in conjunction with the exclusion of other conditions, such as Wilson's disease, alpha-1-antitrypsin deficiency, viral hepatitis, genetic haemochromatosis and drug-induced hepatitis. The work-up of a patient with suspected AIH therefore begins with a detailed history, including family, social and drug history. In determining the presence of characteristic features, a liver biopsy is mandatory. Serum aminotransferases and immunoglobulin levels do not correlate with biopsy findings, including cirrhosis. In addition, the non-organ specific autoantibodies seen in AIH can also be present in other liver diseases, hence their presence alone cannot be diagnostic of AIH.

The criteria for the diagnosis of AIH were agreed in 1993 by a group of experts who convened to form the International Autoimmune Hepatitis Group (IAHG). The system divides the diagnosis into definite or probable AIH (Johnson and McFarlane, 1993). Criteria were updated in 1999 (Table 10.2). A scoring system was devised for use with individual patients to ascertain the strength of the

Table 10.2 Descriptive criteria for diagnosis of autoimmune hepatitis.

Features	Definite AIH	Probable AIH
Liver histology	Interface hepatitis. No biliary lesions, granulomas or other prominent changes suggestive of a different aetiology	Same as for definite
Laboratory features	Predominant serum aminotransferase abnormality. Globulin, γ-globulin or IgG concentrations >1.5 × upper normal limit	Predominant serum aminotransferase abnormality Hypergammaglobulinaemia of any degree
Serum autoantibodies	ANA, SMA or anti-LKM-1 antibodies at titres ≥1:80. No AMA	As for definite but at titres ≥1:40, or other autoantibodies
Viral markers	No markers of current infection with hepatitis A, B and C viruses	Same as for definite
Alcohol and drug exposure	Average alcohol consumption <25 g/day. No recent use of hepatotoxic drugs	As for definite but alcohol intake <50 g/day
Genetic liver disease	Normal α-1-antitrypsin phenotype. Normal serum caeruloplasmin, iron and ferritin levels	Partial α-1-antitrypsin deficiency. Non-specific serum copper, caeruloplasmin, iron and/or ferritin abnormalities

diagnosis, giving weight to those factors considered to be more characteristic of AIH, and taking points away for features which might favour an alternative diagnosis. A pretreatment score of greater than 15 indicates a definite diagnosis and 10–15 a probable diagnosis. Post-treatment, a score of greater than 17 indicates a definite diagnosis and 12–17 a probable diagnosis (Table 10.3) (Alvarez et al., 1999).

These diagnostic criteria and scoring system have been criticised for: a) being of limited value in everyday clinical practice; b) containing inaccuracies for the diagnosis in children; and c) being overly complicated and therefore not user-friendly. Attempts to simplify the diagnostic criteria were presented in abstract form in 2005 (Table 10.4). However, this has yet to be adopted in clinical practice (Hennes et al., 2005).

Histology

A diagnosis of definite AIH requires the assessment of liver histology by performing a liver biopsy. The histological features are those of a chronic hepatitis. There are no histological lesions that are absolutely diagnostic of AIH, but certain features are considered to be typical. Characteristic findings include a periportal infiltrate of inflammatory cells often with an abundance of plasma cells. This is also referred to as interface hepatitis (Figure 10.1, Plate 10). In more severe cases this may progress to include a lobular hepatitis. Fibrosis is seen even in mild cases, but becomes extensive in advanced disease and culminates in architectural distortion and nodular regeneration, signifying the development of cirrhosis.

It is also common for patients with classical AIH to have bile duct damage identified histologically and, in one report, 24% of patients with classical AIH had

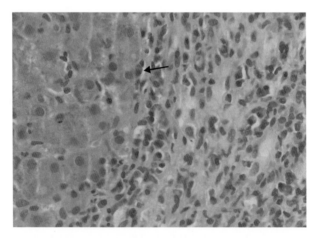

Figure 10.1 Photomicrograph of a liver biopsy specimen from a patient with autoimmune hepatitis, showing interface hepatitis with plasma cell infiltrate (arrowed). Photomicrograph provided by Dr Alberto Quaglia. For a colour version of this figure, please see Plate 10 in the colour plate section.

Table 10.3   Scoring system for diagnosis of autoimmune hepatitis.

Parameters/features	Score
Female sex	+2
ALP:AST (or ALT) ratio:	
<1.5	+2
1.5–3.0	0
>3.0	−2
Serum globulins or IgG above normal:	
>2.0	+3
1.5–2.0	+2
1.0–1.5	+1
<1.0	0
ANA, SMA or LKM-1	
>1:80	+3
1:80	+2
1:40	+1
<1:40	0
AMA positive	−4
Hepatitis viral markers:	
Positive	−3
Negative	+3
Drug history:	
Positive	−4
Negative	+1
Average alcohol intake:	
<25 g/day	+2
>60 g/day	−2
Liver histology:	
Interface hepatitis	+3
Predominantly lymphoplasmacytic infiltrate	+2
Rosetting of liver cells	+1
None of the above	−5
Biliary changes	−3
Atypical features	−3
Other autoimmune disease(s)	+2
Optional additional parameters:	
Seropositivity for other defined antibodies	+2
HLA DR3 or DR4	+1
Response to therapy:	
Remission alone	+2
Remission with relapse	+3
Interpretation of aggregate scores:	
Pre-treatment: Definite AIH	>15
Probable AIH	10–15
Post-treatment: Definite AIH	>17
Probable AIH	12–17

Table 10.4 Simplified diagnostic criteria for autoimmune hepatitis.

Parameter	Level/feature	Score
ANA or SMA	>1:40	1 pt
	>1:80	2 pts
IgG or gammaglobulins	>upper normal limit	1 pt
	>1.156 × upper normal limit	2 pts
Liver histology	Compatible with AIH	1 pt
	Typical AIH	2 pts
Absence of viral hepatitis	No	0 pt
	Yes	2 pts
		≥6 pts: probable AIH
		≥7 pts: definite AIH

bile duct changes on biopsy. These patients were found to have lower diagnostic scores for AIH based on the scoring system described in Table 10.3, but none of the patients had a cholestatic clinical syndrome and the response to corticosteroid treatment was no different compared with those with no bile duct damage. These bile duct changes are not clinically relevant and should not alter management (Czaja and Carpenter, 2001).

The appearance of acute-onset AIH differs from that of insidious-onset disease. There is less fibrosis, due to the acute nature of the illness, but both interface and lobular hepatitis are present, along with often significant hepatic necrosis.

Patients in remission demonstrate histological features of normality or only minor portal inflammation. If cirrhosis was present, this can become histologically inactive and fibrosis may regress or even disappear altogether in rare instances.

Complications

Early reports described mortality in untreated severe disease of 40%, at 6 months post diagnosis. Of those who survive, 40% develop cirrhosis and 54% of these develop oesophageal varices within 2 years of being found to be cirrhotic. Twenty percent of those with oesophageal varices die from variceal haemorrhage. Even in patients with less severe disease, cirrhosis develops in 50% within 15 years, and 10% of these patients die from liver failure (De Groote et al., 1978; Czaja and Freese, 2002). In patients who go on to develop cirrhosis the complications are the same as those associated with chronic liver disease of any aetiology, and include the development of ascites, episodes of hepatic encephalopathy and the presence of portal hypertension resulting in varices and the potential for massive gastro-intestinal haemorrhage. Although less common than in chronic viral hepatitis, primary hepatocellular carcinoma (HCC) is an important complication of AIH. A prospective study showed that based on annual assessment of alpha-fetoprotein and liver ultrasound one patient (0.5%) developed HCC in 1732 patient-years of follow-up and one of 88 patients with cirrhosis (1%) developed HCC in 1002 patient-years of follow-up after being diagnosed cirrhotic (Park et al., 2000). More recent reports suggest that the development of HCC in AIH is not as rare as these results would imply and that it can also follow an aggressive course.

Variant syndromes

The major autoimmune liver diseases aside from AIH are primary biliary cirrhosis (PBC) and primary sclerosing cholangitis (PSC), although whether PSC has a true autoimmune basis is debated. It is not uncommon for patients to present with AIH and features of either PBC or PSC. It is not clear whether these cases represent a distinct clinical entity or fall within a spectrum of autoimmune hepatopathies. The diagnosis of each of these conditions requires the presence of a pattern of characteristic features, rather than any one individual diagnostic criterion. These entities have been designated as overlap syndromes or outlier syndromes and as yet there are no standardised diagnostic criteria. It is common for autoimmune conditions to occur together in the same individual and the presence of co-existing features of AIH and those of PBC, for example, has been likened to type 1 diabetes and autoimmune thyroiditis existing in the same patient.

AIH–PBC overlap

Initially thought to be rare, more recent studies identified AIH–PBC overlap in 8–9% of patients with PBC. Studies vary in the criteria used to determine what is classified as AIH–PBC overlap. Generally, one expects to see raised AST and ALT with markers of cholestasis (raised ALP and GGT), a rise in IgG and IgM, positive AMA (PBC-specific AMA) and histology compatible with AIH, described elsewhere.

There are no controlled trials of treatment in this group. A suggested approach to management is to determine whether the hepatitic or cholestatic component predominates (Woodward and Neuberger, 2001). In a patient with high aminotransferases, serum ALP less than twice the upper limit of normal and moderate to severe interface hepatitis on biopsy the use of corticosteroid therapy in the form of prednisolone may be appropriate. In those with more cholestatic features, biochemical remission is often achieved with a combination of steroids and ursodeoxycholic acid (UDCA) 13–15 mg/kg daily (Ben-Ari and Czaja, 2001). The use of azathioprine has not been determined in this group, but its effectiveness in the long-term management of AIH may make it a plausible alternative for long-term immunosuppression, and the maintenance of remission in AIH–PBC overlap. Liver transplantation should be considered for end-stage disease.

One German study also identified a group with typical features of PBC but a more hepatitic component, with good response to corticosteroids and genetic susceptibility markers of AIH such as HLA DR3 and DR4. The name PBC, hepatitic form was suggested (Lohse et al., 1999). Similarly there are patients with PBC who have positive ANA, but no other markers of AIH. As the features are predominantly those of PBC this would not be considered by most to be an overlap syndrome. These variants, however, do serve to demonstrate what a heterogeneous group of disorders the autoimmune liver diseases are.

AIH–PSC overlap

Cases of an overlapping syndrome where features of both AIH and PSC are present have also been reported. AIH–PSC overlap may be suspected in cases where cholangitis is identified histologically, inflammatory bowel disease is present (based on its strong association with PSC) or where corticosteroid therapy fails. Cholangiography is indicated in these patients. Studies have identified the presence of AIH–PSC overlap in 6% of patients with AIH based on review of the liver biopsy and in 8% of 113 PSC patients by applying the internationally agreed scoring system for the diagnosis of AIH (Czaja, 1998). In studies from the 1980s and 1990s, most overlapping cases were originally diagnosed as AIH, and cholangiography showing bile duct changes diagnostic of PSC was only carried out after follow-up liver biopsies on these patients revealed bile duct abnormalities. It was therefore presumed that in these cases AIH had evolved to develop features of sclerosing cholangitis. Without the benefit of cholangiography at the time of presentation it is impossible to say whether there may have been overlapping features present from the time of the initial diagnosis.

A 16-year prospective study in children carried out in one unit investigated the biliary anatomy of patients presenting with features of AIH. Those with cholangiopathy were labelled as having autoimmune sclerosing cholangitis (ASC). They found that half of the 55 children studied had abnormal cholangiography and, of these, 35% had no evidence of bile duct damage on liver biopsy. Thus the sclerosing cholangitis component of their disease would not have been suspected had endoscopic retrograde cholangiopancreatography (ERCP) not been performed. Follow-up of these patients showed that the two groups are very similar in their mode of presentation and response to immunosuppressive treatment, the only difference being the involvement of the biliary tree (Gregorio et al., 2001).

Some studies have shown a good response to standard immunosuppressive regimens of prednisolone and azathioprine, but reports of efficacy vary. The combination of immunosuppressive agents and UDCA is appropriate in this situation, and in end-stage disease, liver transplantation should be considered, although the disease may occur again in the transplanted liver.

Sequential presentation of overlap/PSC

In addition to patients who present with features of both AIH and PBC, or PSC at first presentation, there is also a phenomenon of cases, in which an existing diagnosis of classical PBC evolves to exhibit features of AIH (this can also occur with AIH and PSC) (Poupon et al., 2006). In those cases they have been termed sequential syndromes rather than overlap syndromes. It is suggested that AIH superimposed on pre-existing PBC, if not recognised early, can progress rapidly to end-stage liver failure.

Treatment

Since the 1970s, when the immunosuppressant drugs azathioprine and 6-mercaptopurine were seen to be effective in autoimmune diseases, and the benefit from corticosteroids was proven in randomised controlled trials, AIH has been considered a treatable condition. Studies show that 65–80% of patients have a successful response to treatment, and modern data suggest that 10-year survival is greater than 90% in patients receiving treatment, although 20-year survival may be less than 80%. In patients with cirrhosis at diagnosis, survival is less than 40% at 20 years (Roberts et al., 1996). In a disease affecting often a young population these are significant figures, and therefore liver transplantion may need to be considered.

Treatment indications

There have been three randomised controlled trials that have shown clinical and histological improvement with the use of corticosteroids in severe AIH. Later studies have shown that patients with cirrhosis respond just as well. Trials have not looked at response rates in milder disease so the indications to treat in this group are not so clear. Fifty percent of patients with mild to moderate disease develop cirrhosis in 15 years and 17% of those with interface hepatitis develop cirrhosis in 5 years, but have a normal 5-year life expectancy. Hence the risk/benefit ratio of treatment in this group is not stratified and treatment recommendations are made on an individual basis (Table 10.5).

Table 10.5 Indications for treatment.

Absolute	Relative
Serum AST ≥10 × upper normal limit	Symptoms (fatigue, joint pains, jaundice)
Serum AST ≥5 × upper normal limit and γ-globulin level ≥2 × normal	Serum AST and/or γ-globulin less than absolute criteria
Bridging necrosis or multiacinar necrosis on histological examination	Interface hepatitis

Treatment regimens

Prednisolone and azathioprine are the two agents most commonly used in the treatment of AIH. The results from initiating prednisolone (40 mg/day) on its own or when compared with a combination of lower dose prednisolone (20 mg/day) and azathioprine are similar in terms of clinical, biochemical and histological remission in cases of severe AIH. There are less corticosteroid side effects from the combination regimen (10% vs. 44%), hence combination therapy is often preferred. Using corticosteroids, 80% get cosmetic side effects, such as Cushingoid appearance (moon face) and acne, after 2 years. Severe side effects, such as psychosis, vertebral compression due to osteoporosis and diabetes can occur after 18 months of prednisolone at a dose of >10 mg daily. Thirteen percent of patients on corticosteroids experience side effects which require dose reduction or cessation of therapy (Heneghan and McFarlane, 2002).

The complications arising from azathioprine toxicity include nausea, vomiting, bone marrow suppression, cholestatic hepatitis, veno-occlusive disease, pancreatitis and skin rashes. These occur in less than 10% of those receiving a dose of 50 mg daily. Azathioprine is a pro-drug for 6-mercaptopurine which is eliminated via the enzyme thiopurine methyltransferase (TPMT). This enzyme is encoded by a highly polymorphic gene. Low enzyme activity is prevalent in 0.3% of the population, resulting in a build-up of drug metabolites and increased toxicity. Intermediate activity is prevalent in 11% of the population. Pre-treatment testing for TPMT activity may therefore predict the potential for toxicity and should be considered in all patients, especially those with pre-treatment cytopenia. In addition there is a risk of cancers developing in relation to immunosuppressant treatment. The frequency of extrahepatic malignancy is 5% with a median treatment duration of 42 months. No specific cell type is affected (Johnson et al., 1995; Heneghan and McFarlane, 2002).

Patients receiving long-term corticosteroids should be monitored for the development of cataracts and glaucoma and bone densitometry should be considered if there are concerns regarding osteoporosis. Patients receiving long-term prednisolone at a dose of 7.5 mg or more daily, particularly post-menopausal women, may benefit from treatment with calcium and vitamin D to prevent bone loss. Patients on azathioprine require close monitoring of leucocyte and platelet counts, particularly within the first few months of therapy. A regimen for therapy is given in Table 10.6.

Treatment end-points

Treatment for AIH continues until either remission is achieved, treatment fails, there is an incomplete response or until drug toxicity stops further treatment with the same regimen. Ninety percent of patients have some improvement in their AST, bilirubin and gamma-globulins within 2 weeks, although it usually takes at least

Table 10.6 Treatment regimens for adults.

	Prednisolone only (mg/day)	Combination	
		Prednisolone (mg/day)	Azathioprine (mg/day)
Week 1	60	30	50
Week 2	40	20	50
Week 3	30	15	50
Week 4	30	15	50
Maintenance until end-point	20	10	50
Reasons for preference	Cytopenia TPMT deficiency Pregnancy Malignancy Short course (≤6 months)	Post-menopausal state Osteoporosis Brittle diabetes Obesity Acne Emotional lability Hypertension	

12 months to achieve complete remission. The chance of achieving remission declines after 2 years of treatment. Histological improvement usually lags 6 months behind clinical and biochemical improvement, which should be taken into account when making decisions about attempting treatment withdrawal (Czaja and Freese, 2002).

Remission

Remission is defined as the absence of symptoms, normal AST, normal bilirubin and gamma-globulins, and histology which has reverted to normal, portal hepatitis only or inactive cirrhosis. Sixty-five percent achieve remission in 18 months with treatment and 80% achieve remission in 3 years. Maintenance doses of prednisolone and/or azathioprine should remain stable until remission is achieved.

Withdrawal of treatment

A liver biopsy may be performed prior to withdrawing therapy in a patient suspected to be in remission, but this is not essential. Fifty-five percent of patients with a normal AST and gamma-globulins will still have interface hepatitis on biopsy and they will invariably relapse if treatment is stopped. If histological assessment is not carried out, it is wise to wait for at least 6 months after normalisation of aminotransferases before stopping treatment to account for the lag in histological improvement. Withdrawal of treatment involves gradually reducing the dose of prednisolone over a period of 6 weeks or more and then stopping azathioprine. Symptoms and laboratory results should be monitored frequently during treatment withdrawal and for 3 months afterwards, following which patients require careful outpatient follow-up.

Relapse

Relapse denotes an increase in disease activity after induction of remission and cessation of therapy. If relapse occurs there is an increased risk of progression to cirrhosis, and its complications. The reported risk of relapse varies widely between studies: 20% of those with normal liver histology prior to treatment withdrawal will relapse, compared with 50% who relapse at 6 months in those patients with portal hepatitis. Those who progress to cirrhosis during treatment or have interface hepatitis frequently relapse. In reality most patients require long-term maintenance therapy.

There are two main approaches to the management of relapse. The first is the indefinite low-dose prednisolone strategy, where the steroid dose is reduced by 2.5 mg per month until such stage as there are no symptoms and the AST is less than five times the upper limit of normal. This approach may be considered more appropriate in women of childbearing age. The second regimen is the indefinite azathioprine strategy, which avoids glucocorticoid-related complications. The azathioprine dose is increased to 2 mg/kg/day then prednisolone is tapered off by 2.5 mg/month. A large study showed that 87% of patients on long-term azathioprine maintenance remained in remission for a median follow-up period of 67 months. The disadvantages of this strategy include the presence of joint pains on steroid withdrawal, which occurred in 63% of patients, and the risk of myelosuppression and the development of malignancy (Johnson et al., 1995).

Treatment failure

Treatment failure denotes the situation where a patient never enters remission and where worsening of clinical, laboratory and histological features are seen, despite compliance with medication. This occurs in less than 10% of cases. A suggested treatment regimen for this group is to use high-dose prednisolone (60 mg daily) or prednisolone 30 mg with azathioprine 150 mg daily for 1 month, then to reduce the steroid by 10 mg and azathioprine by 50 mg each month until a maintenance level is achieved. Seventy percent will improve in 2 years using this approach, although most remain on treatment long term with the ensuing risk of drug toxicity and disease progression. Hepatic decompensation during therapy for treatment failure may be an indication for liver transplantation.

Alternative agents

In cases of incomplete response, where there is improvement with treatment but no remission after 3 years, and cases where drug toxicity necessitates cessation of medication, alternative agents may be considered. Ursodeoxycholic acid (UDCA) has been used, as have budesonide, cyclosporin, 6-mercaptopurine, methotrexate, cyclophosphamide, mycophenolate mofetil and tacrolimus (Heneghan and McFarlane, 2002).

Pregnancy and autoimmune hepatitis

It was previously felt that pregnancy was a rare occurrence in patients with AIH, due to reduced fertility in association with other endocrine conditions, or due to amenorrhoea secondary to hypothalamic–pituitary dysfunction (Heneghan et al., 2001). In the presence of cirrhosis, amenorrhoea and anovulation are common, thus pregnancy remains uncommon in this group. Several studies show that with less active disease, or disease well controlled by treatment, uncomplicated pregnancy and delivery of a healthy child is a realistic expectation. Chapter 16 provides further discussions in relation to pregnancy in AIH.

Liver transplantation

In patients with AIH who progress to end-stage liver disease, the indications for liver transplantation are similar to those for chronic liver disease of any aetiology. These include complications of cirrhosis, such as recurrent ascites, spontaneous bacterial peritonitis, hepatic encephalopathy and recurrent variceal bleeding, and the development of hepatocellular carcinoma. In the Child-Pugh grading system of cirrhosis, where grades A, B and C denote increasing severity of symptoms and diminishing liver synthetic function, transplantation may be considered when a patient with slowly progressive disease reaches Child-Pugh grade B cirrhosis. Other indications for liver transplantation more specific to AIH include failure to achieve remission. Inability to induce remission with corticosteroids after 4 years predicts the likely need for liver transplantation, which should be considered at the first episode of decompensation (Devlin and O'Grady, 1999).

An important indication for liver transplantation in AIH is patients presenting with acute liver failure (ALF), which may require the patient to be listed for transplantation with 'super-urgent' priority. Some physicians advocate that even these patients should receive a trial of steroids, as there are reports of treatment being successful and avoiding the requirement for transplantation, but the issue is debated. Chapter 13 provides a more comprehensive discussion of the management of ALF.

The five-year patient and graft survival rates in patients transplanted for AIH are reported at 83–92% with 10-year survival of 75%. Autoantibodies and immunoglobulins usually normalise within 1 year. Disease recurrence in the allograft occurs in around 42% of patients transplanted for AIH. Recurrence is usually mild and responds well to corticosteroid treatment, however, cirrhosis and graft failure do occur. Patients transplanted for AIH are also at greater risk of developing acute and chronic graft rejection, compared with patients transplanted for other aetiologies, and are therefore at greater risk of graft loss. Care is taken in these patients to keep immunosuppressant levels robust, particularly in the early post-transplant period, to prevent rejection of the graft (Neuberger, 2002).

De novo AIH

A syndrome of post-transplant graft dysfunction resembling AIH has been identified in patients grafted for all causes of liver disease. No specific risk factors for
this have been identified, although some studies have suggested the presence of
autoantibodies, which may be directed to an antigen not present in the recipient,
i.e. a donor-derived antigen. Most patients respond to increased immunosuppression and steroids, but graft failure can occur (Czaja, 2002).

Chapter summary

In summary, AIH is a progressive condition characterised by abnormal liver biochemistry, raised serum globulins and circulating non-organ specific autoantibodies with portal and periportal inflammation. The cause is unknown, but is likely
to be due to an environmental trigger in a genetically susceptible individual. Standard treatment is with corticosteroids with or without azathioprine and most
patients respond well, although long-term maintenance therapy is often required.
There are groups of patients who present acutely, present late or with progressive
disease, or who are refractory to or intolerant of drug treatment in whom liver
transplantation may be considered.

Illustrative case study

A 26-year-old woman presented to her doctor complaining of a 6-week history
of fatigue, lethargy and mild joint pains. On examination she had evidence of
hepatomegaly and appeared mildly jaundiced. Screening blood tests confirmed
abnormalities in the liver function tests, and she was referred urgently to a local
gastroenterologist.

Further history elicited at the time of her initial hospital outpatient assessment
revealed that she had had similar symptoms 2 years previously, which were mild,
and for which she did not seek medical advice. She was otherwise previously fit
and well. There was no history of recent exposure to any prescribed or over-the-
counter medications or herbal remedies. Her mother was on long-term thyroxine
replacement for hypothyroidism and her sister had recently been diagnosed with
coeliac disease. She consumed up to 10 units of alcohol per week, had no history
of blood transfusions or body tattoos and had never abused recreational drugs.
Ear piercing had been performed with sterile equipment. Physical examination
confirmed mild hepatomegaly and jaundice, with no evidence of active synovitis
or cutaneous stigmata of chronic liver disease.

Initial laboratory investigations revealed (normal laboratory values in brackets): bilirubin 105 μmol/L (<17 μmol/L), ALP 240 IU/L (35–115 IU/L), ALT 2570 IU/L (3–30 IU/L), albumin 36 g/L (36–54 g/L), globulin 73 g/L (25–35 g/L), IgG 40.6 g/L (7.00–18.60 g/L), ANA +ve (titre 1:640), anti-SMA +ve (titre 1:320), hep A-C and E negative, liver ultrasound scan normal. On the basis of these results a liver biopsy was performed. The findings were reported as showing interface hepatitis with an abundance of plasma cells, and some spill-over into the lobule. Moderate portal fibrosis was noted. By the IAHG scoring system she was calculated to have a pre-treatment score of +19, suggesting a 'definite' diagnosis of AIH.

Treatment was commenced with prednisolone 40 mg daily, which was tapered by 10 mg every 2 weeks until maintaining a dose of 20 mg daily. After 4 weeks the bilirubin had fallen to 35 μmol/L and ALT to 157 IU/L with an IgG of 21 g/L. At this stage azathioprine was introduced at a dose of 50 mg daily, with the prednisolone dose being reduced by 5 mg weekly from this point until achieving maintenance doses of azathioprine 50 mg plus prednisolone 10 mg daily. The patient continued to make good clinical improvement with normalisation of the bilirubin, ALT, globulin and IgG fractions, and after 6 months prednisolone was gradually withdrawn.

References

Alvarez F, Berg PA, Bianchi FB, Bianchi L, Burroughs AK, Cancado EL, Chapman RW, Cooksley WG, Czaja AJ, Desmet VJ, Donaldson PT, Eddleston AL, Fainboim L, et al. (1999) International Autoimmune Hepatitis Group report: review of criteria for diagnosis of autoimmune hepatitis. *Journal of Hepatology* **31**:929–938

Ben-Ari Z, Czaja AJ (2001) Autoimmune hepatitis and its variant syndromes. *Gut* **49**:589–594

Czaja AJ (1998) Frequency and nature of the variant syndromes of autoimmune liver disease. *Hepatology* **28**:360–365

Czaja AJ (2002) Autoimmune hepatitis after liver transplantation and other lessons of self-tolerance. *Liver Transplantation* **8**(6):505–513

Czaja AJ, Carpenter HA (2001) Autoimmune hepatitis with incidental histological features of bile duct injury. *Hepatology* **34**:659–665

Czaja AJ, Freese DK (2002) Diagnosis and treatment of autoimmune hepatitis. *Hepatology* **36**(2):479–497

Czaja AJ, Homburger HA (2001) Autoantibodies in liver disease. *Gastroenterology* **120**:239–249

Czaja AJ, Manns MP (1995) The validity and importance of subtypes of autoimmune hepatitis: a point of view. *American Journal of Gastroenterology* **90**: 1206–1211

Czaja AJ, Strettell MDJ, Thomson LJ, Santrach PJ, Breanndan Moore S, Donaldson PT, Williams R (1997) Associations between alleles of the major histocompatibility complex and type 1 autoimmune hepatitis. *Hepatology* 25(2):317–323

De Groote J, Fevery J, Lepoutre L (1978) Long-term follow-up of chronic active hepatitis of moderate severity. *Gut* 19:510–513

Devlin J, O'Grady J (1999) Indications for referral and assessment in adult liver transplantation. *Gut* 45(Suppl VI):VI1–VI22

Djilali-Saiah I, Renous R, Caillat-Zucman S, Debray D, Alvarez F (2004) Linkage disequilibrium between HLA class II region and autoimmune hepatitis in pediatric patients. *Journal of Hepatology* 40:904–909

Gregorio GV, Portmann B, Karani J, Harrison P, Donaldson PT, Vergani D, Mieli-Vergani G (2001) Autoimmune hepatitis/sclerosing cholangitis overlap syndrome in childhood: a 16-year prospective study. *Hepatology* 33:544–553

Heneghan MA, McFarlane IG (2002) Current and novel immunosupressive therapy for autoimmune hepatitis. *Hepatology* 35:7–13

Heneghan MA, Norris SM, O'Grady JG, Harrison PM, McFarlane IG (2001) Management and outcome of pregnancy in autoimmune hepatitis. *Gut* 48:97–102

Hennes EM, Zeniya M, Czaja AJ, Parés A, Dalekos GN, Krawitt EL, Bittencourt PL, et al. (2005) Simplified diagnostic criteria for autoimmune hepatitis. *Hepatology* 42:295A

Johnson PJ, McFarlane IG (1993) Meeting report: International Autoimmune Hepatitis Group. *Hepatology* 18:998–1005

Johnson PJ, McFarlane IG, Williams R (1995) Azathioprine for long-term maintenance of remission in autoimmune hepatitis. *New England Journal of Medicine* 333:958–963

Krawitt EL (2006) Autoimmune hepatitis. *New England Journal of Medicine* 354:54–66

Lohse AW, zum Buschenfekle KH, Franz B, Kanzler S, Gerken G, Dienes HP (1999) Characterisation of the overlap syndrome of primary biliary cirrhosis (PBC) and autoimmune hepatitis: evidence for it being a hepatitic form of PBC in genetically susceptible individuals. *Hepatology* 29:1078–1084

Neuberger J (2002) Transplantation for autoimmune hepatitis. *Seminars in Liver Disease* 22:379–386

Park SZ, Nagorney DM, Czaja AJ (2000) Hepatocellular carcinoma in autoimmune hepatitis. *Digestive Diseases and Sciences* 45(10):1944–1948

Poupon R, Chazouilleres O, Corpechot C, Chretien Y (2006) Development of autoimmune hepatitis in patients with typical primary biliary cirrhosis. *Hepatology* 44:85–90

Reuben A (2003) A sheep in wolf's clothing. *Hepatology* 38:1596–1601

Roberts SK, Therneau T, Czaja AJ (1996) Prognosis of histological cirrhosis in type 1 autoimmune hepatitis. *Gastroenterology* 110:848–857

Woodward J, Neuberger J (2001) Autoimmune overlap syndromes. *Hepatology* 33:994–1002

11
Primary biliary cirrhosis and primary sclerosing cholangitis

Danielle Fullwood

Introduction

This chapter will discuss two autoimmune disorders that affect the biliary tree and ultimately lead to liver cirrhosis. Primary biliary cirrhosis (PBC) and primary schlerosing cholangitis (PSC) affect different genders and ages, however both have various hypothesised causes and are associated with other autoimmune and inflammatory diseases. The aetiology and presentation of these are considered, as well as the diagnostic criteria and management of the diseases and their symptoms.

Primary biliary cirrhosis

PBC is a chronic and progressive autoimmune disease, characterised by inflammation and destruction of the interlobal bile ducts, leading to biliary cirrhosis (Levy and Lindor, 2003). Up to 90% of patients with PBC are women aged between 40 and 60 years; however case studies have reported extreme variations of this. Disease prevalence ranges from 100–200/million and it is found worldwide amongst all ethnic groups (Poupon and Poupon, 2006).

There is no cure for PBC and therefore treatment is aimed at slowing disease progression and controlling symptoms such as osteoporosis, pruritis (itching) and portal hypertension, until liver transplantation.

Pathophysiology

As with most autoimmune diseases, the aetiology remains unknown. However there are several hypotheses, including genetic, immune and environmental.

There may be a genetic element as studies have shown that patients with PBC have a 4–6% prevalence of the disease in first-degree relatives (Levy and Lindor, 2003). However the focus has been on immune factors as the likely cause. Patients with PBC have a 3–15 times higher occurrence of co-existing autoimmune disorders such as Sjögren's syndrome, Raynauld's syndrome, or autoimmune thyroid disease than their siblings (Talwalker and Lindor, 2003).

Patients with PBC have a variety of immune disturbances with the presence of increased cytokines, T-cell infiltration of the biliary tree, a plethora of circulating antibodies and increased immunoglobulin M. Autoantobodies found in the serum include anti-smooth muscle, anti-thyroid, anti-platelet, anti-acetylcholine, lymphotoxic and anti-nuclear antibodies (ANA). The latter are found in up to half of people with PBC (Kaplan and Gershwin, 2005).

It is thought that 96% of people with PBC have anti-mitochondrial antibodies (AMAs) in their serum. Many see this as an indication or at least a precursor of PBC. AMAs can be detected in the serum before any symptoms are apparent (Kaplan and Gershwin, 2005). AMAs are present in all nucleated cells of the body although their action is only directed against the intrahepatic bile ducts. It is possible, therefore, that there are differences in the biliary epithelium of people with PBC causing it to react to the presence of AMA, which elicits an immune reaction (Kaplan and Gershwin, 2005).

This difference may be the release of pyruvate dehydrogenase E2 complex (PDC-E2) from the biliary cells. AMAs target this and react to the PDC-E2 and a response from T- and B-cells is seen. The infiltration of T-cells increases cytokine production, possibly resulting in destruction of the intrahepatic bile ducts. People with early PBC have evidence of a T-cell response to PDC-E2, showing an impaired tolerance to this complex (O'Donohue and Williams, 1996).

Both bacteria and viruses have been suggested as possible trigger factors. Urinary tract infections (UTIs) caused by *Escherichia coli* are found significantly more in people with PBC than those without the disease, and are associated with elevated serum levels of AMAs (Gershwin et al., 2005). Other hypothesised pathogens have included myobacteria gordonae and *Salmonella typhimurium* (Sherlock and Dooley, 2002). It may be possible that these bacteria mimic the PDC-E2 complex causing an immune response (Poupon and Poupon, 2006).

Presentation

In the early stages of PBC patients are often asymptomatic, a phase that is estimated to last 15–20 years (Mahl and O'Grady, 2006). Consequently the disease is often detected by the presence of abnormal liver function tests such as elevated ALP, as shown in Table 11.1. However, most asymptomatic patients will eventually develop symptoms of PBC.

Table 11.1 Laboratory findings on presentation of PBC and PSC.

Biochemical marker	PBC	PSC
Alkaline phosphatase	Increased	Increased
Gamma-glutamyltranferase	Increased	Increased
Aminotransferases (AST or ALT)	Normal or mildly increased	Normal or mildly increased
Bilirubin	Normal	Increased
Cholesterol	Increased	Normal
Immunoglobulins		
IgM	Moderate to marked increase	Normal or mildly Increased
IgG	Normal or mildly increased	Mild or moderately increased
IgA	Normal or mildly increased	Normal or mildly increased
INR	Normal	Normal
Autoanitibodies (% with titres >1:40)		
ANA or SMA	30–40%	20%
AMA	90%	0

Findings on clinical examination are primarily independent of the stage of the disease and may be normal in asymptomatic patients. However the most common presenting symptoms include pruritus and fatigue, which do not necessarily correlate with either laboratory or histological findings. Jaundice may never develop, but in the majority of patients it appears within 6 months to 2 years after the onset of pruritis and is indicative that the disease is in its final stages (Sherlock and Dooley, 2002). Patients with end-stage PBC may present with spider naevi, ascites, oedema and proximal wasting (Kaplan and Lee, 2004).

Prolonged cholestasis leads to cholesterol deposits under the skin resulting in xanthelasma around the inner eye and xanthoma on the palms and buttocks, which are seen in 10–20% of patients (Figure 11.1, Plate 11). However, the development of xanthoma does not correlate with either the serum cholesterol or triglyceride concentrations. Skin hyperpigmentation that resembles tanning due to melanin can be seen in early stages of PBC (Kaplan and Lee, 2004).

Diagnosis

Laboratory findings

The common laboratory findings in patients with PBC are demonstrated in Table 11.1, however, these will vary between asymptomatic and symptomatic patients. A diagnosis of PBC can be made if there is evidence of serum AMA in titres greater than 1:40, a cholestatic liver profile in the absence of any other explanation and an elevated IgM (Heathcote, 2000). Hepatic synthetic function is usually well preserved until the later stages therefore serum albumin and prothrombin time (PT) are usually normal (Neuberger, 2000).

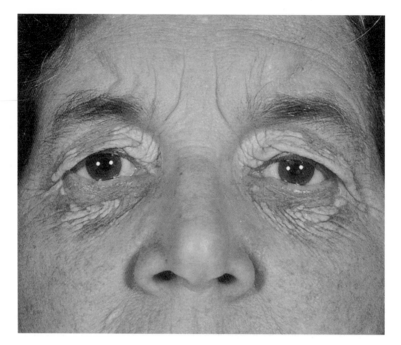

Figure 11.1   Both xanthelasma and pigmentation in a patient with primary biliary cirrhosis. Reproduced with permission from Sherlock S, Dooley J (2002) *Diseases of the Liver and Biliary System*, 11th edn. Blackwell Publishing. For a colour version of this figure, please see Plate 11 in the colour plate section.

Radiology

Radiology has little part to play in the diagnosis of PBC (Neuberger, 2000). However an abdominal ultrasound scan may be useful to rule out bile duct obstruction. Endoscopic retrograde cholangiopancreatography (ERCP) is usually not needed but may be useful in AMA-negative patients to exclude conditions such as PSC.

Histology

A liver biopsy is not always considered necessary for diagnosis, but considered useful for disease staging. Histological lesions are divided into four stages as demonstrated in Table 11.2, however overlap between stages and non-uniform changes are common (Sherlock and Dooley, 2002).

Table 11.2   Histological staging of PBC and PSC.

Stage	Histological findings in PBC	Histological findings in PSC
1	Damage to the lining of the bile ducts causes them to shrink and to become inflamed. At this stage the inflammation is isolated to the portal triads	Portal oedema, inflammation of ductal proliferation, abnormalities do not extend beyond limiting plate
2	There is a reduction in the number of normal bile ducts and the inflammation spreads to the liver tissue	Periportal fibrosis with or without inflammation extending beyond the limited plate
3	Fibrous tissue builds up between the portal triads	Septal fibrosis, bridging necrosis or both
4	Nodular cirrhosis is seen	Biliary cirrhosis

Complications of primary biliary cirrhosis

Fatigue

Fatigue is thought to affect up to 85% of patients with PBC, which has a significant impact on quality of life (Neuberger, 2000). Although the aetiology of fatigue is poorly understood, it is thought to be as a result of a decrease in corticotropic-releasing hormone, altered serotonin neurotransmission and the presence of cytokines (Jorgenson, 2006). There is no treatment for fatigue but it is imperative to exclude any other causes, e.g. hypothyroidism, depression, altered sleeping patterns, exercise and caffeine and alcohol intake (Swain, 1999).

Pruritis

Pruritus is a common presenting symptom, occurring in 65% of patients with PBC. In most cases the pruritus is moderate; however pruritus can be severe in approximately 5–10% of cases (Poupon and Poupon, 2006). The pathogenesis of pruritus in PBC is unknown but increased deposits of bile acids and endogenous opioid accumulation are found in people with the disease, which may be contributing factors (Swain, 2000). When cholestasis occurs, opioid receptors are also thought to be upgraded, increasing the opioid effect. Most treatments are directed towards either reducing bile acids or reversing the opioid effect.

The itching typically starts at the feet and palms of the hands before becoming more generalised, and can be exacerbated by numerous factors. Therefore education plays an important role. As heat can exacerbate pruritus, patients should be advised to take tepid showers or a cool bath, and to avoid spicy foods. Because pruritus is often associated with dry skin, health care professionals should do a detailed examination to assess the hydration status of the patient and the dryness of their skin. Keeping the skin moist with emollient (moisturiser) is imperative. Whilst several products are available, aqueous cream BP is usually adequate when applied twice daily (Twycross et al., 2003). Patients should be advised to avoid soap and any perfumed products, which dry the skin, and to be aware of the impact

Table 11.3   Pharmacological treatments for pruritus.

Drug	Method of action	Dosing and administration	Other information
Cholestyramine	Resin not absorbed in the gastrointestinal tract. Able to join with bile acids to form an insoluble complex in the intestine	Recommended for pruritus associated with PBC in doses of 4–16 mg/day	Binds other oral drugs therefore they should be taken 1 hour before or 4–6 hours after Cholestryamine to avoid any interference with absorption
Colestipol	Bile acid resin	5 mg orally	
Rifampicin	Competes with bile acids for hepatic uptake	150 mg, twice daily	Side effects include liver disturbance and toxicity
Naloxone, nalmephene, naltraxate	Opioid antagonists		Not yet licensed for use in pruritus

of a dry environment. The use of room humidifiers may be of benefit (Bosonnet, 2003). Topical irritants such as wool or synthetic fabrics should be avoided, and patients should be encouraged to wear loose clothing, particularly at night when the itching can be worse.

Repeated scratching can result in damage to the skin, therefore nails should be kept short in order to minimise harm. Patting the skin in a circular motion can also provide relief from the itch without causing skin breakage.

Medical treatments for pruritus are summarised in Table 11.3, however cholestyramine (Questran®) or colestipol are the mainstay in therapy and are successful in 90% of patients with mild to moderate pruritus. Depending on the severity of the cholestasis, it takes 1–4 days from the initiation of cholestyramine before the itching reduces (Kaplan and Lee, 2004). Side effects include altered bowel habits and bloating, though colestipol is less constipating than cholestyramine. Rifampicin is the second line of therapy but this has been associated with hepatotoxicity. Antihistamines have little effect on pruritus and can make patients drowsy.

Other treatments such as albumin dialysis and plasmapharesis have been studied with some suggested benefits, although further research is necessary to prove their efficacy.

Metabolic bone disease

Osteoporosis is frequently noticed before the diagnosis of PBC. The pathophysiology of this is relatively unknown, however it may be caused by a decrease in osteoblast activity and an increase in osteoclast activity, which have been found to occur in PBC (Neuberger, 2000). The standard treatment for osteoporosis is calcium and vitamin D supplements (Levy and Lindor, 2003). Patients should be encouraged to abstain from smoking to reduce the risk of osteoporosis. Dietary management plays a significant role and is discussed further in Chapter 14.

Fat-soluble vitamin deficiency

Cholestasis can lead to malabsorption of fat-soluble vitamins (A, D, E and K), but this is normally in advanced or severe PBC (Sherlock and Dooley, 2002). Patients therefore should have their vitamin levels monitored and low levels treated accordingly. Dietary advice regarding fat-soluble vitamin deficiency is discussed further in Chapter 14.

Steatorrhoea

Steatorrhoea is normally treated with a low-fat diet and supplements of medium chain triglycerides (MCT) to maintain a reasonable caloric intake (Kaplan and Lee, 2004).

Disease management

The main drug therapy currently used for the treatment of PBC is ursodeoxycholic acid (UDCA). UDCA is a hydrophilic bile acid found endogenously in the body. There are multiple mechanisms of action suggested, some of which include (Sherlock and Dooley, 2002):

- Stimulates excretion of toxic bile acids
- Increases anion exchange in the liver
- Reduces HLA class 1 expression on bile ducts therefore decreasing cytolytic attack of T-cells on bile ducts
- Inhibits the production of nitric oxide synthase

Liver biochemistry, levels of IgM, fatigue and pruritus have all been found to improve with the administration of UDCA. However there is limited evidence that UDCA prolongs survival or decreases the need for liver transplantation (Palmer, 2004; Mahl and O'Grady, 2006).

UDCA should be given to early cases of PBC in doses of 13–15 mg/kg/day after an evening meal. If cholestyramine is being administered for pruritus, then UDCA should be given several hours after the ingestion of this drug (Heathcote, 2000). The systematic reviews of other pharmacological treatment trials that have been tested in patients not responding to UDCA monotherapy are demonstrated in Table 11.4.

Prognosis

The prognosis of individual PBC patients is important to establish the optimum time of liver transplantation. A serum bilirubin >100 μmol/L (6 g/dL), is associated with a survival of less than 2 years (Sherlock and Dooley, 2002). Other considerations relate to signs of advanced liver disease and portal hypertension, severe pruritus or osteoporosis, or complications such as hepatocellular carcinoma.

Table 11.4   Systematic reviews of other pharmacological therapies tested in PBC.

Drug name	Proposed action	Systematic review findings	Reviewers
D-penicillamine	Reduction of hepatic copper and immunomodulatory effects	Numbers of adverse incidents significantly increased with use of D-penicillamine. Did not improve survival	Gong et al. (2004)
Colchicine	Immunomodulatory and antifibrotic effects	No effect on outcome, mortality, biochemistry or histology	Gong and Gluud (2004)
Glucocorticoids	Immunosupressive effects	Improved liver inflammatory markers and histology seen. BMD lowered	Prince et al. (2005)
Methotrexate	Immunosuppresive effects	Increased mortality seen	Gong and Gluud (2005)

Several prognostic models can be applied. The Mayo model takes into account factors such as age, total bilirubin, albumin, PT and the presence or absence of oedema and ascites (Poupon and Poupon, 2006). This model can predict life expectancy and is independent of liver biopsy.

Liver transplantation

One-year survival after transplantation in PBC is about 85–90% and 75% at 5 years (Poupon and Poupon, 2006). There is evidence that PBC recurs in the donor graft after transplantation. Studies have shown that around 14% of patients will go on to get some evidence of disease recurrence, although it is usually a very slow progression. Often it is completely asymptomatic and only evident on liver biopsy (Jacob et al., 2006).

Primary sclerosing cholangitis

PSC is a chronic cholestatic disorder of unknown aetiology that is characterised by diffuse inflammation and fibrosis that involves the entire biliary tree. The pathological process obliterates intra- and extrahepatic bile ducts, which leads to biliary cirrhosis, portal hypertension and liver failure (Narayanan Menon and Wiesner, 2006). There is no cure for PSC and treatment involves the management of symptoms until the damage progresses, necessitating liver transplantation.

Pathophysiology

Despite advances in the understanding of PSC, the pathophysiology of the disease remains relatively unknown; however there are growing indications that immune mechanisms are involved. Other postulated theories have suggested genetic influences and viral or bacterial infections.

PSC is very strongly associated with inflammatory diseases affecting the large bowel, including ulcerative colitis and, to a lesser extent, Crohn's disease. Inflammatory bowel disease (IBD) is seen in 80% of patients with PSC and up to 7.5% of patients with ulcerative colitis have PBC (Narayanan Menon and Wiesner, 2006). However, PSC may exist without any evidence of IBD.

The most accepted theory for the pathogenesis of PSC is that it is caused by immune-mediated damage of the bile ducts (Narayanan Menon and Wiesner, 2006). Support for this theory comes from the immunological abnormalities reported, which include the presence of increased titres of perinuclear anti-neutrophilic cytoplasmic antibodies (pANCA), and anti-neutrophil cytoplasmic antibodies (ANCA), which are found in people with PSC and which persist after liver transplant (Sherlock and Dooley, 2002).

There is a strong genetic predisposition to the development of PSC. Both family clustering and an association between certain human leucocyte antigen (HLA) haplotypes (HLA-B8, HLA DR2, HLA-DR3, HLA-DR6) have been reported, suggesting genetic susceptibility (Narayanan Menon and Wiesner, 2006). However, there is no evidence that PSC can be inherited as a single gene disorder (Sherlock and Dooley, 2002). Bacterial and viral infections have been implicated but there is limited evidence supporting this theory.

Presentation

Seventy percent of patients with PSC are men, where it commonly presents in the fourth decade of life. Disease prevalence is thought to be 8.5 cases per 100 000 population (Wiesner, 2004).

Patients can be asymptomatic, but present with abnormal liver biochemistry on routine investigation. A cholestatic picture is commonly seen with a rise in ALP and GGT (Table 11.1), usually in the early stages of the disease. Asymptomatic elevation of ALP and a history of ulcerative colitis are highly suggestive of PSC.

However, the majority of patients present in the symptomatic phase, characterised by pruritus, fatigue, abdominal pain, intermittent jaundice and weight loss which occurs in 75% of patients (Narayanan Menon and Wiesner, 2006). Other signs and symptoms include bacterial cholangitis and those associated with portal hypertension (oesophageal varices, splenomegaly and ascites).

Diagnosis

Imaging

An ultrasound scan is useful to exclude other causes of cholestasis. Imaging of the biliary tree with either a percutaneous transhepatic cholangiogram (PTC) or endoscopic retrograde cholangiopancreatograph (ERCP) is considered the gold standard to make a diagnosis of PSC (Wilkinson, 1992). The disease is characterised by both dilation and stricturing of the entire bile duct, which gives the impression of a bead-like effect (DeSouza, 1997). However, it has been suggested that magnetic resonance cholangiography may avoid the necessity of an invasive cholangiography when a diagnosis is the overall aim of the procedure (Angulo and Lindor, 1999).

Histology

Even after a cholangiogram has established the diagnosis of PBC, a liver biopsy is necessary for disease staging (Angulo and Lindor, 1999). The histological staging of the disease can be made into four categories depending on disease severity, as shown in Table 11.2.

Complications of primary sclerosing cholangitis

Several complications are seen in both PSC and PBC, which are related to cholestasis, as previously discussed. However there are some complications that are unique to this disease.

Biliary strictures

Up to 15–20% of patients with PSC will develop a dominant stricture in the extrahepatic bile ducts, and 30% may form small hepatic stones or pigmented debris (Levy and Lindor, 2003). Strictures are treated at ERCP with dilatation or stents, which have been associated with an improvement in quality of life (Narayanan Menon and Wiesner, 2006). However, these procedures are associated with the occurrence of bacterial cholangitis and although prophylactic antibiotics are given, their effectiveness has been found to be limited in some studies (Pohl et al., 2006). If there are many small strictures in the intrahepatic ducts then dilatation may not be effective.

Biliary reconstruction is also an option for patients with strictures. Survival rates, for those without cirrhosis after reconstructions, have been found to be significantly higher than for those patients who had stenting. However, if cirrhosis is present then neither stenting nor reconstruction has proved successful. Transplantation is therefore recommended if cirrhosis has occurred (Ahrendt et al., 1998).

Cholangitis

Bacterial cholangitis is rare in the absence of biliary obstruction. Infection is presumed to ascend from the gut, in which the presence of biliary strictures results in the overgrowth of enteric organisms in the upper small intestine (Sherlock and Dooley, 2002). Signs and symptoms usually include those of biliary obstruction (jaundice, dark urine, pale stool), pain and fever. Management is primarily aimed at fluid and pain management and treatment with broad-spectrum antibiotics after blood cultures have been taken. ERCP and stenting or dilatation may also be indicated. The associated mortality is 5–10%.

Cholangiocarcinoma

Patients with PSC have a higher incidence of developing cholangiocarcinoma than the normal population, with a reported prevalence of 10–20% (Figure 11.2). The

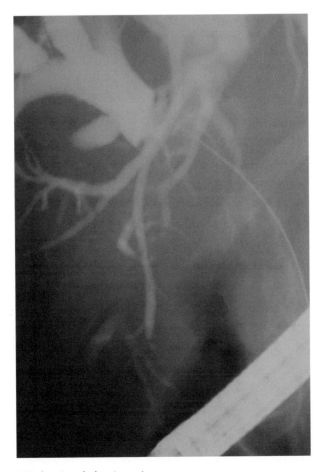

Figure 11.2 ERCP showing cholangiocarcinoma.

reasons for this are relatively unknown, but have been associated with smoking, older age and longer duration of IBD (Angulo and Lindor, 1999). Once diagnosed with cholangiocarcinoma, survival is less than 10% in 2 years (Narayanan Menon and Wiesner, 2006). A diagnosis of cholangiocarcinoma is also a contraindication to transplantation, due to the high recurrence rate of this cancer in the donor organ (Mahl and O'Grady, 2006). The risk of pancreatic cancer is increased by 14-fold compared to the normal population, and colon cancer is reported as ten times higher in PSC patients (Levy and Lindor, 2003).

Prognostic survival models

The mean survival from diagnosis is 10–12 years. Predictive survival is based on clinical, biochemical and histological features which are considered useful for both the evaluation of therapeutic interventions and the timing for liver transplantation (Narayanan Menon and Wiesner, 2006). Several models have been proposed and include the Mayo PSC model, which is based on the patient's bilirubin, age, histological staging, haemoglobin, and the presence of inflammatory bowel disease, and is thought to be useful in early disease stages (Sherlock and Dooley, 2002). Alternatively the Child-Pugh or MELD scores are also frequently used.

Disease management

Trials have failed to demonstrate any significant benefits of several pharmacological therapies in disease progression, including immunosuppressants (cyclosporin, azathioprine, methotraxate, and tacrolimus), corticosteroids and antifibrotic agents (colchicine) (Narayanan Menon and Wiesner, 2006).

The success of using UDCA in patients with PBC has led to trials being conducted to test the drug efficiency and safety in PSC patients (Levy and Lindor, 2003). Doses are normally prescribed at 15–20 mg/kg, and whilst some improvements in liver biochemistry have been found, they make no difference in the time from diagnosis to transplantation.

Sigmoidoscopy and rectal biopsy should be performed in all patients who have not previously been diagnosed with ulcerative colitis. In patients with PSC and ulcerative colitis, proctocolectomy is frequently performed due to indications relevant to inflammatory bowel disease and bowel cancer (Narayanan Menon and Wiesner, 2006).

Symptoms of the disease can be managed but at present no treatment is available to slow the disease progression. Liver transplantation is indicated for end-stage liver disease if hepatic encephalopathy, oesophageal varices, recurrent bacterial cholangitis or refractory ascites are present (Lee and Kaplan, 1995). Survival rates post liver transplantation are reported to be 90–97% at 1 year and 85–88% at 5 years (Narayanan Menon and Wiesner, 2006).

Recurrence of PSC in the donor graft has been found to be 8–15% and is occasionally a cause of significant graft dysfunction (Mahl and O'Grady, 2006). This recurrence is associated with the patient being male and having an intact colon before or during transplantation. Patients who have a colectomy before or during the transplant procedure are less likely to get a recurrence of the disease and there is a prolonged time before transplantation is needed in these patients (Vera et al., 2002). However, it should be noted that histological appearances of PSC are difficult to distinguish from graft rejection (Sherlock and Dooley, 2002).

Chapter summary

This chapter has discussed two autoimmune disease processes that cause the destruction of part or the entire biliary tree. The diseases are characterised by raised levels of particular autoantibodies and immunoglobulins. The resulting liver damage causes debilitating symptoms, such as profound lethargy and pruritus, as well as stigmata of chronic liver disease in advanced stages. Health care professionals should be aware of the pathophysiology of these diseases and educate patients and their relatives regarding the management of symptoms associated with them. Despite advancement in pharmacological therapies, transplantation is still required by many patients.

Illustrative case study

A 37-year-old white male presented to his GP with a 2-month history of altered bowel habits, experiencing six to eight episodes of diarrhoea per day, some with bright blood flecks. On examination his abdomen was soft and non-tender and his rectal examination was normal. He was referred for a colonoscopy and blood taken for full blood count and biochemistry.

Six weeks later the patient was experiencing regular diarrhoea up to 10 times per day and had lost 3 kg in weight. The colonoscopy report showed red, ulcerated areas of colon, which were biopsied. The laboratory investigations revealed an increase in liver enzymes with an ALP 262 IU/L and a GGT 86 IU/L. All other results were within normal ranges.

Results of the biopsies showed ulcerative colitis, for which he was prescribed prednisolone. An ultrasound was ordered which demonstrated a dilated common bile duct, which was confirmed on CT.

Due to the patient's age, gender, diagnosis of IBD, cholestatic biochemistry and dilated bile ducts, an ERCP was performed due to the suspicion of PSC. This confirmed PSC with multiple intra- and extrahepatic biliary strictures.

The patient was commenced on UDCA at 15 mg/kg. A subsequent liver biopsy found evidence of stage 2 disease progression. Twelve months later the patient was experiencing intermittent bouts of jaundice with presence of a dominant stricture on ERCP. This was treated with dilation and stenting. Histological findings revealed the disease had progressed to stage 3, and the patient was experiencing both pruritus, and fatigue. He was additionally commenced on cholestyramine.

References

Ahrendt SA, Pitt HA, Kalloo AN, Venbrux AC, Klein AS, Herlong HF, Coleman J, Lillemoe KD, Cameron JL (1998) Primary sclerosing cholangitis: resect, dilate or transplant? *Annals of Surgery* **227**(3):412–423

Angulo P, Lindor KD (1999) Primary sclerosing cholangitis. *Hepatology* **30**(1): 325–332

Bosonnet L (2003) Pruritus: scratching the surface. *European Journal of Cancer Care* **12**:162–165

DeSouza P (1997) Primary sclerosing cholangitis: a case study. *Gastroenterology Nurse* **20**(6):219–220

Gershwin ME, Selmi C, Worman HJ, Gold EB, Watnik M, Utts J, Lindor KD, Kaplan MM, Vierling JM, USA PBC Epidemiology Group (2005) Risk factors and comorbidities in primary biliary cirrhosis: a controlled interview-based study of 1032 patients. *Hepatology* **42**(5):1194–1202

Gluud C, Christensen E (2002) Ursodeoxycholic acid for primary biliary cirrhosis. *Cochrane Database of Systematic Reviews*, Issue 1. Art. No.: CD000551. DOI: 10.1002/14651858.CD000551

Gong Y, Frederiksen SL, Gluud C (2004) D-penicillamine for primary biliary cirrhosis. *Cochrane Database of Systematic Reviews*, Issue 4. Art. No.: CD004789. DOI: 10.1002/14651858.CD004789.pub2

Gong Y, Gluud C (2004) Colchicine for primary biliary cirrhosis. *Cochrane Database of Systematic Reviews*, Issue 2. Art. No.: CD004481. DOI: 10.1002/14651858.CD004481.pub2

Gong Y, Gluud C (2005) Methotrexate for primary biliary cirrhosis. *Cochrane Database of Systematic Reviews*, Issue 3. Art. No.: CD004385. DOI: 10.1002/14651858.CD004385.pub2

Heathcote J (2000) Management of primary biliary cirrhosis. *Hepatology* **131**(4): 1005–1013

Jacob DA, Neumann UP, Bahra M, Klupp J, Puhl G, Neuhaus R, Langrehr JM (2006) Long-term follow-up after recurrence of primary biliary cirrhosis after liver transplantation in 100 patients. *Clinical Transplantation* **20**:211–220

Jorgenson R (2006) A phenomenological study of fatigue in patients with primary biliary cirrhosis. *Issues and Innovations in Nursing Practice* **55**(6): 689–697

Kaplan MM, Gershwin ME (2005) Primary biliary cirrhosis. *New England Journal of Medicine* **353**(12):1261–1273

Kaplan MM, Lee YM (2004) Primary biliary cirrhosis. In: Freidman LS and Keeffe EB (eds) *Handbook of Liver Disease*, 2nd edn. Churchill Livingstone, Philadelphia

Lee YM , Kaplan MM (1995) Primary sclerosing cholangitis. *New England Journal of Medicine* **332**(14):924–933

Levy C, Lindor KD (2003) Current management of primary biliary cirrhosis and primary sclerosing cholangitis. *Journal of Hepatology* **38**:S24–S37

Lindor KD (1997) Ursodiol for primary sclerosing cholangitis. *New England Journal of Medicine* **336**(10):691–695

Mahl T, O'Grady JG (2006) *Fast Facts: Liver Disorders*. Health Press, Oxford

Narayanan Menon KV, Wiesner RH (2006) Primary sclerosing cholangitis. In: Bacon BR, O'Grady JG, Di Bisceglie AM, Lake JR (eds) *Comprehensive Clinical Hepatology*, 2nd edn. Mosby Elsevier, Philadelphia, pp. 289–308

Neuberger J (2000) Primary biliary cirrhosis. In: O'Grady JG, Lake JR, Howdle PD (eds) *Comprehensive Clinical Hepatology*. Mosby Elsevier, London, pp. 17.1–17.14

O'Donohue J, Williams R (1996) Primary biliary cirrhosis. *Quarterly Journal of Medicine* **89**:5–13

Palmer M (2004) *Hepatitis and Liver Disease*. Avery, New York

Pohl J, Ring A, Stremmel W , Stiehl A (2006) The role of dominant stenosis in bacterial infections of bile ducts in primary sclerosing cholangitis. *European Journal of Gastroenterology and Hepatology* **18**(1):69–74

Poupon R, Poupon RE (2006) Primary biliary cirrhosis. In: Bacon BR, O'Grady JG, Di Bisceglie AM, Lake JR (eds) *Comprehensive Clinical Hepatology*, 2nd edn. Mosby Elsevier, Philadelphia, pp. 277–288

Prince M, Christensen E, Gluud C (2005) Glucocorticosteroids for primary biliary cirrhosis. *Cochrane Database of Systematic Reviews*, Issue 2. Art. No.: CD003778. DOI: 10.1002/14651858.CD003778.pub2

Sherlock S, Dooley J (2002) *Diseases of the Liver and Biliary System*, 11th edn. Blackwell Publishing, Oxford

Swain MG (1999) Pruritus and lethargy in the primary biliary cirrhosis patient. In: Neuberger J (ed) *Primary Biliary Cirrhosis*. West End Studios, Eastbourne

Talwalker JA, Lindor KD (2003) Primary biliary cirrhosis. *The Lancet* **362**:53–61

Twycross R, Greaves MW, Handwerker H, Jones EA, Libretto SE, Szepietowski JC, Zylicz Z (2003) Itch: scratching more than the surface. *Quarterly Journal of Medicine* **96**:7–26

Vera A, Moledina S, Gunson B, Hubscher S, Mirza D, Olliff S, Neuberger J (2002) Risk factors for recurrence of primary sclerosing cholangitis of liver allograft. *The Lancet* **360**:1943–1944

Wiesner RH (2004) Primary sclerosing cholangitis. In: Friedman LS, Keefe EB (eds) *Handbook of Liver Disease*, 2nd edn. Churchill Livingstone, Philadelphia

Wilkinson MM (1992) Primary sclerosing cholangitis: what are the nursing implications? *Gastroenterology Nursing* 14:215–218

12

Metabolic liver disease

Rachel Taylor and Teresa Corbani

Introduction

There are several liver diseases caused by enzyme defects in the body's metabolic pathways. A large proportion of these present in childhood and, with advances in medical care, including transplantation, children are surviving into adulthood. While nurses may meet patients with a number of paediatric metabolic diseases, such as glycogen storage disease or Crigler Najjar, the focus of this chapter is on the metabolic liver diseases most commonly seen in adulthood. The chapter will discuss presentation, diagnosis and clinical management of patients with Wilson's disease, haemochromatosis, alpha-1-antitrypsin deficiency, cystic fibrosis liver disease and porphyria.

Wilson's disease

Wilson's disease (WD) is a rare but treatable disorder with an estimated incidence of 1 : 30 000 (Schilsky, 1996). Patients present from childhood to late adulthood with a diverse range of symptoms including acute and chronic liver disease and neuropsychiatric manifestations. WD was first described in 1912 by Kinnear Wilson, who noted progressive degeneration of lenticular nuclei with associated liver cirrhosis during a review of a series of autopsies. WD is attributed to a gene mutation coding for ATPase copper transporting beta polypeptide (ATP7B), which is located on chromosome 13 and expressed predominantly in the liver (Das and Ray, 2006). Over 300 mutations have been identified, the most common in central, eastern and northern Europe being H1069Q (Ferenci, 2006). No single mutation predominates, therefore genetic testing in not a diagnostic tool for index cases. However, as an autosomal recessive disorder, there is a 25% chance of siblings being affected therefore ATP7B mutation analysis is important for confirming diagnosis and family screening (Brewer and Askari, 2005)

The body requires 1–2 mg of copper a day which is obtained through dietary intake. It is absorbed mainly in the duodenum by binding to the protein metallo-thionein in the enterocytes. The copper-containing molecules bind with amino acids, polypeptides and albumin and are transported to the liver. Copper in the liver cells aids various enzyme processes and excess copper is excreted from the liver in bile. About 50% of metabolisable copper is stored in the muscles and bone, 15% in the liver and the remainder in the brain, heart and kidneys. The liver is central to copper homeostasis, which is regulated by hepatocytes mainly through biliary excretion or by binding the copper to caeruloplasmin. Caeruloplasmin is a glycoprotein synthesised by hepatocytes independent of the amount of copper. Copper binds to caeruloplasmin, which enables renal excretion. Excretion through the biliary system depends on glutathione and the ATP7B protein. Bound copper in the bile cannot be reabsorbed in the intestine, ensuring faecal excretion (Steinberg and Sternlieb, 1996; Loudianos and Gitlin, 2000).

The exact pathogenesis of copper accumulation in WD is unknown but the main hypotheses are:

- Diminished synthesis of caeruloplasmin by the liver. As a singular cause, this does not explain the accumulation of copper because 5–25% of patients with WD have normal caeruloplasmin. Furthermore, patients with acaeruloplasmi-naemia, a congenital deficiency, have no excess copper
- A block in transfer at the site of the hepatocyte uptake to the lyosomes. This might involve a deficiency or abnormality in a copper-binding protein or enzyme required for intracellular transport of the metal
- Reduced biliary excretion as a result of mutations in ATP7B

Clinical presentation

The most common presentation of WD is hepatic and/or neuropsychiatric but none of the presenting features are typical or diagnostic. A summary of the clinical manifestations of WD is shown in Table 12.1.

Acute hepatic Wilson's disease

Acute or fulminant liver failure occurs in approximately 5% of WD patients, 6–12% of all acute liver failure (ALF) patients in adults. There is an increased

Table 12.1 Clinical manifestations of Wilson's disease. Adapted from Ala et al. (2007); Das and Ray (2006)

Hepatic
    Increased transaminases
    Chronic hepatitis
    Cirrhosis
    Acute liver failure

Neurological
    Tremor
    Choreiform movements
    Parkinsonism or partial Parkinsonism
    Gait disturbances
    Dysarthria
    Pseudobulbar palsy
    Rigid dystonia
    Seizures
    Migraine headaches
    Insomnia

Ophthalmic
    KF rings
    Sunflower cataracts

Psychiatric
    Depression
    Neuroses
    Personality changes
    Psychosis

Haematological
    Acute non-immunological haemolytic anaemia
    Epistaxis

Orthopaedic
    Chondrocalcinosis
    Osteoarthritis
    Metabolic bone disease
    Juvenile polyarthritis
    Recurrent fracture and dislocation

Cardiovascular
    Arrythmias
    Rheumatic fever-like manifestations

Renal
    Renal tubular acidosis
    Hypercalciuria
    Microscopic haematuria and/or minimal proteinuria

Dermatological
    Hyperpigmentation

Gynaecological
    Primary or secondary amenorrhoea

preponderance in females (3:1) although the reason for this is unclear. The onset is rapid with typical features of ALF: coagulopathy and hepatic encephalopathy (see Chapter 13). There are usually no neurological symptoms and there can be an absence of Kayser-Fleischer (KF) rings, therefore rapid diagnosis is often not possible. Often diagnosis is made following transplantation or death. During this acute phase there is a large amount of copper released from the necrotic hepato-cytes causing severe Coombs-negative haemolytic anaemia. Liver histology shows massive necrosis (Das and Ray, 2006; Ala et al., 2007).

Chronic hepatic Wilson's disease

Chronic presentation is usually with chronic hepatitis or cirrhosis. Symptoms are non-specific: hepatosplenomegaly, ascites and jaundice. The younger the patient is at the time of diagnosis the greater the severity of liver disease. Disease progression depends on the effectiveness of treatment. Patients who develop end-stage liver disease have all the associated complications, such as portal hypertension, oesoph-ageal varices etc. An increased risk of developing hepatocellular carcinoma (HCC) in later adulthood has been noted in WD, more often in males (Gollan and Zakko, 2004; Brewer and Askari, 2005; Ala et al., 2007).

Neuropsychiatic Wilson's disease

Approximately 40–50% of patients with WD have neuropsychiatric symptoms. These usually present between the second and third decade, however neurological and behavioural problems can be present in younger WD patients and have been noted in patients up to 72 years of age. In those who have neuropsychiatric symp-toms, behavioural symptoms occur prior to neurological symptoms in 50% of cases. Neurological abnormalities can be classified as: akinetic–rigid symptom similar to Parkinson's disease; pseudosclerosis-dominated tremor; ataxia; or dys-tonic syndrome (Ala et al., 2007). However, there is varied neuropsychiatric pre-sentation (Table 12.1), which contributes to the difficulty in diagnosis. MRI is a valuable diagnostic instrument. Typically lesions are found in the putamen, globus pallidus, caudate, thalamus, midbrain, pons and cerebellum. Cortical atrophy and white matter changes can also be seen on MRI in WD patients.

Diagnosis

Diagnosis of WD is based on a number of clinical and laboratory abnormalities but no single test confirms WD (Ferenci, 2004). A summary of the diagnostic tests of WD is shown in Table 12.2.

Caeruloplasmin

Caeruloplasmin is an acute-phase reactant so levels may be elevated because of other inflammatory causes (Scheinberg and Sternlieb, 1996).

Table 12.2 Diagnostic tests of Wilson's disease. Adapted from Ferenci et al. (2003).

Test	Diagnostic range	Limitations
Serum caeruloplasmin	<0.2 g/L	Low levels seen in protein-losing enteropathy, nephritic syndrome, Kwashiorkor
24-hour urinary copper excretion	>1 μmol/24 hours	Elevated urine copper levels in autoimmune hepatitis, sclerosing cholangitis, chronic active hepatitis and nephritic syndrome
Hepatic copper	>250 μg/g dry weight	Acute cholestasis, Alagille syndrome and sclerosing cholangitis
KF rings	Present	Present in patients with prolonged cholestasis, primary biliary cirrhosis

Urinary copper

Urinary copper excretion in WD is inconsistent, varying from normal in asymptomatic patients to >157 μmol/24 hours in symptomatic patients and those with acute liver failure (Gollan and Zakko, 2004). Penicillamine promotes the urinary excretion of copper therefore a penicillamine challenge can be made (da Costa et al., 1992). D-Penicillamine 0.5 gm is administered prior to the 24-hour urine collection. However Gollan and Zakko (2004) advocate that this does not reliably distinguish WD from other liver diseases.

Liver biopsy

The normal hepatic copper content of the liver is less than 50 μg/g dry weight. A hepatic copper concentration >250 μg/g dry weight when accompanied by low caeruloplasmin is usually indicative of WD. However, high values of liver copper are seen in other liver conditions (Table 12.2). Ferenci et al. (2003) proposed an algorithm to aid the diagnosis of WD as no test is specific (Figure 12.1) and subsequently a score has been developed (Table 12.3). A score ≥4 is indicative of WD, 2–3 is probable but more tests are required and WD is unlikely with a score 0–1 (Ferenci, 2004).

Kayser-Fleischer rings

Kayser-Fleischer (KF) rings are a greenish brown ring on the cornea, present in 90% of symptomatic WD patients (Figure 12.2, Plate 12). The ring is caused by granular deposits of copper on the membrane of the cornea. KF rings can occasionally be seen by the naked eye or ophthalmoscope, however a slit lamp examination is usually required (Ferenci, 2003).

Table 12.3   Scoring system for the diagnosis of Wilson's disease. (ULN = upper limit of normal)

Parameter	Score
Symptoms	
KF rings (slit lamp examination)	
Present	2
Absent	0
Neuropsychiatric symptoms or typical brain MRI	
Present	2
Absent	0
Coombs negative haemolytic anaemia plus high serum copper	
Present	1
Absent	0
Laboratory investigations	
Urine copper in the absence of acute hepatitis	
Normal	0
1–2 × ULN	1
>2 × ULN	2
Normal but >5 × ULN after penicillamine challenge	2
Liver copper	
Normal	0
Up to 5 × ULN	1
>5 × ULN	2
Serum caeruloplasmin	
Normal	0
0.1–0.2 g/L	1
<0.1 g/L	2
Mutation analysis	
Disease causing mutations on both chromosomes	4
Disease causing mutations on one chromosome	1
No disease causing mutations	0

Family screening

WD is a genetic disorder therefore once it has been diagnosed in an index case evaluation of the family is important as there is a 1 in 4 chance siblings could be affected (Ferenci, 2004). Screening involves clinical examination, liver function test, caeruloplasmin and 24-hour urinary copper levels. If WD is present in asymptomatic siblings, chelation therapy (see below) is needed for life.

Management

Diet

A low-copper diet is not usually necessary, however patients should be advised to avoid foods with a high copper content. These include nuts, chocolate,

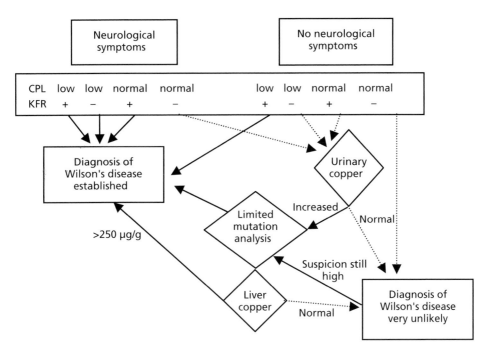

Figure 12.1 Algorithm for diagnosing Wilson's disease. Adapted from Ferenci (2003). (CPL = caeruloplasmin; KFR = Kayser-Fleischer rings)

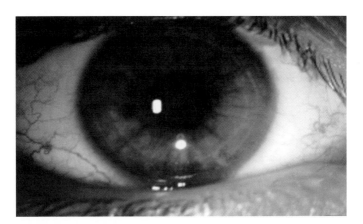

Figure 12.2 Kayser-Fleischer ring in a patient with Wilson's disease. Reproduced with permission from Ryder SD, Beckingham IJ (2001) ABC of diseases of liver, pancreas, and biliary system: Other causes of parenchymal liver disease. *British Medical Journal* **322**:290–292. For a colour version of this figure, please see Plate 12 in the colour plate section.

mushrooms, shellfish, liver and kidneys. A patient's drinking water source may also need to be checked if supplied through copper piping as this can increase dietary copper intake (Roberts and Schilsky, 2003).

Pharmacological therapy

Life-long pharmacological therapy is required to treat patients with WD. The aim of treatment is to 'decopper' the liver, i.e. promote excretion of excess circulating copper. Pharmacological agents currently used in WD are summarised in Table 12.4. The American Association for the Study of Liver Disease (AASLD) practice guidelines on WD state initial treatment of all symptomatic patients should include the chelating agents, penicillamine and trientine. In the UK only penicillamine has a licence for initial use. Trientine is licensed for use in patients who develop toxic side effects to penicillamine.

Penicillamine reduces the copper bound to protein, and therefore increases urinary excretion. Excretion can be as much as 1000–3000 μg/day. However, penicillamine is associated with numerous side effects (Table 12.4), which occur in approximately 20% of patients (Sherlock and Dooley, 2002). In order to prevent the occurrence of side effects, penicillamine is introduced at a lower dose and gradually increased until the patient tolerates a full dose. If patients are unable to tolerate penicillamine they can be converted to trientine, which has a similar action. Both penicillamine and trientine are potentially teratogenic. In an early publication, Walshe (1986) reported 11 normal pregnancies in seven patients with WD, all of whom were receiving trientine. Cessation of chelation therapy can be fatal so chelation therapy needs to be continued throughout pregnancy.

Other pharmacological therapies that are currently used are zinc acetate or sulphate and ammonium tetrathiomolybdate (TTM). Both medications interfere with the absorption of copper in the intestine. TTM is currently not available in the UK. Zinc has been advocated for use in pre-symptomatic patients identified through family screening. Zinc can also be given with penicillamine as it has a different action of eliminating copper. Zinc is chemically similar to copper therefore should never be administered together with penicillamine or it will be chelated in the same way. Future therapies include antioxidants (vitamin E and N-acetylcysteine) to reduce the oxidant damage in the liver, and gene therapy (Ryder and Beckingham, 2001; Brewer, 2005).

Liver transplantation

Liver transplantation is the treatment of choice in patients presenting with fulminant WD, in those in whom medical therapy is ineffective or for patients with decompensated cirrhosis. Survival rates are as high as 87% but total reversal of all neurological symptoms is not always possible (Roberts and Schilsky, 2003).

Table 12.4 Drugs used in the treatment of Wilson's disease.

Drug	Action	Dose	Side effects
Penicillamine	Chelator, promotes cupuresis	Initial therapy: 1.5–2 g in divided doses before food for 1 year. Maintenance dose: 0.75–1 g a day	Nausea, anorexia, skin reaction, leucopenia, thrombocytopenia, aplastic anaemia, proteinuria
Trientine	Chelator, promotes cupuresis	1.2–2.4 g/day in two to four divided doses	Nausea, rash, rarely anaemia
Zinc	Reduces copper absorption from the gastrointestinal tract	Maintenance dose: 50 mg q8 h	Gastric irritation, less commonly sideroblastic anaemia and leucopenia
Ammonium tetrathiomolybdate	Reduces absorption of copper from the gastrointestinal tract. Renders copper unavailable for celluar uptake	40 mg TDS (dose divided to during and post meal times)	Anaemia, bone marrow depression

Haemochromatosis

Haemochromatosis is 'an iron-loading disorder caused by genetically determined failure to prevent unneeded dietary iron from entering the circulatory pool and is characterised by progressive parenchymal iron overload with the potential for multiorgan damage and disease' (Pietrangelo, 2006). While there are five types of haemochromatosis (Table 12.5), 90% of patients have type 1 HFE haemochromatosis, which will be the main focus of this chapter.

Only 10% of dietary iron intake is absorbed in the intestine, which is the body's mechanism of regulating iron metabolism. Iron is stored in the liver and is required for erthyropoesis. The body has difficulty in excreting iron, the only way is through bleeding. This may explain why women tend to present much later than men because of the protective action of menstruation and child birth. Defects in the genes associated with iron metabolism (Table 12.5) result in increased absorption of iron. Excess is stored in the hepatocytes but iron deposits can also accumulate in endocrine glands and heart. The time for symptoms to develop depends on the mutation. HFE and TfR2 mutations occur in a milder form mostly in middle age, whereas patients with the more severe forms (hemojuvelin gene (HJV) and hepcidin antimicrobial peptide (HAMP)) present and often die before 30 years of age (McFarlane et al., 2000; Mahl and O'Grady, 2006).

Presentation

Similarly to WD, haemochromatosis does not have any specific symptoms but it needs to be suspected in middle-aged men with cirrhosis, bronze skin, diabetes, joint inflammation and heart disease (Pietrangelo, 2006). The most common symptoms are fatigue, malaise, arthralgia and hepatomegaly, therefore haemochromatosis might not be suspected until there is significant, irreversible organ damage. While the liver is the primary site of damage, iron deposits in other organs can lead to a number of other conditions, such as diabetes, heart failure, arthritis, hypothyroidism and increased pigmentation (bronze skin).

Table 12.5 Types of haemochromatosis.

Type	Mutation
1	HFE gene
2: juvenile (type a and b)	HJV or HAMP genes
3	Transferrin receptor 2 (TfR2) gene
4	Mutation of ferroportin gene
5	Rare forms due to mutations in caeruloplasmin, transferrin or divalent metal transporter 1 (DMT1) gene

Diagnosis

Standard liver function tests are of limited use in the initial diagnosis of haemochromatosis as these are only mildly elevated and give no indication of the underlying condition (McFarlane et al., 2000). If haemochromatosis is undetected the elevation in liver function tests will correlate with the development of cirrhosis. Brissot and de Bels (2006) suggest a four-stage process in diagnosing haemochromatosis:

1. Investigate transferrin saturation level (serum iron divided by total iron binding capacity (TBC) × 100), the earliest biochemical indicator. Haemochromatosis would be suspected if this was elevated >80%
2. Perform genetic tests, typically C282Y mutation
3. Quantify the iron overload using plasma ferritin level. Mild overload <500 µg/L, moderate 500–1000 µg/L and severe >1000 µg/L (this would be accompanied by severe clinical complications)
4. Stage the phenotypic manifestion:
   - Stage 0: no biochemical or clinical symptoms
   - Stage I: increased transferrin, normal ferritin, no clinical symptoms
   - Stage II: increased transferrin, increased ferritin, no clinical symptoms
   - Stage III: increased transferrin, increased ferritin, clinical symptoms
   - Stage IV: increased transferrin, increased ferritin, clinical symptoms causing organ damage, i.e., cirrhosis

Management

The reduction of systemic iron overload is key to the management of haemochromatosis, therefore the main treatment involves removal of accumulated iron through therapeutic phlebotomy. This should be started when the patient is at stage II. Significant quantities of blood need to be removed to achieve a ferritin level of <50 µg/L. One unit of blood (approximately 400–500 mL) removes 250 mg of iron. Patients may have 200 times this amount (Sherlock and Dooley, 2002) therefore weekly or twice weekly venesection with the removal of one unit of blood is necessary to achieve the desired serum ferritin level and transferrin saturations of <30% (EASL, 2000). Due to fluctuations in ferritin levels, it is advised these are checked every 10–12 venesections. Haemocrit should be checked before each session with the target range being no lower than 20% below the previous level (Tavill, 2001). It may take 2–3 years to adequately reduce stored iron to a ferritin level of <50 µg/L (Pietrangelo, 2004). Once iron stores have been mobilised, maintenance phlebotomy will vary depending on the individual, ranging from once a month to three or four times a year to prevent re-accumulation (Tavill and Kowdley, 2004). Chelation with desferrioxamine is only used if venesection is contraindicated, i.e. anaemia.

Therapeutic phlebotomy will relieve symptoms such as malaise, fatigue, skin pigmentation and abdominal pain, and improve liver function tests. Cirrhosis, diabetes, hypogonadism and arthritis cannot be reversed but the disease progression can be slowed. In addition improvements in fibrosis and insulin requirements have been noted (Pietrangelo, 2004). It is important nurses caring for patients with haemochromatosis with diabetes take into consideration blood glucose levels whilst patients are undergoing venesection therapy. This requires careful monitoring and adjustment of insulin or tablet therapy (Clayton and Holt, 2006). Patients may benefit from being referred to an endocrinologist or diabetic nurse specialist for advice and effective management during this phase of treatment.

The risk of HCC is increased 200-fold in patients with cirrhotic haemochromatosis; therefore it is important patients are screened every 6–12 months with ultrasonography and measurement of alpha-fetoprotein (AFP) levels. After the de-ironing process HCC can still occur (see Chapter 17 for further information).

Dietary management

Patients need to be educated to avoid food with a high iron content, e.g. red meat, fortified cereals etc., therefore a dietetic referral is important. Patients also need to avoid high doses of ascorbic acid, citric acid and vitamin C because ascorbic acid increases the absorption of iron. Dietary supplements containing iron are also not recommended (Tavill and Kowdley, 2004). There is evidence to suggest that alcohol can accelerate disease progression and increase iron absorption therefore reduced alcohol intake is recommended.

Liver transplantation

Survival post liver transplant for end-stage liver disease due to haemochromatosis is known to be poorer than other conditions, with a 50–60% survival at 1 year (Tavill and Kowdley, 2004). Over time the allograft may be at risk of iron re-accumulation (Bacon, 2006). Cardiac- or infection-related complications can also arise, particularly in patients who are not diagnosed or treated prior to transplantation (Tavill, 2001).

Screening

Screening is recommended in two target populations: in patients with unexplained liver disease or diabetes with hepatomegaly; and in patients who are asymptomatic but are first-degree relatives of haemochromatosis sufferers with unexplained abnormal liver function tests (Tavill, 2001). It has been advocated that all first-degree relatives should be screened (Bacon, 2006).

Alpha-1-antitrypsin deficiency

Alpha-1-antitrypsin deficiency (A1ATD) is a common autosomal disease predominantly in Caucasian people. It results in pulmonary disease and to a lesser extent liver disease, being the most common paediatric metabolic disorder requiring liver transplantation (Abusriwil and Stockley, 2006; Bonkovsky and Reichheld, 2006). The disease prevalence varies geographically with disease incidence ranging from 1:1700 in northern Europe to 1:1800–2000 in the USA (Quist et al., 2000).

Alpha-1-antitrypsin (AAT) is a serine protease inhibitor, which is secreted primarily in the liver parenchymal cells and to a lesser extent in macrophages. It is present in tears, duodenal fluid, saliva, nasal secretions, cerebrospinal fluid, pulmonary secretions and milk (Morrison and Kowdley, 2000). AAT protects tissues by inactivating a variety of proteases including trypsin, neutrophil elastase, collagenase and chymotrypsin. The pathogenesis of chronic liver disease associated with A1ATD remains controversial, with several postulated theories which include: proteolytic imbalance due to decreased serum AAT; secondary to an abnormal immune response; and overaccumulation of protein within the hepatocytes causing direct hepatocyte injury (Quist et al., 2000). Pulmonary injury occurs due to the diminished protection of AAT from the damage of neutrophil elastase, which leads to the degradation of elastic tissue and the eventual development of emphysema (Abusriwil and Stockley, 2006).

The gene encoding for AAT is located on chromosome 14q3, however more than 90 genetic variants (allele) have been identified by studying electrophoretograms of serum AAT. The alleles (phenotypes identification: Pi) are named alphabetically according to the alleles migration speed on isoelectric focus gel. Consequently the letter A is indicative of a fast migration, whereas the letter Z is indicative of a slower migration (Abusriwil and Stockley, 2006; Bonkovsky and Reichheld, 2006). M is the most common allele, accounting for 95% of those found in Caucasian people, whilst S and Z are the most common mutant alleles (Bonkovsky and Reichheld, 2006). Liver disease is primarily associated with the PiZZ phenotype in which the risk of homozygous offspring inheriting the disorder is 1 in 4 if both parents are carriers of the Z mutation. PiZZ phenotype is associated with the development of liver disease in about 15–30% and affects both children and adults (Quist et al., 2000). Hepatic manifestations of A1ATD in children are coagulopathy, protracted jaundice and neonatal hepatitis. Adults present with chronic hepatitis, cirrhosis and HCC (Mahl and O'Grady, 2006).

Diagnosis

A1ATD should be a differential diagnosis in jaundiced neonates, infants who have failure-to-thrive or poor feeding, and any patient who presents with unexplained, asymptomatic hepatomegaly, elevated transaminases, chronic hepatitis, cirrhosis, portal hypertension or HCC of unknown aetiology (Rosen and Schwartz, 2004). Diagnosis can be confirmed by:

- Serum alpha-1 phenotype determination (Pi typing) by isoelectric focusing or immunofixation

- Serum levels of AAT <25% of lower normal limit (normal range 800 mg/L)
- Liver biopsy

It is important to note that as an acute phase reactant, false high AAT levels may be seen in patients with an acute inflammatory state (Bonkovsky and Reichheld, 2006).

Management

In the absence of chronic liver disease, the management of A1ATD is primarily supportive and patients should be encouraged to: avoid smoking, avoid secondary smoke and air pollution, maintain an adequate nutritional intake, take oral supplements of fat-soluble vitamins and avoid alcohol (Quist et al., 2000). Additional strategies should include genetic counselling and phenotype identification of relatives and patients with A1ATD to ascertain those at high risk. Other experimental treatments for both pulmonary disease and hepatic disease include infusions or inhalation of purified plasma AAT and gene therapy (Bonkovsky and Reichheld, 2006).

Liver transplantation

Liver transplantation is advocated for patients with progressive liver failure and portal hypertension although the disease progression is relatively slow. Survival rates following transplant are 80% at 1 year and 70% at 5 years. Importantly, the donor liver synthesises normal protein, therefore the condition will not recur in new graft (Bonkovsky and Reichheld, 2006).

Cystic fibrosis

Cystic fibrosis (CF) is an inherited, autosomal recessive disease of epithelial cell ion transport. It affects approximately 1:2000 newborn Caucasian babies, with an estimated 5% carrier rate (Sherlock and Dooley, 2002; Rosen and Schwartz, 2004). Although CF is more commonly associated with pulmonary disease and pancreatic and sweat gland insufficiency, hepatobiliary abnormalities of varying severity occur in over a third of CF patients. This is the second leading cause of death (Bonkovsky and Reichheld, 2006). Additionally, as treatment for CF has improved life expectancy beyond 30 years of age, there has been a rise in the prevalence of CF-related liver disease (McFarlane et al., 2000).

The gene responsible for CF is located on chromosome 7 and encodes for the cystic fibrosis transmembrane regulator (CFTR). More than 200 mutations of the gene responsible for CF have been reported. A defective CFTR results in diminished chloride channel conductance, causing the inability to maintain sufficient lumen fluid, which leads to thick viscous secretions and abnormal bile composition and flow (Rosen and Schwartz, 2004; Bonkovsky and Reichheld, 2006; Colombo et al., 2006). Intrahepatic bile ducts collect plugs of inspissated biliary secretions, leading to progressive periportal fibrosis and cirrhosis. The reason only a third of patients with CF develop liver disease is unclear but factors such as nutrition, antioxidants and non-adherence have been suggested as triggers.

Presentation

Patients often present when hepatosplenomegaly is found during routine clinical examination. This can be with or without abnormal biochemistry. Abnormal liver function tests are not usually seen, however, patients can present with a cholestatic profile (elevated GGT and ALP). If there is neonatal cholestasis or end-stage biliary cirrhosis the patient will be jaundiced. The most common presentation is portal hypertension and oesophageal varices. If patients have end-stage liver disease they will also present with severe malnutrition, osteodystrophy and reduced pulmonary status.

Diagnosis

Liver disease in patients with CF is often subclinical therefore it is often under-diagnosed. Similar to patients with chronic liver disease, diagnosis is made on the basis of physical clinical examination, conventional liver biochemistry, liver biopsy and ultrasonography (Colombo et al., 2006).

Management

Management is based on treating the symptoms accompanying cirrhosis, such as portal hypertension and oesophageal varies. Patients with CF are at greater risk of developing malnutrition than patients with other liver disorders because of an increased energy expenditure, anorexia, fat malabsorption (cholestasis and pancreatic insufficiency) and abnormal nutrient metabolism. Referral to a dietician and careful monitoring of nutritional status are therefore important (Colombo et al., 2006). Bile acid replacement therapy (ursodeoxycholic acid) has been proposed as supportive treatment in patients with CF liver disease because it reduces bile duct proliferation, inflammation and fibrosis. Patients have improved essential fatty deficiency and liver biochemistry. The impact on the natural history of liver disease has yet to be determined (Paumgartner and Beuers, 2002).

Liver transplantation

Liver transplantation is a treatment option for patients with CF with end-stage liver disease if pulmonary dysfunction is mild. Survival at 1 year is approximately

80% and transplantation has the added benefit of improving not only liver function but also pulmonary function and nutritional status (Colombo et al., 2006).

Porphyria

Most people have the image of the 'madness of King George' when they think of porphyria. However it is a disorder accompanied with photosensitivity, hepatic disease as well as neuropsychiatric symptoms. Porphyria is a group of disorders caused by a deficiency in enzyme activity of the haem biosynthesis pathway (Figure 12.3). Most are inherited but not all carriers of the gene develop clinical disease (McFarlane et al., 2000). There are over 400 different mutations of the gene therefore it is not useful for clinical diagnosis in an index case but is important for family screening. There are seven types of porphyria, which are classified as

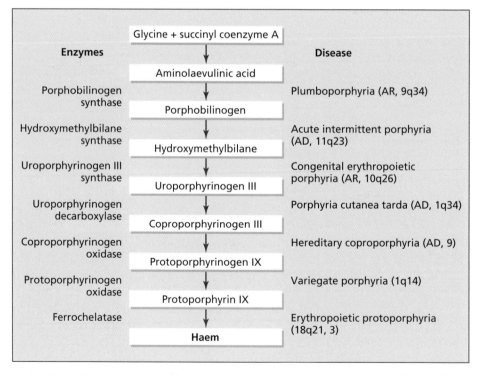

Figure 12.3 Pathway of haem synthesis. Blocks at various parts of the pathway result in different porphyrias. Reproduced with permission from Thandani et al. (2000) Diagnosis and management of porphyria. *British Medical Journal* **320**:1647–1651. (AR = autosomal recessive; AD = autosomal dominant)

Table 12.6 Types of porphyria. Adapted from Peters and Sarkaney (2005). (ALA = δ-aminolaevulinic acid; PBG = porphobilinogen; GI = gastrointestinal)

Type	Main clinical features	Diagnosis
Erythropoietic		
Congenital erythropoietic porphyria (CEP)	Severe skin lesions Haemolytic anaemia	Normal ALA and PBG ↑ urinary and faecal porphyrins ↑ red cell protoporphyrins
Erythropoietic protoporphyria (EPP)	Acute photosensitivity Mild anaemia	↑ red cell protoporphyrin IX
Acute hepatic		
ALA dehydratase porphyria (ADP)	Abdominal pain	↑ urinary ALA and copro III Normal faecal porphyrins
Acute intermittent porphyria (AIP)	Abdominal pain Motor neuropathy GI disturbances Neuropsychiatric features	↑ ALA and PBG ↑ urinary porphyrins
Hereditary coproporphyria (HCP)	Neuropsychiatric features Vesicular skin lesions	↑ ALA and PBG ↑ urinary and faecal copro III
Variegate porphyria (VP)	Neuropsychiatric features Vesicular skin lesions	Characteristic plasma fluorescence ↑ faecal protoporphyrins
Chronic hepatic		
Porphyria cutanea tarda (PCT)	Marked skin lesions	Normal ALA and PBG ↑ urinary and faecal porphyrins especially carboxylic porphyrins
Hepatoerythropoietic porphyria (HEP)	Blistering skin lesions Hypertrichosis Red urine	

erthyropoietic, acute hepatic porphyria or chronic hepatic porphyria (Table 12.6) (Sassa, 2006).

Presentation

Erythropoietic porphyrias are the most severe and present in childhood. Patients with acute hepatic porphyrias present with similar symptoms, the differential diagnosis depends on the diagnostic test. The most common complaints in the acute hepatic porphyrias are: abdominal pain, vomiting, constipation, muscle weakness, mental symptoms, pain (limb, head, neck and chest), hypertension, tachycardia, convulsions, sensory loss, fever, respiratory paralysis and diarrhoea. Patients with acute intermittent porphyria (AIP) can have 'port-wine' reddish urine which is due to the presence of porphobilin (the oxidised product of porphobilinogen (PBG)). Patients with chronic hepatic porphyria present with significant cutaneous photosensitivity, including blistering on exposed skin in the sun, facial hypertrichosis and hyperpigmentation (Peters and Sarkany, 2005; Sassa, 2006).

Diagnosis

The diagnosis of porphyria is based on the presence of porphyrin prescursors δ-aminolaevulinic acid (ALA) and/or PBG (Table 12.6).

Management

The mainstay of management is avoiding precipitating factors. These include a number of medications, reduced calorie intake, smoking, infection, surgery, stress, and in those with photosensitivity, the sun. In acute attacks in patients with acute hepatic porphyria, intravenous glucose (approx 400 g/day) is required. Intravenous haematin, such as Normosang (Orphan-Europe Ltd) can be given to curtail the urinary excretion of ALA and PBG. Porphyria cutanea tarda (PCT) and hepato-erythropoietic porphyria (HEP) are treated with repeated phlebotomy to normalise serum ferritin levels. If this is ineffective chloroquine therapy can used. Chloro-quine is thought to chelate porphyrins promoting urinary excretion (Thadani et al., 2000; Soonawalla et al., 2004; Sassa, 2006).

Chapter summary

This chapter has provided a brief overview of pathophysiology, presentation and disease management of some of the more commonly found metabolic diseases that lead to complex complications and hepatic manifestations. However, it is only the advancement of molecular biology that has allowed us to identify the genetic defects responsible for some of these conditions thus enabling us to ascertain a greater understanding of the disease processes. Treatment varies due to the under-lying disease pathogenesis, with the aim of slowing or treating the disease process. Cirrhosis and end-stage liver disease can potentially complicate most of these metabolic conditions.

Illustrative case study

A 21-year-old female presented with a febrile illness, diarrhoea, dark urine and jaundice. She had no previous medical or relevant family history. Laboratory investigations suggested haemolysis and pantocytopenia: haemogloblin 8.5 g/L, red cell count 2.32×10^{12}/L, platelets 71×10^{9}/L. The patient had a PT of 0.16 seconds, serum bilirubin 284 µmol/L, AST 73 IU/L, ALT 31 IU/L, GGT 61 IU/L and ALP 55 IU/L. An abdominal ultrasound scan revealed normal biliary tract, small nodular liver suggesting cirrhosis, enlarged spleen and no ascites or focal lesions.

An upper gastrointestinal endoscopy showed grade II oesophageal varices. Autoantibodies and viral serology were negative but serum ferritin was elevated (638 g/L) and caeroplasmin decreased (0.17 g/L). Further investigation demonstrated a serum copper level of 17.2 µmol/L and urinary copper excretion of 13.2 µmol/24 hours. KF rings were detectable on slit lamp examination therefore a diagnosis of Wilson's disease was made. The patient was commenced on D-penicillamine 1.2 g daily and discharged home with a planned elective admission in 8 weeks for further assessment.

However, within 6 weeks the patient re-presented with lower abdominal pain, and rapidly deteriorating hepatic function. She developed advanced hepatic encephalopathy (grade III/IV), coagulopathy (INR 3.7), renal failure (serum creatinine 395 µmol/L) and frequent episodes of hypoglycaemia. Her remaining laboratory investigations revealed a platelet count of 35×10^9/L, serum bilirubin 700 µmol/L, AST 45 IU/L, ALT 13 IU/L, ALP 25 IU/L and albumin 22 g/L. A further ultrasound scan showed patent vessels and mild ascites. After elective endotracheal intubation the patient was transferred to a liver transplant centre. Fulfilling King's poor prognosis criteria, the patient was super-urgently listed for liver transplantation and received an orthotopic liver transplant 48 hours later. The patient made a good postoperative recovery regaining spontaneous renal function.

This example shows the importance of taking chelation therapy. There is the possibility that the patient deteriorated because she was non-adherent.

References

Abusriwil H, Stockley RA (2006) Alpha-1-antirypsin replacement therapy: current status. *Current Opinion in Pulmonary Medicine* **12**(2):125–131

Ala A, Walker AP, Ashkan K, Dooley JS, Schilsky AL (2007) Wilson's disease. *The Lancet* **369**:397–408

Bacon BR (2006) Hereditary hemochromatosis. In: Bacon B, O'Grady J, Di Bisceglie A, Lake J (eds) *Comprehensive Clinical Hepatology*, 2nd edn. Mosby Elsevier, Philadelphia

Bonkovsky HL, Reichheld JH (2006) The porphyrias, α1-antitrypsin deficiency, cystic fibrosis and other metabolic diseases of the liver. In: Bacon B, O'Grady J, Di Bisceglie A, Lake J (eds) *Comprehensive Clinical Hepatology*, 2nd edn. Mosby Elsevier, Philadelphia

Brewer GJ (2005) Neurologically presenting Wilson's disease: epidemiology, pathophysiology and treatment. *CNS Drugs* **19**:185–192

Brewer GJ, Askari FK (2005) Wilson's disease: clinical management and therapy. *Journal of Hepatology* **42**(Suppl):13–21

Brissot P, de Bels F (2006) Current approaches to the management of haemochromatosis. *Hematology* 36–41

Clayton M, Holt P (2006) Hereditary haemochromatosis and diabetes – implications for practice. *Gastrointestinal Nursing* 4(8):22–26

Colombo C, Russo M, Zazzeron L, Romano G (2006) Liver disease in cystic fibrosis. *Journal of Pediatric Gastroenterology and Nutrition* 43:S49–S55

da Costa M, Baldwin D, Portmann B, Lolin Y, Moat AP, Mieli-Vergani G (1992) Value of urinary copper excretion after penicillamine challenge in the diagnosis of Wilson's disease. *Hepatology* 15:609–615

Das SK, Ray K (2006) Wilson's disease: an update. *Nature: Clinical Practice Neurology* 2(9):482–493

European Association of the Study of the Liver (2000) EASL International consensus conference on haemochromatosis: Part II expert document. *Journal of Hepatology* 33:487–496

Ferenci P (2004) Review article: diagnosis and current therapy of Wilson's disease. *Alimentary Pharmacology & Therapeutics* 19(2):157–165

Ferenci P (2006) Wilson disease. In: Bacon B, O'Grady J, Di Bisceglie A, Lake J (eds) *Comprehensive Clinical Hepatology*, 2nd edn. Mosby Elsevier, Philadelphia

Ferenci P, Cac K, Loudianis G, Mieli-Vergani G, Tanner S, Sternlieb I, Schilsky M, Cox D, Berr F (2003) Diagnosis and phenotypic classification of Wilson disease. *Liver International* 23:139–142

Gollan J, Zakko WF (2004) Wilson Disease and related disorders of copper. In: Friedman LS, Keeffe E (eds) *Handbook of Liver Disease*, 2nd edn. Elsevier, Philadelphia

Loudianos G, Gitlin JD (2000) Wilson's disease. *Seminars in Liver Disease* 20:353–364

Mahl T, O'Grady J (2006) *Fast Facts: Liver Disorders*. Health Press, Oxford

McFarlane I, Bomford A, Sherwood R (2000) *Liver Disease and Laboratory Medicine*. ACB Venture Publications, London

Morrison ED, Kowdley KV (2000) Genetic liver disease in adults. *Postgraduate Medicine* 107(2):147–159

Paumgartner G, Beuers U (2002) Ursodeoxycholic acid in cholestatic liver disease: mechanisms of action and therapeutic use revisited. *Hepatology* 36: 525–531

Peters TJ, Sarkany R (2005) Porphyria for the general physician. *Clinical Medicine* 5:275–281

Pietrangelo A (2004) Hereditary haemochromatosis: a new look at an old disease. *New England Journal of Medicine* 350(23):2383–2397

Pietrangelo A (2006) Hereditary haemochromatosis. *Annual Review of Nutrition* 26:251–71

Quist RG, Baker AJ, Dhawan A, Bass NM (2000) *Metabolic Liver Disease in Comprehensive Clinical Hepatology*. Mosby Press, London

Roberts WA, Schilsky ML (2003) A practice guideline on Wilson disease, AASLD Practice Guideline. *Hepatology* 37(6):1475–1492

Rosen HR, Schwartz J (2004) Alpha-1 antitrypsin deficiency and other metabolic liver diseases. In: Friedman LS, Keeffe E (eds) *Handbook of Liver Disease*, 2nd edn. Elsevier, Philadelphia

Ryder SD, Beckingham IJ (2001) ABC of diseases of liver, pancreas, and biliary system: Other causes of parenchymal liver disease. *British Medical Journal* **322**:290–292

Sassa S (2006) Modern diagnosis and management of porphyrias. *British Journal of Haematology* **135**:281–292

Scheinberg IH, Sternlieb I (1996) Wilson disease and idiopathic toxicosis. *American Journal of Clinical Nutrition* **63**:842s–845s

Schilsky ML (1996) Wilson disease: genetic basis of copper toxicity and natural history. *Seminars in Liver Disease* **16**:83–95

Sherlock S, Dooley J (2002) *Disease of the Liver and Biliary System*, 11th edn. Blackwell Publishing, Oxford

Soonawalla ZF, Orug T, Badminton MN, Elder GH, Rhodes JM Bramhall SR, Elias E (2004) Liver transplantation as a cure for acute intermittent porphyries. *The Lancet* **363**:705–706

Tavill AS (2001) Diagnosis and management of haemochromatosis. AASLD Practice Guidelines. *Hepatology* **33**(5):1321–1328

Tavill AS, Kowdley KV (2004) Hemochromatosis. In: Friedman LS, Keeffe E (eds) *Handbook of Liver Disease*, 2nd edn. Elsevier, Philadelphia

Thadani H, Deacon A, Peters T (2000) Diagnosis and management of porphyria. *British Medical Journal* **320**:1647–1651

Walshe JM (1986) The management of pregnancy in Wilson's disease treated with trientine. *Quarterly Journal of Medicine* **58**:81–87

13

Acute liver failure

Zebina Ratansi

Introduction

Acute liver failure (ALF) or fulminant hepatic failure (FHF) are interchangeable terms used to describe a rare condition that is characterised by severe liver injury, jaundice and hepatic encephalopathy, usually in the absence of pre-existing liver disease (Benhamou, 1991). ALF has many causes and, despite improvement in critical care management, morbidity and mortality remain high. Orthotopic liver transplantation (OLT) remains the only effective treatment for those patients who are unlikely to recover spontaneously (Shakil et al., 2000; Gill and Sterling, 2001). ALF invariably leads to multi-organ failure and all patients have some degree of hepatic encephalopathy, which, when advanced, results in a high incidence of cerebral oedema and intracranial hypertension (Sargent and Fullwood, 2006), making this group of patients extremely challenging to manage. Therefore appropriate nursing and medical management of these patients are imperative to ensure successful bridging to liver transplantation.

Definition

ALF can be defined as sudden onset of liver impairment rapidly leading to encephalopathy and multi-organ dysfunction (Bernal and Wendon, 2000). However this definition alone does not reflect differences in clinical features and prognosis which

Table 13.1 Classification of acute liver failure (O'Grady et al., 1993).

Definition	Interval jaundice to encephalopathy	Cerebral oedema	Prognosis (survival)
Hyperacute	<7 days	Common >70%	Moderate (36%)
Acute	8–28 days	Common >55%	Poor (7%)
Subacute	5–12 weeks	Low <15%	Poor (14%)

has led to a reclassification depending on the onset of jaundice to the development of encephalopathy (Table 13.1). In hyperacute liver failure, encephalopathy occurs within 7 days of the onset of jaundice. This group of patients has a high likelihood of surviving with supportive management only, despite the high incidence of cerebral oedema. ALF, on the other hand, has a poorer prognosis without transplantation. Jaundice occurs 8–28 days after the onset of encephalopathy. In this group the incidence of cerebral oedema is also high. In subacute liver failure the interval between the onset of jaundice and the development of encephalopathy ranges from 5–12 weeks. This group also has a high mortality rate, despite a very low incidence of cerebral oedema (O'Grady et al., 1993; O'Grady, 2006).

Aetiology

The aetiology of ALF varies considerably worldwide, there are differences between the developing and developed world (Figure 13.1, Plate 13). Viral infection (hepatitis A, B and E) is the most common cause of ALF in the developing world, whereas drug-induced hepatotoxicity, especially acetaminophen (paracetamol), is the most common cause of ALF in the USA and western Europe (Bernal and Wendon, 2000). Seronegative or non A-E hepatitis is the most common presumed viral cause of ALF, in the UK it accounts for 56% of such cases (O'Grady, 2006). Other rare viral causes of ALF include infection with cytomegalovirus, Epstein-Barr virus, herpes virus, varicella zoster virus, adenovirus and paramyxoma virus (Gill and Sterling, 2001).

Idiosyncratic drug reaction can culminate in acute or subacute liver failure and carry a poor prognosis without liver transplant (Gill and Sterling, 2001). Certain herbal preparations and other nutritional supplements have also been found to cause liver injury (Polson and Lee, 2005). In addition, the recreational drug, ecstasy, has also been implicated as a cause of ALF, either through direct hepatotoxic effect or after fulminant hyperthermia and rhabdomyolysis (Bernal and Wendon, 2000).

Mushroom poisoning, usually *Amanita phalloides*, is most commonly found in the west coast of the USA, central Europe and South Africa. Other hepatotoxins include yellow phosphors, carbon tetrachloride, aflotoxin and some herbal medicines. Acute fatty liver of pregnancy, HELLP syndrome (haemolysis, elevated liver enzymes, low platelets), autoimmune hepatitis, Wilson's disease and Budd-Chiari

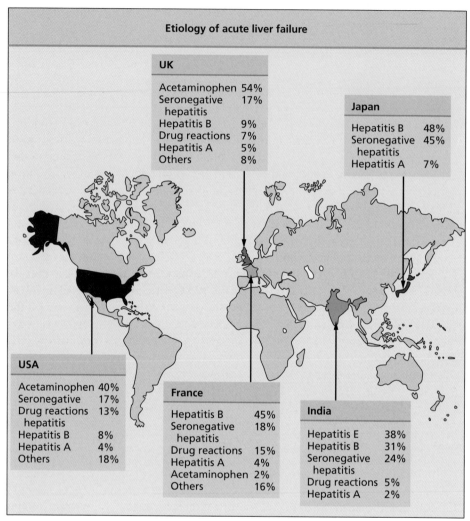

© Elsevier 2006. Bacon, O'Grady, Di Bisceglie and Lake: Comprehensive Clinical Hepatology, 2nd edition

Figure 13.1 Worldwide aetiology of acute liver failure. Reproduced from Bacon et al. (2006) with permission from Elsevier. For a colour version of this figure, please see Plate 13 in the colour plate section.

syndrome can all cause ALF (Gill and Sterling, 2001; Polson and Lee, 2005; O'Grady, 2006).

Presentation

The most common clinical features of ALF are abnormal biochemistries, jaundice, coagulopathy and hepatic encephalopathy. The normal histological pattern seen in ALF is hepatocellular necrosis with or without preservation of hepatic architecture. Jaundice is present in most patients, but some cases of hyperacute liver failure, such as acetaminophen poisoning, develop encephalopathy before jaundice becomes clinically apparent. Most other signs of liver failure are absent. Liver cell necrosis will lead to elevation of aminotransferase (AST), but relatively normal AST may be found and this usually signifies that massive necrosis has already occurred, particularly if associated with deep jaundice. Bilirubin concentrations that are persistently >300 μmol/L also suggest that disease is severe. ALP concentrations are rarely elevated above three times the upper limit of normal (ULN). The PT or international normalised ratio (INR) is usually grossly prolonged. In general if the PT is prolonged by 4–6 seconds in the presence of hepatic encephalopathy, a diagnosis of ALF is made. In ALF profound hypoglycaemia can occur and disturbances of acid–base balance are frequent.

The high mortality rates associated with ALF are caused by the complications of ALF, which include the development of cerebral oedema, renal failure, sepsis and cardiopulmonary collapse that result in multi-system organ failure (Gill and Sterling, 2001; Jalan, 2005; Polson and Lee, 2005; O'Grady, 2006). These patients require close monitoring and organ support in an intensive care environment.

Transfer criteria

The main strategy for patients presenting with ALF is to support liver regeneration or support the failing liver. Early discussion with the local liver transplant centre is imperative. Time is of the essence in the management of patients with ALF because rapid deterioration is commonly seen (Jalan, 2005). Two key factors need to be considered when assessing patients with ALF: the need to refer patients to a specialist centre and the selection of these patients for liver transplantation. The Kings College Hospital referral criteria are divided into two groups, one following acetaminophen (paracetamol) hepatotoxicity (Table 13.2) and the other for patients with non-acetaminophen aetiologies (Table 13.3) (O'Grady, 2006).

If the patient is referred to a specialist centre, it is critical to ensure clear communication between all teams, the intensive care unit (ICU) team, transfer team and the referral unit, to enable all parties to prepare adequately for safe transportation of the patient.

Table 13.2   Referral to specialist units following (paracetamol) acetaminophen ingestion (O'Grady, 2006). Any of these criteria should prompt referral.

Day 2	Day 3	Day 4
Arterial pH <7.30	Arterial pH <7.30	INR >6 or PT>100 seconds
INR >3.0 or PT >50 seconds	INR >4.5 or PT >75 seconds	Progressive rise in PT to any level
Oliguria	Oliguria	Oliguria
Creatinine >200 µmol/L (1.5 mg/dL)	Creatinine >200 µmol/L (1.5 mg/dL)	Creatinine >300 µmol/L (2.3 mg/dL)
Hypoglycaemia	Encephalopathy	Encephalopathy
	Severe thrombocytopenia	Severe thrombocytopenia

Table 13.3   Referral to specialist units in non-acetaminophen aetiologies (O'Grady, 2006). The presence of any of the following criteria should prompt referral.

Hyperacute	Acute	Subacute
Encephalopathy	Encephalopathy	Encephalopathy
Hypoglycaemia	Hypoglycaemia	Hypoglycaemia (less common)
PT >30 seconds	PT >30 seconds	PT >20 seconds
INR >2.0	INR >2.0	INR >1.5
Renal failure	Renal failure	Renal failure
Hyperpyrexia		Serum sodium <130 mmol/L
		Shrinking liver volume

Management during transfer

Once a decision to transport the patient to the liver unit has been made, it is necessary to ensure a controlled environment for transfer, and that adequate personnel specifically trained to deal with the emergent situation that a patient with ALF may present during transfer, are present. Airway management is important as the patient can rapidly develop grade 3 or 4 hepatic encephalopathy, which will render them unable to protect their airway. Specialist advice may include elective intubation and artificial mechanical ventilation of the patient prior to transfer. ALF causes a hyperdynamic state, with high cardiac output (CO), low mean arterial pressure (MAP) and low systemic vascular resistance (SVR). This reduction in MAP may require vasopressors, such as noradrenaline (norephinephrine) to improve MAP and SVR. Fluid resuscitation is also necessary, the choice of fluid is not crucial and usually a mixture of crystalloids and colloids is used. Close attention to acid–base balance and correction of hyperlactataemia are important because they can impact upon circulatory function and also aggravate cerebral hyperaemia. Glucose levels need to be monitored for the effects of hypoglycaemia (Jalan, 2005; O'Grady, 2006). Where possible the patient and family should be informed of the transfer and possible treatment pathway.

Disease management

The care and treatment for patients with ALF is best achieved in a monitored environment, such as a high dependency unit (HDU) or an ICU depending upon the severity of illness and the requirement for invasive monitoring and treatment. A multidisciplinary approach is essential, involving hepatologists, intensivists, nurses, liver transplant surgeons, radiologists, physiotherapists and pharmacists. The clinical management of these patients is complex and intricate. Patients generally need close monitoring and often progress rapidly to multi-organ failure. Good critical care management is essential to successfully bridge to liver transplant.

Hepatic encephalopathy and cerebral oedema

One of the most serious complications of ALF is the development of hepatic encephalopathy, which may be associated with cerebral oedema and eventual brainstem herniation and death (Bernal and Wendon, 2000). All patients with ALF have some degree of encephalopathy (O'Grady, 2006). Hepatic encephalopathy is an altered neuropsychiatric state. The severity of hepatic encephalopathy is classified according to the West Haven criteria from grades 1 to 4, where patients with grade 1 or 2 encephalopathy exhibit degrees of drowsiness or disorientation. Extreme agitation and severe confusion are normally seen in grade 3 encephalopathy. At this point the patients are very vulnerable to self-injury and agitation could lead to inadvertent removal of invasive lines, such as arterial or central venous catheter (CVC). Grade 4 encephalopathy signifies deep coma with the patient being unresponsive. Again patients are extremely vulnerable here as they cannot protect their airway and intubation and mechanical ventilation are necessary (Ong and Mullen, 2001; O'Grady, 2006).

Cerebral oedema is a unique feature of ALF that is not usually seen in chronic liver disease. Cerebral oedema develops in 70% of hyperacute liver failure (O'Grady, 2006). The pathogenesis of cerebral oedema is poorly understood and is described in Chapter 6.

In addition to cerebral oedema, autoregulation is lost in many patients with ALF. Cerebral autoregulation ensures flow of blood in the brain is constant despite variation in blood pressures. When this fails any increase in MAP will increase intracranial pressure (ICP); if the pressure in the brain is sustained for long periods of time, this can lead to hypoperfusion resulting in cerebral hypoxia or brainstem herniation (O'Grady, 2006).

Cerebral monitoring and management of intracranial hypertension

The principles of management of elevated ICP in ALF are similar to those for ICP of any other cause, such as traumatic brain injury. The main aims are to monitor, prevent, and treat any increases in ICP.

In support of the hyperammonaemia theory, arterial ammonia levels will need to be measured regularly. Normal ammonia levels within the blood circulation with functioning liver are 15–45 µmol/L. In one study, an arterial ammonia level of greater than 150 µmol/L has correlated with hepatic encephalopathy and increase in ICP (Clemmesen et al., 1999; Jalan et al., 2004). However it is important to note that there is poor sensitivity with ammonia testing and the test may give false-negative results.

Jugular bulb venous saturations are used to monitor cerebral oxygen delivery and utilisation. The jugular bulb saturations are measured using a catheter placed in the jugular bulb, blood samples are withdrawn and analysed. The normal range of jugular bulb saturations (Sj02) is 55–70%. If the Sj02 falls below 55%, this could indicate high cerebral oxygen extraction and may be caused by increased metabolic activity, such as fitting or cerebral ischaemia related to inadequate cerebral blood flow. Conversely, if the Sj02 is high, this indicates low oxygen consumption and could suggest cerebral hyperaemia and/or decrease in metabolic activity (Harry and Wendon, 2001). In addition to Sj02, mixed venous saturations (Sv02) are also simultaneously assessed. The comparison between the two samples could indicate whether the abnormalities are global or cerebral related. Low or high Sj02 may indicate the need for intracranial pressure monitoring (Jalan, 2005).

An ICP monitoring catheter allows continual monitoring of ICP and is a way of guiding nursing care and therapy to prevent brain injury. The main aim of monitoring ICP is to ascertain cerebral perfusion pressure (CPP); this can be done by subtracting ICP from MAP. One of the complications of insertion of an ICP catheter in ALF is intracranial bleeding as the patients have coagulopathy. This risk can be minimised by administering clotting factors (Jalan, 2005).

Normal ICP range is between 4 and 15 mmHg (Hickey, 1986). Although there is some debate about the use of ICP bolt and jugular bulb catheter insertion in ALF (O'Grady, 2006), Wendon and Larsen (2006) argue that without ICP monitoring the effect of interventions cannot be examined. ICP monitoring allows an ICP trigger to be established, and efficacy of treatment to be determined. They further suggest that ICP monitoring coupled with jugular bulb saturation measurement allows clinicians to make informed decisions as to the most appropriate treatment and the benefits and duration of such treatment on ICP.

There are several pharmacological and nursing strategies used to maintain stable ICP or to treat surges in ICP.

Surges in ICP can be treated with bolus doses of mannitol up to 1 g/kg (O'Grady, 2006). Mannitol is an osmotic diuretic which increases water extraction through osmotic processes. The differences in osmolality between the plasma and brain shifts water from lower osmolality to one that is higher (Rang et al., 1996). The patient's urine output needs to be closely monitored for diuresis, but the prevalence of renal failure in ALF necessitates extracorporeal renal support. It is important to ensure that the fluid removal from haemofiltration is three times the amount of administered mannitol to avoid hyperosmolarity and fluid overload. Additionally it is essential to maintain serum osmolality less than 320 mOsm, as the equilibrium in osmolality will render the drug ineffective (Harry and Wendon, 2001).

Intracranial hypertension can also be reduced by hyperventilation as this induces vasoconstriction and reduces cerebral blood volume, however its effects cannot be sustained (Sherlock and Dooley, 2002). Therefore, hyperventilation may be useful for reducing ICP surges but should not be used over a prolonged period (Jalan, 2005).

Hypertonic saline creates as osmotic gradient between intravascular and interstitial compartments, in the presence of an intact blood–brain barrier, leading to shrinkage in brain tissue and therefore a reduction in ICP (White et al., 2006). The use of hypertonic saline in ALF is based on the findings of one clinical trial in which hypertonic saline (30%) was administered via continuous intravenous infusion to maintain serum sodium levels of 145–155 mmol/L. The study found the hypernatraemic group had decreased incidences of surges in ICP and a reduction in ICP values above 25 mmHg (Murphy et al., 2004). However, Jalan (2005) suggests that due to the potential adverse side effects, these findings necessitate further validation.

In some studies, intravenous indomethacin has been shown to reduce ICP in traumatic brain injury. Indomethacin causes cerebral vasoconstriction and a reduction in cerebral blood flow, and thereby a decrease in ICP. One study has described low-dose indomethacin normalising intracranial pressure in ALF and refractory ICP. However the use of non-steroidal drugs in patients with ALF with coagulopathy and renal dysfunction excludes it from routine use without further validation (Clemmensen et al., 1997; Slavik and Rhoney, 1999; Richardson and Bellamy, 2002; Jalan, 2005).

Hyperthermia in patients with head injuries increases the brain's metabolic rate causing an increase in cerebral blood flow and an increase in ICP. Therefore moderate hypothermia is thought to reduce these effects. Some studies have also shown hypothermia to reduce arterial ammonia levels, but research is not conclusive. Consequently hyperthermia should be avoided in such cases (Jalan et al., 1999; Roberts and Manas, 1999; Jalan, 2005).

Thiopentone sodium causes cerebral vasoconstriction, thereby reducing blood volume and decreasing ICP. Thiopentone is not used routinely in ALF due to its haemodynamic effects, prolonged sedative action and increased risk of infection. Therefore it is only used in catastrophic increase in ICP that is unresponsive to all other therapies (O'Grady, 2006).

Respiratory

Most patients with grade 3 or 4 hepatic encephalopathy are intubated and mechanically ventilated. The complications of artificial mechanical ventilation for patients with ALF are the same as with any other patients requiring ventilatory support. These complications include ventilator-associated pneumonia (VAP), pleural effusion, atelectasis and acute lung injury (ALI). In one study the incidence of ALI in patients with acetaminophen-induced ALF was found to be high (Baudouin et al., 1995), however a more recent study showed 25% of patients with all types of ALF showed signs of ALI but this was not associated with increased mortality (Auzinger et al., 2004).

ALI and its more severe form, acute respiratory distress syndrome (ARDS), are results of various direct and indirect insults to the lungs. A low tidal volume (6 mL/kg) and optimum level of positive end expiratory pressure (PEEP) are standard ventilatory strategies for these patients. Adequate PEEP will increase the lungs' functional residual capacity and enable the lungs to be inflated in the presence of poor lung compliance. The cornerstone of treatment is to avoid overdistension of the lungs by limiting tidal volume and recruitment of recruitable lung tissue (MacIntyre, 2005). Part of ALI/ARDS ventilatory strategy is permissive hypercarbia, however this is problematic in patients with ALF due to the high incidence, intracranial hypertension; carbon dioxide levels are therefore maintained at 4–4.5 kPa (30–40 mmHg).

Ventilated patients are routinely sedated, usually with propofol or benzodiazepines. Propofol has been shown to reduce cerebral blood flow through metabolic suppression in patients with ALF (Jalan, 2005). However, it is important to note that such sedative agents can induce hypotension and often have a negative inotropic effect, therefore close monitoring of arterial blood pressures is important to ensure adequate cerebral perfusion pressure. An opiate such as fentanyl is also used in conjunction with sedation to aid patient comfort and reduce ICP. Daily sedation holds may not be appropriate in patients with ALF and hepatic encephalopathy awaiting liver transplantation.

In order to prevent or treat atelectasis, patients may be nursed tilted on their sides to aid postural drainage. It has been suggested that positioning the patient with neutral head alignment and elevated head up to 20–30° will aid venous drainage from cerebral circulation and reduce ICP. It is also important to ensure that the tapes used to secure the endotracheal tube should not obstruct venous drainage (Hickey, 1986; Davenport et al., 1990). Additionally this position is also recommended in ventilator care bundle for the reduction of VAP (Berenholtz et al., 2002). As with all mechanically ventilated patients, clearance of endotracheal secretions is necessary and is generally applied when there is evidence of secretions on chest auscultation, increased airway pressure and reduction in peripheral oxygen saturations; it is normal practice to pre-oxygenate patients. However, endotracheal suctioning should be undertaken with great care in patients with ALF, as this activity can increase ICP. It is important to monitor for ICP surges and pupillary reactions during this phase and it may be necessary to administer bolus sedation to suppress coughing during this intervention.

Cardiovascular

The cardiovascular changes seen in ALF are characterised by peripheral vasodilatation which results in hypotension, a decrease in afterload and an increase in cardiac output leading to a hyperdynamic circulation (Harry and Wendon, 2001). This mimics sepsis and is thought to be caused by increased levels of circulating endotoxins (Gill and Sterling, 2001). These changes also result in a decrease in effective circulating volume. Fluid resuscitation as first-line treatment of arterial hypotension can alone normalise blood pressure and correct acidosis. Patients should therefore be managed with the early insertion of a central venous catheter (CVC) and monitoring of central venous pressure (CVP) and central venous saturation to guide volume loading. There is no specific guideline as to the type of resuscitation fluid used in ALF.

When volume resuscitation is not effective at restoring blood pressure, inotropic support may be necessitated. In ALF, a decrease in SVR, rather than cardiac dysfunction, is usually responsible for hypotension, therefore vasocontrictors such as noradrenaline (norepinephrine) are used. Noradrenaline causes an increase in MAP and oxygen delivery in patients with ALF (Jalan, 2005). It is important to measure and monitor blood pressure continuously via an arterial line. In addition to arterial and CVP measurements, the use of an advanced haemodynamic monitoring system, such as transpulmonary thermodilution technique, may be useful in providing information on cardiac output, cardiac index, stroke volume, cardiac function index and calculated measurements of extravascular lung water (EVWL) and intrathoracic blood volume (ITBV) (Cholley and Payen, 2005).

Renal failure

Acute kidney injury is a frequent complication in patients with ALF and may be due to dehydration, hepatorenal syndrome or acute tubular necrosis (Polson and Lee, 2005). Extracorporeal renal support may be required in 75% of acetaminophen-induced ALF and 30% of other aetiologies that have progressed to grade 3 or 4 encephalopathy (O'Grady, 2006). Extracorporeal renal support also provides the opportunity to manage cerebral oedema, via induction of hypothermia, and allows removal of fluid and reduction of ammonia concentration (Jalan, 2005). Continuous rather than intermittent renal replacement therapy (RRT) should be used, as this has been shown to improve stability in cardiovascular and ICP parameters compared with intermittent modes of dialysis (Davenport et al., 1993; Polson and Lee, 2005). Recent studies in acute renal failure and multi-organ dysfunction suggest that increase in the rate of ultrafiltration is associated with haemodynamic improvement. The ultrafiltraton rate of 35 mL/kg/h is considered to have a better overall outcome compared to lower rates (Ronco et al., 2000). Due to severe coagulopathy in patients with ALF, prostacyclin infusion of 2–5 ng/kg/min may be used as an alternative anticoagulant for haemofiltration to increase filter life and to reduce the risk of bleeding complications (O'Grady, 2006).

Coagulopathy

The liver is responsible for the synthesis of most of the coagulation factors. ALF results in an abrupt and profound decrease in the synthesis of these proteins, which is manifested by the prolongation of PT (Gill and Sterling, 2001). The PT is widely used as an indicator of the severity of liver damage (O'Grady, 2006). The patient may exhibit signs of disseminated intravascular coagulation (DIC). Serial measurements of PT or INR have prognostic implications (O'Grady, 2006). Routine use of fresh frozen plasma is not recommended unless spontaneous bleeding occurs (this is not common) or an invasive procedure is undertaken (Gill and Sterling, 2001). As these patients will have multiple invasive lines, the care of line dressings is important. Additionally oral care of the patient will need to be used judiciously to prevent gum bleeding.

Infection

All patients with ALF are at risk of bacterial and fungal infection and/or systemic inflammatory response syndrome (SIRS) (Polson and Lee, 2005). Impaired immune function in ALF leads to an increased susceptibility to infections. Studies have demonstrated that 80% of patients with ALF have bacterial and 32% have fungal infections (Rolando et al., 1996). Surveillance of infections should be performed to detect and treat bacterial and fungal infections early. Prophylactic antibiotics are used widely and have been shown to lower infection rates (Stadlbauer and Jalan, 2007). Most ICUs will choose an antibiotic and fungal regimen according to the local microbiological and resistance data. Good infection control practices by all health care personnel dealing with these patients are important.

Metabolic

In ALF, the capacity of the liver to metabolise lactate may be compromised. Indeed the liver may become a net producer of lactate during ALF. Hyperlactataemia is common in critical illness and has been shown to have prognostic significance in septic and trauma patients and those with ALF. The cause of hyperlactataemia in critical illness is not fully understood, but recent evidence has challenged the view that lactic acidosis is always the result of cellular hypoxia or hypoperfusion with resulting anaerobic metabolism, particularly in sepsis or SIRS (Murphy et al., 2001). A study by Bernal et al. (2002) demonstrated blood lactate concentration was a significant predictor of survival in patients with acetaminophen-induced ALF. The study suggests patients with early lactate concentration >3.0 mmol/L, following fluid resuscitation, can be viewed as being at high risk of subsequently meeting liver transplantation criteria and early listing for transplantation should be considered.

Hypoglycaemia is a common complication of ALF, found in 40% of patients. Hypoglycaemia is caused by high plasma insulin levels owing to a reduced hepatic uptake and reduced gluconeogenesis in the failing liver. Hypoglycaemia worsens cerebral oedema in patients with ALF (Jalan, 2005; O'Grady, 2006). Close monitoring of blood sugar and correction of hypoglycaemia are important. At the same time it is imperative to prevent hyperglycaemia. Recent studies by Van de Berghe et al. (2001) showed that tight blood glucose control (4–6 mmol/L) with intensive insulin therapy can lower mortality by 43%, the incidence of polyneuropathy by 44% and blood stream infections by 46%. Many ICUs have developed local flow charts and protocols for the maintenance of tight glucose control.

Additional monitoring

Indocyanine green (ICG) is a dye with infra-red absorbing and fluorescent properties. After intravenous administration, ICG is nearly exclusively eliminated by the liver into the bile. ICG removal depends on liver blood flow, liver parenchymal and cellular function and biliary excretion (Sakka, 2007). ICG clearance is measured by the percentage plasma disappearance rate (PDR), which detects alteration in liver function and may be used as a non-invasive determinant of hepatic reserve. PDR of <5% has been shown to be a significant predictor of irreversible liver damage (Quintero et al., 2007). The normal value for ICG clearance is 700 mL/min/m^2 and for PDR is over 18%/min (Sakka, 2007).

Intra-abdominal hypertension (IAH) and abdominal compartment syndrome (ACS) as a result of elevated intra-abdominal pressure (IAP), affect perfusion and function of every organ system in the body. The normal values of IAP at subatmospheric level is 0 mmHg; values above 12 mmHg are considered elevated. Post-abdominal surgery IAP usually ranges from 2–15 mmHg. When IAP is >10 mmHg it is likely to drop cardiac output; IAP >15 mmHg compromises renal and splanchnic perfusion, and IAP >20–25 mmHg increases peak alveolar pressures. ACS is defined as IAP >20–30 mmHg, which is associated with organ dysfunction and is an emergency situation. ACS is a pathological state caused by an acute increase in IAP that adversely affects cardiopulmonary function and impairs splanchnic perfusion. It can also lead to serious wound complications in surgical patients (Malbrain, 2000; Malbrain et al., 2005). There is increasing awareness of the harmful effects of IAH and ACS on end-organ function in critically ill patients. IAH decreases hepatic artery flow and portal venous blood flow while portocollateral flow increases, lactate clearance drops, glucose metabolism diminishes and PDR for ICG rate decreases (Malbrain et al., 2005). The implication of IAH and ACS in renal, cardiovascular and respiratory systems is well reported, however, knowledge of its complications in ALF is limited despite incidences of significant elevations in IAP in ALF (Wendon and Larsen, 2006).

Because the abdomen acts as a fluid compartment, IAP can be measured via multiple routes, such as intraperitoneal route, via bladder, uterus, inferior vena cava, rectum or stomach. Measurement of IAP by an indwelling catheter in the urinary bladder has been suggested as the method of choice (Malbrain, 2000). This method of measuring IAP is relatively quick and easy to perform by using a commercially available manometer which can be attached between the urinary catheter and urine collection bag. IAP is normally measured every 4–6 hours.

Nutrition

Generally patients with ALF are well nourished at the onset of the illness; however as with any other critically ill patients protein energy malnutrition is a major problem with hypercatabolic state. Early initiation of enteral nutrition has proved to be beneficial, with significant reduction in septic complications, and has been shown to improve outcome when compared with parenteral nutrition (van der Voort and Zandstra, 2001; O'Grady, 2006). Among other beneficial effects, enteral feeding stimulates mucosal blood flow, and maintains gut barrier function and mucosal integrity (Binnekade et al., 2005). Normally enteral feed is instituted via nasograstic or nasojejunum tube. Most ICUs have protocols regarding enteral feeding regimes and prokinetics are used when necessary.

Gastrointestinal ulcer prophylaxis is another important consideration in these patients due to the increased risk of bleeding from stress ulceration (O'Grady, 2006).

Critical illness polyneuropathy and myopathy

Critical illness polyneuropathy (CIP) and myopathy (CIM) are neuromuscular disorders that occur in critically ill patients. Clinical features often consist of difficulty in weaning from mechanical ventilation, tetraparesis and muscle wasting of the limbs. Patients with weakness acquired in the ICU are often sedated and mechanically ventilated, and have unreliable sensory and motor examinations, and so diagnosis can be difficult. It is believed that the development of CIP and CIM is associated with multi-organ dysfunction, sepsis and SIRS, probably by the same basic mechanisms that lead to organ dysfunction. Complete recovery may occur after successful treatment of the original insult, but impairments in physical function and health status may persist, even 1 year after of discharge from ICU (Bird and Rich, 2002; Kerbaul et al., 2004; Young and Hammond, 2004).

Additional considerations

One of the main principles of nursing care is to minimise ICP surges and this can be achieved by minimal intervention and in taking extreme care when moving patients (Jalan, 2005). O'Neil et al. (2006) found that the term minimal intervention was used in regional liver units, as a means to minimise rises in ICP. However, they found no formal nursing or medical guidelines which defined what the term minimal intervention meant in relation to patient care. Audit and research, such as control trials in this area, are difficult due to the potential risk of causing intracranial hypertension and brainstem herniation.

Nursing care can be guided by the monitoring of ICP and/or measuring jugular bulb saturations to ensure increases in ICP are not sustained during nursing care. The following are considered to be minimal interventions:

■ Patients should be nursed on a dynamic mattress to prevent pressure ulcerations and should not be turned
■ Patients may be tilted on to their sides to aid postural chest drainage and prevent atelectasis
■ Oral and other hygiene care should be applied judiciously and only when essential

Throughout these interventions, ICP should be monitored closely.

Liver transplantation

The only therapy of confirmed benefit in patients with advanced ALF is emergency liver transplantation. ALF accounts for 5% of all liver transplants in the USA and 11% in Europe (O'Grady, 2006). In the UK 15.6% of all transplants in 2005/2006 were for super-urgent liver transplants (UK Transplant, 2006) (Figure 13.2, Plate 14). Strict criteria define the population who are likely to benefit from emergency liver transplantation. King's College Hospital transplant criteria have been widely used. UK Transplant has recently updated the criteria for super-urgent liver transplant (Table 13.4). Worldwide survival rates in ALF transplant recipients have been reported as 60–90% (Sherlock and Dooley, 2002).

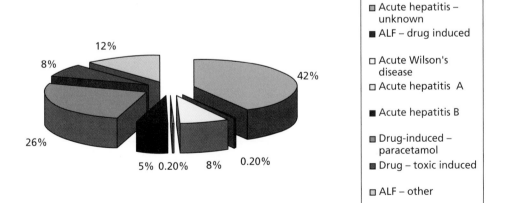

Figure 13.2   UK aetiologies for ALF transplants 2001–2006 (UK Transplant, 2006). For a colour version of this figure, please see Plate 14 in the colour plate section.

Table 13.4 Super-urgent transplant listing criteria for ALF in the UK. National Transplant Database (2005) Guideline for completing the Super-urgent Liver Recipient Registration Form. UK Transplant.

Cause of ALF	Category	Notes
Paracetamol toxicity	Category 1	pH <7.25 more then 24 hours after ingestion and after fluid resuscitation
	Category 2	PT >100 seconds or INR >6.5 with a creatinine >300 µmol/L or anuria with a grade 3–4 encephalopathy
	Category 3	Serum lactate >3.5 mmol/L on admission or >3.0 mmol/L after fluid resuscitation more than 24 hours post ingestion
	Category 4	Two out of three of the criteria from category 2 plus deterioration such as an increase in ICP or increased FiO2 requirements in the absence of clinical sepsis
Hepatitis A, B, idiosyncratic drug reaction or seronegative	Category 5	PTT >100 seconds or INR >6.5 with any grade of encephalopathy
	Category 6	Any grade of encephalopathy plus any three of the following: (a) Unfavourable cause, i.e. drug induced or seronegative (b) Age >40 years (c) Jaundice to encephalopathy time >7 days (d) Serum bilirubin >300 µmol/L (e) PTT >50 seconds (f) INR >3.5
Acute presentation of Wilson's disease or Budd-Chiari	Category 7	Coagulopathy with any grade of encephalopathy
Hepatic artery thrombosis	Category 8	Within 14 days of liver transplantation
Early graft dysfunction	Category 9	At least two of the following: (a) AST >10 000 IU/L (b) INR >3.0 (c) Serum lactate >3 mmol/L (d) Absence of bile production

Chapter summary

Multi-organ failure complicating ALF is one of the most challenging management problems in clinical practice and requires a multi-disciplinary team approach. Early identification and referral of these patients to a liver transplant centre is imperative. Supportive management of multi-organ failure should be initiated expediently. The goal of clinical management is primarily to prevent intracranial hypertension and bridge patients who fulfil criteria to liver transplantation.

Illustrative case study

A 57-year-old woman presented with a short history of generalised abdominal pain and jaundice, anorexia and fatigue. No risk factors for liver disease were identified and there was no history of recent foreign travel. She had been taking non-steroidal anti-inflammatory medication (NSAID). Abdominal examination showed normal liver and spleen on palpations.

On day 14 following hospital admission the patient developed confusion and grade 2 hepatic encephalopathy. The local liver transplant centre was contacted and the patient was transferred. The patient was admitted directly to specialist liver ICU and closely monitored. She was intubated and mechanically ventilated. She was sedated with propofol and fentanyl. Invasive lines were inserted; vascath for renal replacement therapy, PiCCO arterial line for the measurement of pre-load and cardiac output and, due to hepatic encephalopathy, a jugular bulb catheter and an ICP bolt were inserted. She was aggressively fluid resuscitated as her ITBV was low and lactate high. The opening pressure of ICP measured at 23 mmHg, therefore, minimal intervention of care was instituted. Thirty percent hypertonic saline via continuous intravenous infusion was commenced and her sodium level was kept >145 mmol/L. Hepatitis screen was conducted, which was negative. A provisional diagnosis of subacute liver failure NSAID/seronegative hepatitis was made.

The patient fulfilled transplant criteria and received an orthotopic cadaveric liver transplant 3 days later. Table 13.5 presents the trends in biochemistry, lactate, ammonia and ICP values from referral to post liver transplant. Following liver transplantation the patient's ICP reduced to less than 10 mmHg. There was also a reduction in lactate and INR.

Table 13.5 Trends in biochemistry, lactate, ammonia and ICP values from referral to post liver transplant.

	Normal values	On admission	On arrival at the specialist unit	Pre liver transplant	Post liver transplant
INR	0.9–1.2	1.4	3.9 (8 hours later 6.77)	3.86	1.48
Bilirubin (μmol/L)	3–20	135	454	198	87
AST (IU/L)	10–50	1263	1453	400	299
ALP (IU/L)	30–130	216	181	131	109
Creatinine (mmol/L)	45–120	–	71	86	80
pH	7.35–7.45	–	7.48	7.44	7.40
Lactate (mmol/L)	0.2–1.0	–	3.3	2.3	1.03
Ammonia (μmol/L)	15–45	–	189	182	27
ICP (mmHg)	4–15	–	25	17	<10

This case study demonstrates the rapid deterioration of patients with ALF and the need to transfer these patients to a specialist centre early for a successful bridge to liver transplantation.

References

Auzinger G, Sizer E, Bernal W, Wendon J (2004) Incidence of lung injury in acute liver failure: diagnostic role of extravascular lung water index. *Critical Care* 8(suppl 1):40

Bacon B, O'Grady J, Di Bisceglie A, Lake J (eds) (2006) *Comprehensive Clinical Hepatology*, 2nd edn. Mosby Elsevier, Philadelphia

Baudouin SV, Howdle P, O'Grady JR, Webster NR (1995) Acute lung injury in fulminant hepatic failure following paracetamol poisoning. *Thorax* 50(4):399–402

Benhamou JP (1991) Fulminant and subfulminant liver failure: definition and causes. In: William R and Hughes R (eds) *Acute Liver Failure: Improved Understanding and Better Therapy*. Proceedings of the 11th BSG/SK&F International Workshop 1990, Smith Kline & French Laboratories, London, UK

Berenholtz SM, Dorman T, Ngo K, Provonost PJ (2002) Qualitative review of intensive care unit quality indicators. *Journal of Critical Care* 17(1):1–12

Bernal W, Donaldson N, Wyncoll O, Wendon J (2002) Blood lactate as an early predictor of outcome in paracetamol-induced acute liver failure: a cohort study. *The Lancet* 359:558–563

Bernal W, Wendon J (2000) Acute liver failure. *Current Opinion in Anaesthesiology* 13:113–118

Binnekade JM, Tepsake R, Bruynzeel P, Mathus-Vliegen EMH, de Haan RJ (2005) Daily enteral feeding practice on the ICU: attainment of goals and interfering factors. *Critical Care* 9:R218–R225

Bird SJ, Rich MM (2002) Critical illness myopathy and polyneuropathy. *Current Neurological and Neuroscience Reports* 2(6):527–533

Cholley BP, Payen D (2005) Non invasive techniques for measurements of cardiac output. *Current Opinions in Critical Care* 11(5):424–429

Clemmesen JO, Hansen BA, Larsen FS (1997) Indomethacin normalizes intracranial pressure in acute liver failure: a twenty-three-year-old woman treated with indomethacin. *Hepatology* 26(6):1423–1425

Clemmesen JO, Larsen FS, Kondrup J, Hansen BA, Ott P (1999) Cerebral herniation in patients with acute liver failure is correlated with arterial ammonia concentration. *Hepatology* 29(3):648–653

Davenport A, Will EJ, Davison AM (1990) Effects of posture on intracranial pressure and cerebral perfusion pressure in patients with fulminant hepatic failure and renal failure after acetaminophen self-poisoning. *Critical Care Medicine* 18(3):286–289

Davenport A, Will EJ, Davison AM (1993) Effects of renal replacement therapy on patients with combined acute renal failure and fulminant hepatic failure. *Kidney International* **41**:s245–s251

Gill RQ, Sterling RK (2001) Acute liver failure. *Journal of Clinical Gastroenterology* **33**(3):191–198

Harry R, Wendon J (2001) The management of acute liver failure. *CME Journal of Gastroenterology Hepatology and Nutrition* **4**(2):58–61

Hickey JV (1986) *The Clinical Practice of Neurological and Neurosurgical Nursing*, 2nd edn. JB Lippincott Company, Philadelphia, pp. 246–275

Jalan R (2005) Acute liver failure: current management and future prospects. *Journal of Hepatology*, **42**(suppl):S115–S123

Jalan R, Demink SWO, Deutz NEP, Lee A, Hayes PC (1999) Moderate hypothermia for uncontrolled intracranial hypertension in acute liver failure. *The Lancet* **354**:1164–1168

Jalan R, Olde Damink SWO, Hayes PC, Deutz NEP, Lee A (2004) Pathogenesis of intracranial hypertension in acute liver failure: inflammation, ammonia and cerebral blood flow. *Journal of Hepatology* **41**:613–620

Kerbaul F, Brousse M, Collart F, Pellissier J-F, Planche D, Fernandex C, Gouin F, Guidon C (2004) Combinatin of histopathological and electromyographic patterns can help to evaluate functional outcome of critical ill patients with neuromuscular weakness syndromes. *Critical Care* **8**:R358–R366

MacIntyre NR (2005) Current issues in mechanical ventilation for respiratory failure. *Chest* **128**(2):561S-567S

Malbrain MLNG (2000) Abdominal pressure in the critically ill. *Current Opinion in Critical Care* **6**:17–29

Malbrain MLNG, Deeren D, De Potter TRJR (2005) Intra-abdominal hypertension in the critically ill: it is time to pay attention. *Current Opinion in Critical Care* **11**:156–171

Murphy N, Auzinger G, Bernel W, Wendon J (2004) The effect of hypertonic sodium chloride on intracranial pressure in patients with acute liver failure. *Hepatology* **29**(2):464–470

Murphy ND, Kodakat SK, Wendon JA, Jooste CA, Muiesan P, Rela M, Heaton ND (2001) Liver and intestinal lactate metabolism in patients with acute hepatic failure undergoing liver transplantation. *Critical Care Medicine* **29**(11):2111–2118

Murphy N, Wendon J (2004) Fulminant hepatic failure. In: McDonald JWD, Burroughs AK and Feagan BG (eds) *Evidence-Based Gastroenterology and Hepatology*, 2nd edn. Blackwell Publishing, Oxford, pp. 527–543

O'Grady JG (2006) Acute liver failure. In: Bacon BR, O'Grady JG, Di Bisceglie, AM, Lake RJ (eds) *Comprehensive Clinical Hepatology*, 2nd edn. Mosby, Philadelphia, pp. 517–536

O'Grady JG, Schalm SW, William R (1993) Acute liver failure: redefining the syndromes. *The Lancet* **343**:273–275

O'Neil H, Olds J, Webster N (2006) Managing patients with acute liver failure: developing a tool for practitioners. *Nursing in Critical Care* **11**(2):63–68

Ong JP, Mullen KD (2001) Hepatic encephalopathy. *European Journal of Gastro-enterology and Hepatology* **13**(4):325–334

Polson J and Lee WM (2005) AASLD position paper: the management of acute liver failure. *Hepatology* **41**(5):1179–1197

Quintero J, Ortega J, Bueno J, Flores S, Roqueta J (2007) Predictive value of indocyanine green clearance in acute liver failure in children: comparison with King's College and Clichy scores. *Critical Care* **11**(suppl 2):398

Rang HP, Dale MM, Ritter JM (1996) *Pharmacology*, 3rd edn. Churchill Living-stone, Edinburgh, pp. 382–389

Richardson D, Bellamy M (2002) Intracranial hypertension in acute liver failure. *Nephrology Dialysis Transplantation*, **17**:23–27

Roberts DRD, Manas D (1999) Induced hypothermia in the management of cerebral oedema secondary to fulminant liver failure. *Clinical Transplantation* **13**(16):545–547

Rolando N, Harvey FAH, Brahm J (1996) Prospective study of bacterial and fungal infections in acute liver failure: an analysis of fifty patients. *Liver Transplant Surgery* **2**:8–13

Ronco C, Bellomo R, Homel P, Brendolan A, Dan M, Piccinni P, La Greca G (2000) Effects of different doses in continuous veno-venous haemofiltration on outcomes of acute renal failure: a prospective randomised trial. *The Lancet* **356**(9223):26–30

Sakka SG (2007) Assessing liver function. *Current Opinion in Critical Care* **13**: 207–214

Sargent S, Fullwood D (2006) The management of hepatic encephalopathy and cerebral oedema in acute liver failure. *British Journal of Neuroscience Nursing* **2**(9):448–451

Shakil AO, Kramer D, Mazariegos V, Fung JJ, Rakela J (2000) Acute liver failure: clinical features, outcome and analysis, and applicability of prognostic criteria. *Liver Transplantation* **6**(2):163–169

Sherlock S, Dooley J (2002) *Diseases of the Liver and Biliary System*, 11th edn. Blackwell Publishing, Oxford

Slavik RS, Rhoney DH (1999) Indomethacin: a review of its cerebral blood flow effects and potential use for controlling intracranial pressure in traumatic head injured patients. *Neurological Research* **21**(5):491–499

Stadlbauer V, Jalan R (2007) Acute liver failure: liver support therapies. *Current Opinions in Critical Care* **13**(2):215–221

UK Transplant (2006) www.uktransplant.org.uk (Accessed 2nd February 2006 and 19th March 2007)

Van de Berghe G, Wouters PJ, Weekes F, Verwaest C, Bunnynickx F, Schetz M, Vlasserlaesrs D, Ferdinade P, Lauwers P, Bouillon R (2001) Intensive insulin therapy in critically ill patients. *New England Journal of Medicine* **345**:1359–1367

van der Voort PH, Zandstra DF (2001) Enteral feeding in the critically ill: comparison between the supine and prone positions: a prospective crossover study in mechanically ventilated patients. *Critical Care* **5**(4):216–220

Wendon J, Larsen FS (2006) Intracranial pressure monitoring in acute liver failure. A procedure with clear indications. *Hepatology* **44**(2):504–506

White H, Cook D, Venkatesh B (2006) The use of hypertonic saline for treating intracranial hypertension after traumatic brain injury. *Anesthesia and Analgesia* **102**(6):1836–1846

Young GB, Hammond RR (2004) A stronger approach to weakness in the intensive care unit. *Critical Care* **8**:416–418

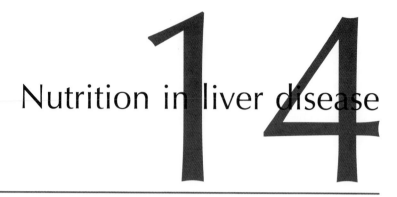

Nutrition in liver disease

Susie Hamlin and Julie Leaper

Introduction

In this chapter the nutritional treatment of patients with liver disease will be discussed. Nutritional therapy has always been recognised as an important part of treatment in people with cirrhosis. Protein calorie malnutrition (PCM) is an increasingly recognised complication of chronic liver disease that has important prognostic implications.

The prevalence of PCM in patients with compensated cirrhosis is reported as 20–40% (Plauth et al., 1997; Johnson, 2003); whereas, the prevalence of PCM is 80–100% in patients with decompensated cirrhosis (McCullough and Bugionesie, 1997; Runyon, 1998). Malnutrition develops in patients with cirrhosis irrespective of the aetiology of disease and the incidence is similar between alcoholic and non-alcoholic patients. However, despite the high incidence of PCM some patients remain obese. Careful management of weight, nutritional support and dietary therapy is necessary to ensure this group of patients is appropriately managed and PCM recognised despite what appears to be a high body mass index (BMI) (Day, 2006).

Malnutrition and nutritional assessment

The cause of malnutrition is multi-factorial and compromises the clinical outcome of patients with end-stage liver disease. The presence of muscle wasting indicates an advanced stage and is associated with poorer survival (Merli et al., 1996). Protein energy malnutrition has also been correlated with worsening ascites, encephalopathy and increased infection rates, hospital re-admissions and increased mortality (Cabre et al., 1990; Mullen and Weber, 1991; Runyon, 1998).

Matos et al. (2002) highlight the reasons why patients with liver disease develop malnutrition, which include:

- Poor dietary intake
- Malabsorption and maldigestion of nutrients
- Metabolic abnormalities including protein, glucose and fat
- Altered metabolism of micronutrients

All of these factors will be discussed in more detail throughout the chapter.

There are many difficulties with regards to nutritional assessment of patients with liver disease as no gold standard exists which can determine the extent of malnutrition (Campos et al., 2002). Assessment of nutritional status should include medical and dietary history, subjective global assessment, anthropometric measurements, biochemistry and body composition analysis, if available. Some of these are difficult to interpret and require specialist knowledge.

Dietary history can give indications of timing of meals, food portions and taste alterations, early satiety and malabsorption. Anthropometric measurements, including triceps skin fold thickness, mid-arm circumference and handgrip, can be used in patients with liver disease. Handgrip strength has been shown to predict clinical outcome in patients with cirrhosis (Alvares-da-Silva and Reverbel da Silveria, 2005). The tool is very non-invasive and can be used in a variety of settings.

For nursing staff, the Malnutrition Universal Screening Tool (MUST) can be a start for screening groups of patients at risk of malnutrition (British Association for Parenteral and Enteral Nutrition, 2003). For liver disease, BMI and weight changes should be calculated using estimated dry body weight. Looking at food portions and meal patterns can give indications of potential poor intakes. For all liver patients with decompensated liver disease one should assume they are at risk of protein energy malnutrition and osteoporosis.

Dietetic management of ascites

The management of ascites is frequently associated with sodium and fluid restrictions, and malnutrition, the need for therapeutic diets and aggressive nutritional support (Fisher et al., 2002; Moore and Aithal, 2006). Ascites can aggravate PCM due to many factors. The nature of the symptoms can severely limit dietary intake due to feelings of early satiety, or the patients may experience abdominal pain, bloating, reflux, constipation, reduced mobility, and reduced ability to shop, cook and prepare meals. Other symptoms can include breathlessness and increased infections such as spontaneous bacterial peritonitis.

For patients being assessed with ascites the primary aim is to ensure nutritional requirements are being met. Secondly, salt and fluid restrictions should be used with caution when appropriate and with close review in order to prevent further compromising the patient's nutritional status.

Nutritional support in ascites management

If patients have fluid restrictions, nutritional support products should be prioritised, within the restriction, above nutritionally poor fluids such as tea, coffee and juices. Milk-based sip feeds have considerably higher protein than juice-based sip feeds and are often the supplements of choice, especially if patients are undergoing therapeutic paracentesis when protein losses per drain can exceed 90 g of protein.

If enteral feeding is necessary then most standard enteral feeds (1 kcal/mL) are suitable as they contain less than 40 mmol sodium per litre of feed. High-energy/protein feeds are often prescribed (1.5–2 kcal/mL) as they provide more kcal/protein in smaller volumes. Sip feeds, if prescribed in addition to the nasogastric feed, can be flushed down the nasogastric tube rather than drunk if the patient is struggling to consume them orally.

Dietary salt restrictions

Dietary salt restrictions have been shown to lower diuretic requirement, resolve ascites faster and reduce hospitalisation in ascitic patients (Soulsby, 1997; Moore and Aithal, 2006). Traditionally patients are advised to follow a 'no added salt' diet, which is 80–100 mmol sodium (4.65–5.8 g salt). The typical UK diet provides approximately 9–10 g of salt per day, despite the recommendation for the general population to be no higher than 6 g/day. Most hospitals provide meals that provide less than 6 g of salt per day so in hospital further restrictions are usually unnecessary. There is no evidence to restrict salt below the recommended amount for the general population in patients with liver disease without ascites or oedema (Moore and Aithal, 2006).

Sodium intakes vary enormously between patients and each patient's intake needs to be assessed individually. Very often reducing a few key foods can have a profound influence on daily net sodium intake whilst maintaining an adequate dietary intake.

Basic advice to all ascitic patients is as simple as:

- No added salt to meals
- Avoid salty snacks such as crisps (20 mmol Na) and soups
- Encourage high-calorie high-protein snacks with a carbohydrate-rich snack in the evening

Table 14.1 General advice and foods to avoid for sodium restrictions in ascitic patients.

General advice	Foods to avoid
No salt added at the table	Bacon, ham, sausages, pate
Pinch only in cooking	Tinned and smoked fish and meat
Avoid salt substitutes	Fish and meat pastes
Up to 100 g cheese/week	Tinned and packet soups
Up to 4 slices bread/day	Sauce mixes, stock cubes, soya sauce, MSG
Avoid all processed foods	Tinned vegetables
	Bottled sauces and chutneys
	Meat and vegetable extracts
	Salted nuts and crisps

It is vital to remember that by the time patients have developed ascites their appetites are frequently so poor that restrictions are unnecessary. However if a full 'no added salt' restriction is required the advice in Table 14.1 should be given.

Assessing dry weight

Correct interpretation of the weight of fluid in patients with ascites and peripheral oedema is vital. Suggested guidelines are detailed below for estimating the amount of fluid present with mild, moderate and severe ascites (Johnson, 2003).

Patients with ascites:

- Minimal 2.2 kg
- Moderate 6.0 kg
- Severe 14.0 kg

Patients with oedema:

- Minimal 1.0 kg
- Moderate 5.0 kg
- Severe 10.0 kg

These figures have limitations and often patients have more fluid than this evidence-based estimate advises. It is important to consider each patient as an individual and use these figures as a guide. Using weight histories and dry weights following paracentesis can be the best estimate that can be obtained of actual flesh weight with adjustment if necessary for peripheral oedema. It is important to stress that dry weight or estimated dry weights must always be used for calculating BMI and calculating nutritional requirements, as BMI can be grossly misleading in interpreting the level of malnutrition if adjustments for dry weight are not made.

Nutrition in hepatic encephalopathy

A definition and pathophysiology of hepatic encephalopathy are discussed in Chapter 6. There is a direct link between PCM and worsening encephalopathy (Mullen and Weber, 1991; Morgan et al., 1995; Kondrup and Muller, 1997).

Historically dietary protein restrictions as low as 20 g per day were used to treat hepatic encephalopathy, as it was thought that nitrogenous waste products from protein metabolism, in particular ammonia, worsened acute hepatic encephalopathy (Phillips et al., 1952). This therapy was not evidence based and therefore is not recommended. Evidence has also shown cirrhotic patients need at least 1.2–1.3 g protein/kg/day to remain in a positive nitrogen balance (De Bruijn et al., 1983). When nutritional requirements are not met, nitrogenous waste products from skeletal muscle breakdown from the resulting catabolism can exacerbate encephalopathy. Hence aggressive nutritional support is necessary.

Nutritional requirements

Nutritional requirements should be met aggressively, aiming for minimum of 1.2 g protein and 35 kcal/kg dry body weight (Plauth et al., 1997; Johnson, 2003). Encephalopathic patients will not meet nutritional requirements via standard hospital diets alone and sip feeds and enteral nasogastric feeding should not be delayed. To avoid large dietary protein boluses, meals should be spaced out throughout the day with a snack between each meal and a late evening snack of at least 50 g of carbohydrate. Periods of fasting should be kept to an absolute minimum. If the patient is being enterally fed, administering the feed overnight breaks the overnight fast and promotes a positive nitrogen balance. If being exclusively enterally fed, the feed should be administered over 24 hours until encephalopathy resolves, and then reviewed.

Chronic encephalopathy

In 'true' chronic hepatic encephalopathy, as described in Chapter 6, which excludes any identifiable precipitating causes, ensure compliance with bowel management therapy and sufficient dietary management. Patients should be assessed for a defined period before considering any protein restriction, as catabolism can worsen HE.

If encephalopathy persists and there is no improvement, a trial of protein restriction may be indicated. If necessary a trial period of 1 g/kg protein, 35 kcal/kg dry body weight should be tried. A trial period should be defined and progress monitored, including neurological status, in consultation with the multi-disciplinary team. Protein intolerance may be a transient phenomenon so periods of restriction should be kept as short as possible.

Malabsorption and steatorrhoea

Malabsorption and maldigestion of gastrointestinal nutrients frequently exist in patients with liver disease, however the extent to which they occur can vary considerably from one person to another. Malabsorption of fat-soluble vitamins is common, especially in patients with cholestatic disease where the reduced absorption of carbohydrates, protein, water-soluble vitamins and minerals has also been demonstrated (Matos et al., 2002). Other reasons for malabsorption may be bacterial overgrowth resulting from impaired small bowel motility, or the administration of medications, e.g. neomycin, lactulose or cholestyramine. This resultant fat malabsorption contributes to malnutrition and deficiency of fat-soluble vitamins (Henkel and Buchman, 2006).

Classically, the subjective diagnosis of steatorrhoea includes symptoms of loose, pale, floating stools with an offensive smell. People will often describe their bowel motions as difficult to flush away. Care needs to be given when considering these symptoms as they are similar symptoms to those of other malabsorptive states, such as Crohn's disease, and further investigation may be warranted.

There has been a move away from severe fat restriction to a more individualised fat modification taking into account the symptoms of the patient and the degree of restriction necessary. There is no evidence for fat restriction in patients with jaundice or gallstones who do not suffer any symptoms related to fat ingestion, i.e. pain, nausea or steatorrhoea (Madden, 1992).

Situations where fat restriction may be necessary are:

- When severe symptoms are causing distress to the patient
- Weight loss is directly related to the steatorrhoea
- Where there is significant nausea or indigestion with fat intake which does not improve with anti-emetics or antacids

The fat content of the diet should be reduced slowly and in stages whilst monitoring the symptoms of steatorrhoea. Small changes may be necessary, e.g. no fried foods, or more significant alterations could be required to alleviate the symptoms. This advice should be carried out by a dietician who can ensure adequate balance of nutrients is maintained whilst meeting energy and protein requirements.

Meeting nutritional requirements

Where fat restriction is needed in patients who are undernourished, energy and protein requirements still need to be met. Fat is a valuable source of energy and therefore alternative sources need to be used:

- Increase the protein content of the diet by enlarging high biological value protein sources if possible, i.e. meat, fish, chicken, eggs, milk
- Increase the carbohydrate content of the diet using Maxijul, Polycal

- Alter supplements to low fat non-milk based ones, i.e. Enlive Plus, Provide Extra, Fortijuice
- Use medium chain triglycerides (MCTs). These are the preferred form of fat supplementation in chronic liver disease with steatorrhoea because they bypass the carnitine pathway and are readily utilised by the tissues (Sarath et al., 2000). They are partially water-soluble and do not require bile salts for emulsification. They are available in either oil (MCT oil) or an emulsion (Liquigen, SHS). The emulsion can be taken as a 'medicine' spaced out three to four times per day or mixed with milk to disguise the flavour. The oil is not as easy to use in cooking as it has a low smoking point. Consideration needs to be given to enteral feeds which either have a high MCT content or are low fat

Fat-soluble vitamins (A, D, E, K)

Plasma concentrations of fat-soluble vitamins can be insensitive markers of fat-soluble vitamin status. Plasma 25-hydroxyvitamin D gives a good indication of vitamin D status and prolonged PT can be taken as a sign of vitamin K deficiency. However, it is essential to first ensure that the prolonged PT is not a sign of decreased hepatic function.

Vitamin A

This is a family of fat-soluble compounds called retinoids, which have vitamin A activity. Retinol is the predominant form and is important for vision, particularly at night. Deficiency is shown by xerophthalmia, night blindness and increased disease susceptibility (Fairfield and Fletcher, 2002).

In primary biliary cirrhosis (PBC) vitamin A deficiency is seen in 20% of cases but is often clinically asymptomatic (Talwalkar and Lindor, 2003). In advanced primary sclerosing cholangitis (PSC) up to 82% of patients will be deficient in vitamin A (Lee and Kaplan, 2002). Oral supplements are available but effectiveness depends on absorption, with water-soluble forms being used where possible (Kennedy and O'Grady, 2002).

Vitamin D

Vitamin D (calciferol) can be synthesised by humans with adequate exposure to sunlight. In adults, vitamin D deficiency leads to secondary hyperparathyroidism, bone loss, osteopenia, osteoporosis and increased fracture risk (Fairfield and Fletcher, 2002).

Vitamin E

Deficiency of this vitamin is rare but can be seen in chronic cholestatic liver disease. Symptoms include muscle weakness, ataxia and haemolysis.

Vitamin K

This vitamin is essential for normal clotting and bone metabolism. Deficiency results in clotting disorders which are frequently found in patients with liver disease. Supplementation can be given as either intramuscular or intravenous injections. However, due to altered coagulopathy most liver centres administer vitamin K intravenously.

Calcium

Calcium malabsorption can be related to vitamin D deficiency and the formation of unabsorbable calcium soaps in the intestinal lumen (Kehayoglou et al., 1968). The level of supplementation is discussed later in this chapter.

Diabetes in liver disease

Liver disease and its subsequent cirrhosis are associated with insulin resistance, pancreatic beta cell dysfunction and diabetes. It is vital that blood glucose levels are monitored in known diabetics and those who are at risk of developing hyperglycaemia due to steroid use or pancreatic insufficiency.

Diabetes is associated with mobilisation of adipose tissue, fatty acids and increased protein catabolism (McCullough and Bugionesie, 1997; Gonzales-Barranco et al., 1998) For this reason, normal glycaemic control is crucial to prevent further muscle wastage. Consideration of the patient's nutritional requirements, rather than reducing intake to achieve normoglycaemia, is vital.

Patients with elevated blood glucose levels (more than 11 mmol/L) are also at risk of nosocomial infections by up to ten fold (McMahon and Rizza, 1996).

The most suitable types of medication regimen should be discussed in line with current diabetic standards and knowledge of the patient's nutritional requirements. It is inappropriate to provide standard healthy eating advice for diabetes to patients with decompensated liver disease. For most patients, the most suitable advice is:

- Reduce intake of simple sugars
- Regular meals and snacks which include protein and especially including a late evening snack with 50 g carbohydrate content
- Enriching food to increase the energy and protein content, e.g. extra cream, butter, cheese
- Use fruit and vegetables in moderation as these have low energy density and can lead to early satiety, thereby omitting vital macronutrients
- Using proprietary supplements which have lower carbohydrate content or advising the patient to sip the supplements slowly over 1–2 hours after meals

For enteral feeding in patients with diabetes, consideration may be given to the content of the feed in conjunction with the dietician in terms of carbohydrate and fibre content. In situations where parenteral feeding is required, insulin doses should be titrated according to the need to achieve as near normal blood glucose levels as possible.

Osteodystrophy

An important complication of chronic liver disease is osteodystrophy, which includes osteoporosis and osteomalacia. These conditions are associated with significant morbidity through fracture, resulting in pain, deformity and immobility (Collier et al., 2002). It was previously thought that patients with PSC or PBC were those with liver disease at risk of osteodystrophy, however it is now accepted that it is a risk in all cirrhotic patients regardless of their underlying condition.

Risk factors for osteoporosis and subsequent fracture irrespective of cirrhosis include:

- Low BMI <19 kg/m^2
- Excess alcohol consumption
- Steroid use (prednisolone 5 mg/day for more than 3 months)
- Physical inactivity
- Previous fragility fracture
- Early maternal hip fracture (<60 years)
- Hypogonadism and premature menopause (<45 years)

Treatment

General measures that should be advised for all patients with chronic liver disease are to stop smoking, reduce alcohol if intake is excessive and participate in regular weight-bearing exercise. Having a low BMI is an independent risk factor for osteoporosis (Collier et al., 2002). Nutritional assessment is necessary, as is ensuring adequate calories and protein are taken daily with nutritional support products if necessary. Calcium and vitamin D intakes are often inadequate in the general population and poorer in any group of patients with chronic diseases including cirrhosis, and therefore most patients require nutritional support advice and medical supplementation of both calcium and vitamin D.

Types of nutritional support in chronic liver disease

Diet therapy is pivotal to the treatment of nutritional failure in liver cirrhosis. The route and type of nutrition must be carefully planned in order to meet their high nutritional requirements.

Table 14.2 Recommendations for nutritional requirements (Johnson, 2003). Adjust requirements for high BMI. If BMI = 30–40 kg/m², use 75–100% of the value estimated from body weight/estimation of dry body weight. If BMI >40 kg/m² use 65–100% of value estimated from body weight.

Condition	Energy kcal/kg/day (dry weight kg)
Compensated liver disease	25–35
Decompensated liver disease	25–45
	Protein g/kg/day (dry weight kg)
Compensated liver disease	1.2–1.3
Decompensated liver disease	1.5–2.0
Post transplant	1.5–2.0
Acute liver failure	1.2–1.5
Chronic encephalopathy	1.0 (minimum for a trial period only)

Table 14.3 Examples of a 50 g carbohydrate snack. Patients generally tolerate most of the supplements drinks better when chilled, sipped slowly and taken between mealtimes.

Examples of a 50 g carbohydrate snack
200 mL milk with two slices of bread/toast with jam
1 Fortijuice/Enlive
1 Fortisip/ Ensure Plus and one slice bread/toast
1 Build Up and one slice bread/toast
1 Fortimel and one scone
1 Fortisip/Ensure Plus and one biscuit/crumpet

Oral

Patients can generally tolerate a normal diet and should not be restricted unless this is specifically indicated. Great care should be taken to meet their individual nutritional requirements (Table 14.2) and liaison with the multi-disciplinary team, especially the dietician, is vital (Morgan et al., 1995; Lochs and Plauth, 1999).

Both the pattern and timing of food intake have been studied (Verboeket-van De Venne et al., 1995; Tsuchiya et al., 2005; Yamanaka-Okumura et al., 2006). The amount of time needed for patients with liver cirrhosis to reach a catabolic state (in which most of the energy is derived from fat) is much shorter than in non-cirrhotic patients. After a short-term fast of only 9 hours, fat is used by the body as an alternative fuel for glucose which cannot be produced sufficiently due to depleted glycogen stores in the liver (Verboeket-van De Venne et al., 1995). Therefore, for patients with cirrhosis a nibbling pattern of food intake of five to six small meals per day is a better way of providing nutritional support. This should include a late evening snack containing 50 g of carbohydrate to improve glucose intolerance in patients with liver cirrhosis; examples of snacks are demonstrated in Table 14.3 (Tsuchiya et al., 2005).

Enteral nutrition

Randomised controlled trials have shown that enteral nutrition in cirrhosis is nutritionally more effective than oral diet (Mendenhall et al., 1985; Cabre et al., 1990) and is associated with improved liver function and prognosis (Plauth et al., 1997; Cunha et al., 2004).

Nasogastric route

Patients with liver cirrhosis should be considered early for artificial nutrition when they are unable to meet their requirements via diet and supplement drinks alone. There can still be some reluctance to pass nasogastric (NG) tubes where there are known oesophageal varices due to the risk of bleeding; however, this is not supported by the evidence (Cunha et al., 2004; Plauth et al., 2006).

High energy density feeds (1.5 kcal/mL or more) are most often required to achieve the high calculated nutritional requirements. Most feeds contain less than 100 mmol/L of sodium in 2000 kcal, which is equivalent to a no added salt diet and therefore can be used for the majority of patients. It is not necessary to dilute feeds when starting regimens; the rate should be built up over 24–72 hours depending on previous oral intake and the local policy on refeeding syndrome.

Encephalopathic patients provide their own challenges for placement of NG tubes. As their confusion increases the risk of dislodged tubes also escalates. The multi-disciplinary team needs to discuss in conjunction with local policies how to manage these patients, which may include increased nursing care, secure taping of the tube, or restraints.

Nasojejunal feeding

There is a lack of evidence regarding NG versus nasojejunal (NJ) feeding in this group of patients but NJ feeding may be used in the following circumstances:

- Poor absorption of NG feed with large gastric aspirates – can occur in patients with ALF or slow gut motility in critically ill patients who fail to respond to prokinetics
- Where there is nausea and vomiting, e.g. ascites, drug overdose
- Early satiety, e.g. ascites, chronic malnutrition

This route of feeding may also be beneficial by providing a continuous infusion of feed thereby reducing fasting periods. The same types of feeds should be used as for the NG route according to individual need.

Gastrostomy and jejunostomy feeding

The placement of percutaneous endoscopic gastrostomy (PEG) tubes is contraindicated in most patients with cirrhosis (Loser et al., 2005), due to the risk of formation of ascites and the increased risk of leakage of fluid around the stoma site and subsequent infection. Jejunostomy tubes may also be at increased risk of infection if ascites is present. They can be used post transplant for extended periods of feeding, however their use is now declining as most patients can be adequately fed via the NG or NJ route.

Parenteral nutrition

Parenteral nutrition should be reserved for patients where there is no enteral feeding route available (Henkel and Buchman, 2006). This form of nutritional support is more expensive, and is associated with a higher incidence of infections and electrolyte imbalance when compared to enteral nutrition (Sanchez and Aranda-Michel, 2006). Hepatic abnormalities (e.g. hepatic steatosis, intrahepatic cholestasis or elevated liver function tests) are relatively common, occurring in up to 75% of adults receiving parenteral nutrition (Guglielmi et al., 2006). When patients develop abnormal or worsening of liver function tests all other treatable causes should be identified and the risks minimised, e.g. sepsis. In most situations only monitoring is required or a small reduction in the energy content of the feed to 25 kcal/kg including nitrogen calories or 20 kcal/kg from non-nitrogen sources (Kumpf, 2006).

Studies suggest that the initiation of a small amount of enteral nutrition, if possible, may minimise complications such as sepsis by preventing changes to the structure and function of the gut and decreasing the risk of bacterial translocation (Guglielmi et al., 2006).

Energy should be provided by glucose and fat sources. Current research recommends 30–50% of the non-protein energy be given as fat, the higher proportion of fat in glucose-intolerant patients. For those who have ascites or peripheral oedema, a fluid restriction may be required. These patients would normally also be sodium restricted at a level of 80–100 mmol/L.

Standard parenteral nutrition bags which would meet most requirements can be used rather than *modular* bags (Klein et al., 1997). In long-term parenteral nutrition, liver function may be improved by the provision of structured lipids, omega-3 fatty acid, intravenous lipid or cyclical feeding (Rubin et al., 2000).

For patients with acute alcoholic hepatitis, aggressive enteral nutrition should be the route of choice. Parenteral nutrition should be considered if this route is not possible. There is no advantage in giving parenteral nutrition to patients with chronic liver disease for perioperative feeding. Again, the enteral route should be tried first. All cases should be referred to either the hospital nutrition team or a suitably trained health professional.

Nutritional support in alcoholic liver disease

Nutritional support in patients who have alcoholic liver disease (ALD) is necessary as some studies report an incidence of PCM of up to 100% in this group of patients

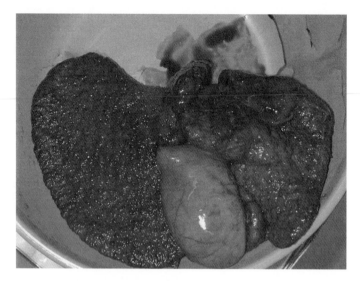

Figure 14.1 Explanted liver demonstrating alcohol-induced liver cirrhosis. For a colour version of this figure, please see Plate 15 in the colour plate section.

(Tome and Lucey, 2004). Malnourishment of patients with alcoholic liver disease is of multi-factorial origin. Poor dietary intake, decreased gastrointestinal use and poor ability to store nutrients all contribute to malnutrition but the mechanisms by which malnutrition worsens ALD are unknown. It has been suggested that protein calorie deficiency could enhance the toxicity of alcohol, partly through the influence of nutritional status on the effect on the immune system integrity and the capacity to respond to infection (MacSween and Burt, 1986). Another explanation is that alcohol inhibits hepatic regeneration and protein synthesis, hence the reason that abstinence is vital to assess how much the liver can compensate without the continued insult of alcohol prior to consideration of transplantation (Figure 14.1, Plate 15).

It is important when assessing a patient with a history of alcohol excess or established ALD that thiamine and vitamin B compound are prescribed as a maintenance prescription due to the increased metabolic need for these vitamins while drinking alcohol. The clinical consequences of thiamine and other B vitamin deficiency can be severely debilitating. Some of the symptoms include peripheral neuropathy, beri beri, cardiomegaly, reduced motility and elasticity of gut lumen, depression, Wernicke's encephalopathy and, should the deficiency continue, the irreversible progression to Korsakoff's psychosis.

For descriptive purposes the three main stages are described as steatosis, acute alcoholic hepatitis and cirrhosis (Baptista et al., 1981). In reality these often overlap and nutritionally it is important to consider each patient on their individual condition.

Steatosis

At this stage the dietary treatment advised is to stop alcohol intake, achieve a body mass index within an acceptable range (BMI 20–25 kg/m^2) and a healthy eating diet with exercise programme.

Alcoholic hepatitis

Most patients who develop alcoholic hepatitis already have an established degree of malnutrition and the mortality as a result of acute alcoholic hepatitis is correlated closely with the severity of protein energy malnutrition (Cabre et al., 1990). Initially medical treatment of gastritis, nausea and vomiting may be necessary to allow nutritional support to commence. Anorexia is common. Nutritional requirements are calculated using 35–45 kcal/kg, 1.2–1.8 g protein/kg/dry body weight per day (Johnson, 2003; Todorovic and Micklewright, 2004). It is unlikely that patients can meet these requirements orally and nutritional support products are essential.

Micronutrient deficiencies are often found, such as vitamin C (ascorbic acid), zinc and B vitamins. All may need additional supplementation. If the enteral route is available it should be used and parenteral nutrition considered only when other feeding routes have been exhausted.

Alcoholic cirrhosis

Studies have reported an incidence of 80–100% of protein energy malnutrition in patients with alcoholic cirrhosis and nutritional support is a vital part of treatment. Enteral nutritional support improves nutritional status and liver function, reduces complications and prolongs survival in cirrhotic patients (Plauth et al., 1997).

Each patient should be assessed on admission to hospital and nutritional treatment is symptom led. Medical treatment of gastritis, nausea and vomiting may be necessary. Complete alcohol abstinence should be advised and thiamine and B vitamins prescribed. Recommended nutritional requirements are 1.5–2.0 g protein/kg dry body weight and 35–40 kcal/kg dry body weight (Johnson, 2003; Todorovi and Micklewright, 2004).

The oral route or nasogastric route should be decided on an individual patient basis. As nutritional support is symptom led, consideration should be given to common symptoms and consequences of cirrhosis, such as ascites, fluid restrictions, early satiety, jaundice and malabsorption. Close systematic monitoring is needed to ensure nutritional requirements are met and hence improve outcome.

Refeeding syndrome

Refeeding syndrome consists of metabolic disturbances that occur as a result of reinstating nutrition to patients who are starved or severely malnourished (Crook et al., 2001; NICE, 2006). Patients can develop fluid and electrolyte disorders, especially hypophosphataemia, hypokalaemia and hypomagnesaemia along with neurological, pulmonary, cardiac, neuromuscular and haematological complications. The effect is due to a sudden shift from fat to carbohydrate metabolism. It can be fatal if not recognised and treated properly. The patients at risk of developing this syndrome have one or more of the following (NICE, 2006):

- BMI less than 16 kg/m^2
- Unintentional weight loss greater than 15% within the last 3–6 months
- Little or no nutritional intake for more than 10 days
- Low levels of potassium, magnesium or phosphate prior to feeding
- Diabetes, hyperglycaemia or increased insulin requirements

Alternatively the patient has two or more of the following:

- BMI less than 18.5 kg/m^2
- Unintentional weight loss greater than 10% within last 3–6 months
- Little or no nutritional intake for more than 5 days
- A history of alcohol abuse or drugs including insulin, chemotherapy, antacids or diuretics

As nutritional support commences patients must have prescribed oral thiamine, vitamin B and a multivitamin preparation, immediately before and during the first 10 days of feeding. Enteral feeding should be commenced at no more than 10 kcal/kg and increased slowly over 7 days to calculated nutritional requirements. Daily monitoring of serum electrolytes, magnesium and phosphate is necessary and medical supplementation should be given as clinically indicated.

Non-alcoholic fatty liver disease

Non-alcoholic fatty liver disease (NAFLD) is an emerging phenomenon which is clearly linked with the increasing prevalence of obesity and metabolic syndrome in the UK, as discussed in Chapter 8.

Dietetic management of metabolic syndrome

Metabolic syndrome is a cluster of risk factors that increase ischaemic heart disease. Abdominal obesity, which is measured by doing a simple waist circumference measurement, is the body fat parameter most closely associated with the metabolic syndrome. This measurement is particularly associated with insulin resistance and is a much stronger predictor of cardiovascular complications and NAFLD than a high BMI (Sanyal and AGA, 2002).

First-line management of the metabolic syndrome consists of lifestyle interventions, weight loss, increased exercise and stopping smoking. Each individual component of the syndrome should be treated medically where appropriate.

Obesity

The UK population is getting fatter and the incidence of type 2 diabetes is dramatically on the increase. Grades of obesity can be defined as:

- Healthy BMI $20–25$ kg/m^2
- Grade 1 obesity $26–30$ kg/m^2
- Grade 2 obesity $30–35$ kg/m^2
- Grade 3 obesity >35 kg/m^2

Weight loss

The value of calorie restriction with exercise in achieving and maintaining weight loss is well established. Weight loss and physical activity improve all components of metabolic syndrome. They improve lipid profiles, insulin sensitivity, hypertension and NAFLD (Sanyal and AGA, 2002). They also further reduce the risk for type 2 diabetes.

To promote weight reduction through caloric restriction, national expert clinical guidelines for weight loss recommend that caloric intake should be reduced by 500–1000 calories per day to produce a weight loss of 0.5–1.0 kg/week (NIDDK, 2004). The goal for patients is to reduce bodyweight by 10% of their baseline weight. Current exercise guidelines recommend 30–60 minutes of moderate-intensity exercise daily (e.g. brisk walking). Dietary changes alone are associated with high failure rate at achieving weight loss due to multi-factorial reasons that are outside the scope of this chapter.

Rapid weight loss should be discouraged to avoid weight loss that exceeds 1.5 kg/week as this can cause worsening steatohepatitis, risk of decompensation and increased risk of gallstones (Sanyal and AGA, 2002). 'Healthy eating' diets as described below should be advised. For people without diabetes advise:

- Balance of Good Health
- British Dietetic Association Healthy Eating Advice
- British Heart Foundation Dietary Advice
- Diet <35% fat, 50% carbohydrate, 15% protein
- 15–20% monosaturates minimal trans fats
- Minimal refined carbohydrate, low gycaemic index (GI) foods
- Fish once or twice per week with one portion being oily
- Lower saturated fat <10% total fat
- Lower total fat
- Increased fruit and vegetables to five portions/day
- Exercise for 30 minutes/day

For people with diabetes advise as above and in line with dietary position statements as described by European Association for the Study of Diabetes and the American Diabetes Association (EASD, 2000; Sanyal and AGA, 2002).

Non-alcoholic steaotohepatitis

'Healthy eating' dietary therapies with exercise and normoglycaemia should be advised with a target weight maintenance of BMI ≤25 kg/m² pre and post transplant, as steatosis (fatty liver) recurs in a majority of patients by 4 years post transplant, with 50% of patients developing recurrent non-alcoholic steatohepatitis (NASH) (Doelle, 2004).

Patients with decompensated NASH

When patients with NASH become cirrhotic the nutritional advice can appear confusing for patients and staff alike. It is important to recognise that these patients are at a high risk of PCM despite what appears to be an elevated BMI. The metabolic changes of cirrhotic liver are present, and to maintain a positive nitrogen balance the patients need 1.5–2 g of protein/kg of dry body weight (Johnson, 2003). Failure to do so results in gross muscle decline and increased mortality.

Muscle mass can be measured objectively using handgrip and mid-arm muscle circumference measurements. It is vital to calculate dry weight BMI adjusting for ascites and oedema as described earlier in the chapter. If weight loss is necessary, to ensure fat and not further muscle mass is lost, advice is given with the aim to lose weight by mobilising fat stores at a rate of 0.5–1 kg dry weight/week. A more rapid loss could cause the liver to decompensate and worsen underlying protein malnutrition. Strict attention to fluid weight adjustments (ascites and oedema) is necessary to distinguish between fluid and dry body weight.

Post-transplant nutrition

The rates of morbidity and mortality post transplant are related to the incidence of pretransplant malnutrition (Hasse, 2006). In the immediate postoperative period, feeding protocols vary between transplant centres. Nonetheless, if the patient requires enteral nutrition this is normally initiated within 12 hours of theatre providing there are no surgical contraindications. All feeds should be started at full strength and increased as per local protocols, and can be continued until an acceptable oral intake is maintained. NG feeding may be reduced to overnight as oral intake increases, in liaison with the dietician caring for the patient.

Once NG feeding has ceased supplementation of the diet will continue to be necessary for the next 2–3 months, depending on the individual, with snacks and/ or supplement drinks as described pre transplant. It is important to continue to be proactive with nutritional support at this stage as the patient may still have

Table 14.4   Long-term complications following liver transplantation and their dietary management.

Complication	Dietary treatment
Diabetes	Continue supplements in the early stages with oral hypoglycaemic agents or insulin being used to maintain normal glucose levels. Simple low sugar advice initially with current guidelines for diabetes being followed longer term
Obesity	Encourage weight maintenance initially with slow weight loss of 0.5–1 kg/week if required longer term
Hyperlipidaemia	Statins can be used under careful monitoring (Massucco et al., 2004). Advise lifestyle modification including weight control, smoking cessation and exercise (Fletcher et al., 2005)
Osteoporosis	See osteoporosis section
Hyperkalaemia	Medical staff may need to reduce immunosuppression doses or start sodium bicarbonate medication in liaison with the transplant unit. Only if this fails should a potassium-restricted diet be advised
Hypertension	Dietary restriction of sodium to no added salt level should be continued

significant wound healing, necessary weight gain and episodes of rejection to overcome. Regular monitoring continues to be essential.

In long-term liver transplant recipients there are six main nutritional problems which may occur, which are shown in Table 14.4.

Chapter summary

Malnutrition is a common complication of liver disease which has important prognostic implications. Nutritional assessment should include a detailed history of symptoms, dietary intake and objective measurements of nutritional status. Dietary advice aims to meet estimated requirements whilst avoiding unnecessary restrictions. Artificial nutrition should be considered early with enteral feeding the route of choice. Some disease aetiologies such as NAFLD are linked to the increasing prevalence of obesity and metabolic syndrome. Dietary treatment consists of lifestyle interventions, weight loss, increased exercise and stopping smoking.

References

Alvares-da-Silva MR, Reverbel da Silveira T (2005) Comparison between handgrip strength, subjective global assessment and prognostic nutritional index in assessing malnutrition and predicting clinical outcome in cirrhotic patients. *Nutrition* **21**(2):113–117

Baptista A, Bianchi L, de Groote J (1981) Alcoholic liver disease: morphological manifestations. Review by an international group. *Lancet* **1**:707–711

British Association for Parenteral and Enteral Nutrition (2003) Malnutrition Universal Screening Tool. BAPEN, Redditch available from www.bapen.org.uk (Accessed 27th September 2007)

Cabre E, Gonzalez-Huix F, Abad-Lacruz A, Esteve M, Acero D, Fernandez-Banares F, Xiol X, Gassull MA (1990) Effect of total enteral nutrition on the short-term outcome of severely malnourished cirrhotics. A randomized controlled trial. *Gastroenterology* **98**(3):715–720

Cabre E, Rodríguez-Iglesias P, Caballería J, Quer JC, Sánchez-Lombraña JL, Parés A, Papo M, Planas R, Gassull MA, Spanish Group for the Study of Alcoholic Hepatitis (2000) Short and long term outcome of severe alcohol induced hepatitis treated with steroids or enteral nutrition, a multicentre randomised trial. *Hepatology* **32**(1):36–42

Campos ACL, Matias JEF, Coelho JCU (2002) Nutritional aspects of liver transplantation. *Current Opinion in Clinical Nutrition and Metabolic Care* **5**(3): 297–307

Collier JD, Ninkovic M, Compston JE (2002) Guidelines on the management of osteoporosis associated with chronic liver disease. *Gut* **50**(Suppl 1): i1–i9

Crook MA, Hally V, Panteli JV (2001) The importance of the refeeding syndrome. *Nutrition* **17**(7–8):632–637

Cunha L, Happi Nono M, Gilbert AL Nidegger D, Beau P, Beauchant M (2004) Effects of prolonged oral nutritional support in malnourished cirrhotic patients: results of a pilot study. *Gastroentérologie Clinique et Biologique* **28**(1):36–39

Day CP (2006) Non alcoholic fatty liver disease: current concepts and management strategies. *Clinical Medicine* **6**(1):9–25

De Bruijn KM, Blendis LM, Zilm DH (1983) Effect of dietary protein manipulation in sub-clinical portal-systemic encephalopathy. *Gut* **24**(1):53–60

Doelle G (2004) The clinical picture of metabolic syndrome. An update on this complex of conditions and risk factors. *Postgraduate Medicine* **116**(1):30–38

European Association for the Study of Diabetes – Dietitian and Nutrition Study Group (2000) Recommendations for the nutritional management for patients with diabetes mellitus. *European Journal of Clinical Nutrition* **54**:353–355

Fairfield KM, Fletcher RH (2002) Vitamins for chronic disease prevention in adults: scientific review. *Journal of the American Medical Association* **287**(23): 3116–3126

Fisher NC, Hanson J, Phillips A, Rao JN, Swarbrick ET (2002) Mortality from liver disease in the West Midlands, 1993–2000. Observational study. *British Medical Journal* **325**:312–313

Fletcher B, Berra K, Ades P, Braun LT, Burke LE, Durstine JL, Fair JM, Fletcher GF, Goff D, Hayman LL, Hiatt WR, Miller NH, Krauss R, Kris-Etherton P, Stone N, Wilterdink J, Winston M, Council on Cardiovascular Nursing, Council on Arteriosclerosis, Thrombosis, and Vascular Biology, Council on Basic Cardiovascular Sciences, Council on Cardiovascular Disease in the Young, Council on Clinical Cardiology, Council on Epidemiology and Prevention, Council on Nutrition, Physical Activity, and Metabolism, Council on Stroke, Preventive

Cardiovascular Nurses Association (2005) Managing abnormal blood lipids: a collaborative approach. *Circulation* **112**(20):3184–3209

Gonzales-Barranco J, Furst P, Schrezenmeir J, O'Dorisio T, Coulston A (1998) Glucose control guidelines: current concepts. *Clinical Nutrition* **17**(suppl 2): 7–17

Guglielmi FW, Boggio Bertinet D, Federico A, Forte GB, Guglielmi A, Loguercio C, Mazzuoli S, Merli M, Palmo A, Panella C, Pironi L, Francavilla A (2006) Total parenteral nutrition-related gastroenterological complications. *Digestive and Liver Disease* **38**(9):623–642

Hasse JM (2006) Examining the role of tube feeding after liver transplantation. *Nutrition in Clinical Practice* **21**(3):299–311

Henkel AS, Buchman AL (2006) Nutritional support in chronic liver disease. *Nature Clinical Practice. Gastroenterology & Hepatology* **3**(4):202–209

Johnson J (2003) Nutritional treatment of liver disease. *Complete Nutrition* **3**(5):9–11

Kehayoglou AK, Holdsworth CD, Agnew JE, Whelton MJ, Sherlock S (1968) Bone disease and calcium absorption in primary biliary cirrhosis with special reference to vitamin D therapy. *Lancet* **1**(7545):715–718

Kennedy PTF, O'Grady JG (2002) Diseases of the liver: chronic liver disease. *Hospital Pharmacist* **9**(5):137–144

Klein S, Kinney J, Jeejeebhoy K, Alpers D, Hellerstein M, Murray M, Twomey P (1997) Nutrition support in clinical practice: review of published data and recommendations for future research directions. *Journal of Parenteral & Enteral Nutrition* **21**(3):133–156

Kondrup J, Muller J (1997) Energy and protein requirements of patients with chronic liver disease. *Journal of Hepatology* **27**:239–247

Kumpf VJ (2006) Parenteral nutrition-associated liver disease in adult and pediatric patients. *Nutrition in Clinical Practice* **21**(3):279–290

Lee YM, Kaplan MM (2002) Management of primary sclerosing cholangitis. *American Journal of Gastroenterology* **97**(3):528–534

Lochs H, Plauth M (1999) Liver cirrhosis: rationale and modalities for nutritional support. The European Society of Parenteral and Enteral Nutrition consensus and beyond. *Current Opinion in Clinical Nutrition and Metabolic Care* **2**(4): 345–349

Loser CHR, Aschl G, Hebuterne X, Mathus-Vliegen EMH, Muscaritoli M, Niv Y, Rollins H, Singer P, Skelly RH (2005) ESPEN guidelines on artificial enteral nutrition – percutaneous endoscopic gastrostomy (PEG). *Clinical Nutrition* **24**(5):848–861

MacSween RN, Burt AD (1986) Histologic spectrum of alcoholic liver disease. *Seminars in Liver Disease* **6**(3):221–232

Madden A (1992) The role of low fat diets in the management of gall-bladder disease. *Journal of Human Nutrition and Dietetics* **5**:267–273

Massucco AG, Bonomo P, Trovati M (2004) Prescription of statins to dyslipidemic patients affected by liver diseases: a subtle balance between risks and benefits. *Nutrition, Metabolism, and Cardiovascular Diseases* **14**(4):215–224

Matos C, Porayko MK, Francisco-Ziller N, DiCecco S (2002) Nutrition and chronic liver disease. *Journal of Clinical Gastroenterology* 35(5):391–397

McCullough AJ, Bugionesie E (1997) Protein-calorie malnutrition and the etiology of cirrhosis. *American Journal of Gastroenterology* 92(5):734–738

McMahon MM, Rizza RA (1996) Nutritional support in hospitalized patients with diabetes mellitus. *Mayo Clinic Proceedings* 71:587–594

Mendenhall C, Bongiovanni G, Goldberg S, Miller B, Moore J, Rouster S, Schneider S, et al. (1985) VA Cooperative Study on Alcohol Hepatitis. III: Changes in protein-calorie malnutrition associated with 30 days of hospitalization with and without enteral nutritional therapy. *Journal of Parenteral and Enteral Nutrition* 9(5):590–596

Merli M, Riggio O, Dally L (1996) Does malnutrition affect survival in liver cirrhosis. *Hepatology* 23(5):1041–1046

Miwa Y, Shiraki M, Kato M, Tajika M, Mohri H, Murakami N, Kato T, Ohnishi H, Morioku T, Muto Y, Moriwaki H (2000) Improvement of fuel metabolism by nonturnal energy supplementation in patients with liver cirrhosis. *Hepatology Research* 18(3):185–189

Moore KP, Aithal GP (2006) Guidelines on the management of ascites in cirrhosis. *Gut* 55(suppl 6):vi1–vi12

Morgan TR, Moritz TE, Mendenhall CL, Haas R (1995) Protein consumption and hepatic encephalopathy in alcoholic hepatitis. *Journal of the American College of Nutrition* 14(2):152–158

Mullen KD, Weber Jr FL (1991) Role of nutrition in hepatic encephalopathy. *Seminars in Liver Disease* 11(4):292–304

National Institute of Diabetes and Diabetic Kidney Disease (2004) Weight Loss Information Network. Available at http://win.niddk.nih.gov (Accessed 2nd October 2007)

National Institute for Health and Clinical Excellence (2006) Nutritional Support in Adults, Clinical Guidelines 32. Available at http://guidance.nice.org.uk/CG32 (Accessed 2nd October 2007)

Phillips GB, Schwartz R, Gabuzda GJ Jr, Davidson CS (1952) The syndrome of impending hepatic coma in patients with cirrhosis of the liver given certain nitrogenous substances. *New England Journal of Medicine* 247:239–246

Plauth M, Cabre E, Riggio O, Assis-Camilo M, Pirlich M, Kondrup J, Ferenchi P, Holme E, Vom Dahl S, Muller MJ, Nolte W (2006) ESPEN guidelines on enteral nutrition: liver disease. *Clinical Nutrition* 25(2):285–294

Plauth M, Merli M, Kondrup J, Weimann A, Ferenci P, Muller MJ. ESPEN Consensus Group (1997) ESPEN Guidelines for Nutrition in Liver Disease and Transplantation. *Clinical Nutrition* 16(2):43–55

Rubin M, Moser A, Vaserberg N, Greig F, Levy Y, Spivak H, Ziv Y, Lelcuk S (2000) Structured triacylglcerol emulsion, containing medium and long chain fatty acids, in long term home parenteral nutrition: a double-blind randomised cross-over study. *Nutrition* 16:95–100

Runyon BA (1998) Management of adult patients with ascites caused by cirrhosis. *Hepatology* 27(1):264–272

Sanchez AJ, Aranda-Michel J (2006) Nutrition for the liver transplant patient. *Liver Transplantation* **12**:1310–1316

Sanyal AJ, American Gastroenterological Association (2002) AGA technical review on non alcoholic fatty liver disease. *Gastroenterology* **123**(5):1705–1725

Sarath G, Shailee S, Raikamal S (2000) Practicalities of nutritional support in chronic liver disease. *Current Opinions in Clinical Nutrition and Metabolism Care* **3**(3):227–229

Soulsby CT (1997) An examination of the effects of dietary sodium restriction on energy and protein intake in the treatment of ascites in cirrhosis. *Proceedings of the Nutrition Society* (abstract) **57**:115A

Talwalkar JA, Lindor KD (2003) Primary biliary cirrhosis. *The Lancet* **362**: 53–61

Todorovic VE, Micklewright A (eds) (2004) *A Pocket Guide to Clinical Nutrition*, 3rd edn. British Dietetic Association, London

Tome S, Lucey MR (2004) Current management of alcoholic liver disease. *Alimentary Pharmacology and Therapeutics* **19**(7):707–714

Tsuchiya M, Sakaida I, Okamoto M, Okita K (2005) The effect of a late evening snack in patients with liver cirrhosis. *Hepatology Research* **31**(2):95–103

Verboeket-van De Venne WPHG, Westerterp KR, Van Hoek B, Swart GR (1995) Energy expenditure and substrate metabolism in patients with cirrhosis of the liver: effects of the pattern of food intake. *Gut* **36**(1):110–116

Yamanaka-Okumura H, Nakamura T, Takeuchi H, Miyake H, Katayama T, Arai H, Taketani Y, Fujii M, Shimada M, Takeda E (2006) Effect of late evening snack with rice ball on energy metabolism in liver cirrhosis. *European Journal of Clinical Nutrition* **60**(9):1067–1072

15

Drug-induced liver injury

Suzanne Sargent

Introduction

The liver is the predominant site of drug metabolism, biotransformation and clearance. Therefore it is not surprising that drug-induced hepatotoxicity accounts for approximately 2% of all inpatient jaundice, and that drug-induced hepatic injury accounts for 10% of all liver disease, with over 1000 drugs and chemical agents being implicated as the cause (McFarlane et al., 2000). In the USA, drug-related hepatotoxicity is now the leading cause of acute liver failure (ALF) amongst patients referred for liver transplantation. Drug-related hepatotoxicity accounts for 50% of all cases of ALF, which is associated with a 90% mortality rate (O'Grady et al., 1989; Navarro and Senior, 2006). However, reliable data of drug-induced hepatotoxicity is difficult to establish. This situation may be compounded by the lack of regulation of herbal remedies which are now used by up to 50% of the western population, and account for as much as 5% of all drug-induced liver disease (Ryder and Beckingham, 2001).

To discuss all aspects of drug-induced hepatic damage is beyond the scope of this chapter, therefore it will focus primarily on the most common type of drug-induced liver injuries, the risk factors for drug-induced hepatotoxicity and the most commonly prescribed and over the counter (OTC) pharmacological preparations and the herbal remedies associated with hepatotoxicity.

Mechanisms of hepatotoxicity

The pathogenesis and clinical presentation of hepatotoxicity varies with each pharmacological agent, and in a large proportion of cases is poorly understood. In general drug-related jaundice can be due to either predictable direct hepato-toxicity, such as paracetamol overdose, or idiosyncratic drug reactions, which make up 20% of all severe liver injury cases requiring hospitalisation (Ryder and Beckingham, 2001).

The liver is central to drug metabolism as the hepatocytes contain all the necessary enzymes to enable this to occur. The enzyme systems responsible for this process are located in the smooth endoplasmic reticulum of the hepatocytes and include mixed function oxidase or mono-oxygenase (MFO), cytochrome c-reductase and cytochrome P450. The main enzymes involved in drug metabolism belong to the cytochrome P450 group (Norris, 2006).

Biotransformation takes place in several stages of biochemical reaction which are classified as phase 1 and phase 2, and are discussed further in Chapter 1. Some drugs undergo just phase 1 or 2 metabolism, however most drugs will undergo sequential metabolism of both phases. Phase 1 reactions are mediated by cyto-chrome P450 and prepare the compound for conjugation by oxidation or hydroxy-lation, therefore making the drug more polar and modifying the structure of the drug (Norris, 2006). There are many differences between patients' ability to perform phase 1 liver metabolism of some drugs, and genetic differences in the activity of P450 isoenzymes which may determine idiosyncratic drug reactions (Norris, 2006). Enzyme inducers such as alcohol, barbiturates and anticonvulsant therapy can alter P450 enzyme activity, therefore increasing the risk of drug toxic-ity (Schiano and Black, 2004).

Phase 2 metabolisms involve conjugation in which the drugs are converted from an active metabolite to a non-toxic more water-soluble product by conjugation with glutathione, sulphate, glucuronide or water. These metabolic processes usually occur in the hepatocyte cytoplasm (Schiano and Black, 2004). Factors which determine whether the metabolised drug will be excreted in bile or urine are mul-tiple and can be dependent on factors such as molecular size, or the polarity of the substances (Sherlock and Dooley, 2002).

Diagnosis of drug-induced liver injury

The clinical manifestations of drug-induced liver injury mirror the signs and symp-toms of most forms of liver disease, therefore this possibility should be considered when taking a patient's history. All drugs taken over the previous 3 months should be recorded, including the dose, route of administration, duration, and any con-comitant medication, including alternative therapies such as herbal and Chinese remedies. Early suspicion of drug-related hepatotoxicity and accurate diagnosis are imperative as the severity of the reaction can be increased if the drug regime is continued, especially after symptoms develop or serum transaminases become elevated.

Other causes of liver disease such as viral hepatitis or autoimmune hepatitis should not be forgotten and need to be excluded by careful assessment of clinical, radiological, biochemical and serological findings. Nonetheless, the possibility of drug injury superimposed on liver disease must always be considered (Schiano and Black, 2004).

Individual susceptibility to hepatic injury is influenced by many factors such as gender, age, genetic predisposition, pregnancy, nutritional status (obesity or malnutrition), pre-existing liver disease and a known history of interactions with other drugs (McFarlane et al., 2000); consequently these facts should always be taken into consideration when suspecting drug-induced liver injury as the primary or differential diagnosis.

Classification of drug injury

Drug-induced liver injury may be either hepatocellular (with liver cell necrosis and/or steatosis), cholestatic (reduced bile flow and jaundiced with little parenchymal damage), or a mixed type with features of parenchymal and cholestatic damage. Often there is overlap between types of liver damage as drugs can cause more than one type of reaction (McFarlane et al., 2000). The presentation of drug-induced liver failure varies and depends on the underlying type of liver injury. Elevation of biochemical tests, such as AST, ALT and GGT, can represent an adaptive response to a drug, but may not be indicative of the true hepatic injury (Watkins and Seeff, 2006). When the diagnosis is difficult to establish, a liver biopsy can be useful with a drug-related reaction suggested by fatty changes, granulomas, bile duct lesions, zonal hepatic necrosis and general hepatocellular 'unrest' (Sherlock and Dooley, 2002).

Hepatocellular drug-induced liver disease

The primary event is caused by hepatocellular necrosis, and the clinical picture varies from subclinical elevations of AST and ALT to acute liver failure. Hepatocyte injury is rarely due to the drug itself and is usually caused by a toxic metabolite or metabolite-mediated immuno-allergic reaction (Norris, 2006). Acute hepatocellular hepatitis generally has no specific features and mimics acute viral hepatitis, and therefore it can be hard to distinguish one from the other. Clinically acute hepatocellular hepatitis is defined by ALT above twice the upper normal limit (ULN) or ALT:ALP ratio of ≥ 5. Prolongation of the INR or PT and hyperbilirubinaemia are all poor prognostic indicators; this is discussed further in Chapter 13.

Drug-induced cholestasis

Cholestasis is the failure of bile to reach the duodenum, and is commonly characterised by jaundice, pruritus, pale stool and dark urine. There are three mechanisms of drug-induced cholestasis which are due to impairment of hepatocellular bile secretion (pure cholestasis or cholestatic hepatitis), obstruction of ductules (cholangiolitis) or interlobular ducts (cholangitis) or extrahepatic obstruction (Erlinger, 1997). Cholestatic injury is associated with serological elevations of ALP, serum bilirubin and GGT (Navarro and Senior, 2006).

Steatosis

Steatosis refers to the accumulation of fat droplets in liver cells, either microvesicular (small droplets of fat within the hepatocytes) or macrovesicular (larger lipid droplets). Examples of drugs that can induce steatosis are shown in Table 15.1.

Fibrosis

Fibrotic damage forms part of most drug reactions, but in some it may the dominant feature. Fibrous tissue is deposited in the Disse space, obstructing the sinusoidal blood flow and causing non-cirrhotic portal hypertension and hepatocellular dysfunction (Sherlock and Dooley, 2002). An example of this is methotrexate-induced hepatic fibrosis.

Hepatic venous damage

Obstruction of both the large (Budd-Chiari syndrome) and small hepatic veins (veno-occlusive disease) can result from adverse drug reactions and is characterised by abdominal pain, ascites and lower limb oedema. In some cases ALF can develop. Diagnosis is usually made with ultrasonography with Doppler studies, CT and hepatic venography for Budd-Chiari syndrome, and liver biopsy in veno-occlusive disease.

Commonly used drugs that cause hepatotoxicity

Over 1000 drugs have been implicated in causing either acute or chronic liver injury, ranging from subclinical elevation of liver function tests to acute liver failure (McFarlane et al., 2000). The commonest drugs that cause hepatotoxicity are demonstrated in Table 15.2, some of which are discussed below.

Table 15.1   Classification of hepatotoxic drug reactions.

Types of hepatotoxic reaction	Examples of drugs
Hepatocellular	Paracetamol (acetaminophen) Halothane Carbon tetrachloride Rifampin Isonizid Ketoconazole Statins Volproic acid NSAIDs
Cholestasis	Amoxicillin–clavulanic acid Anabolic steriods Sex hormones (oestrogen hormone replacement therapy or contraceptive pill) Chlorpromazine Chlororpropamide Flucloxacillin Erythromycin Tricyclics Tamoxifen
Mixed (hepatitis and cholestasis)	Amitriptyline Azathioprine Captopril Phenytoin Verapamil Trimethaprine
Microvesicular steatosis: inhibition of fatty acid mitochondrial beta-oxidation	Sodium valoprate NSAIDs Aspirin Tetracycline
Macrovesicular steatosis: decreased secretions of lipoproteins	Amiodarone Corticosteriods Methotrexate
Fibrosis	Methotrexate Vitamin A Vinyl chloride
Tumours (ademoma and hepatocellular carcinoma)	Oral contraceptive, oestrogen and androgens
Vanishing bile duct syndrome: autoimmune destruction of small bile ducts	Chlorpromazine
Vascular (veno-occlusive disease, hepatic vein obstruction, portal vein obstruction)	Cytotoxics Azathioprine Sex hormones

Table 15.2 Drugs known to cause drug-induced liver injury. Adapted from Norris (2000).

Drug groups	Drugs known to induce liver injury
Anticonvulsants and psychoactive drugs	Phenytoin
	Carbamazine
	Valproic acid
	Chlorpromazine
	Tricyclic antidepressants
	Monoamine oxidase inhibitors
	Cocaine
Antibacterial agents	Tetracyclines
	Erythromycin
	Flucoxacillin
	Amplicillin and amoxycillin
	Sulphonamides
	Nitrofurantoin
Antifungals	Ketoconazole
	Griseofulvin
Antituberculous agents	Isoniazid
	Rifampin
Analgesics and anti-inflammatory drugs	Acetaminophen (paracetamol)
	Salicylates
	Diclofenac
	Phenylbutazone
	Sulindac
	Ibuprofen
	Nimesulide
Cardiovascular agents	Methyldopa
	ACE inhibitors
	Thiazide diuretics
	Hydralazine
	Amiodarone
	Quinidine
	Calcium channel blockers
	Beta-adrenergic blocking drugs
	Perhexilene maleate
	3-Hydroxy-3-methylglutaryl coenzyme A reductase inhibitors
	Clofibrate
Immunomodulatory drugs	Methotrexate
	Antipurines
	Antipyrimidines
	Zidovudine
	Busulfan
	Cyclophosphamide
	Chlorambucil
Naturally occurring immunodulatory agents	L-asparaginase
	Alkaloids
	Adriamycin (doxorubicin hydrochloride)
Anaesthetic agents	Halothane
Industrial and naturally occurring toxins	Carbon tetrachloride
	Yellow phosphorous
	Selenium
	Vinyl chloride
	Pesticides
	Arsenic
	Mushroom poisioning
	Alfatoxins
	Herbal medicines

Paracetamol (acetaminophen)

Paracetamol (acetaminophen) is the most common cause of drug-induced liver injury and ALF in both the UK and USA. Whilst paracetamol hepatotoxicity is often linked to people attempting or achieving suicide, accidental overdose accounts for 8% of cases in the UK to 48% of cases in the USA. The median dose of paracetamol causing ALF in the UK was reported to be 40 g, with the highest mortality seen at doses exceeding 48 g (O'Grady, 2006).

Paracetamol is primarily metabolised by conjugation to glucuronide and sulphate before being excreted in the urine. However approximately 5% is metabolised by the cytochrome P450 pathway, which results in the formation of a highly toxic metabolite N-acetyl-P-benzoquinone imine (NAPQI). This is turned into harmless metabolite by conjugation with glutathione S-transferases (GSTs) before being excreted in the urine as mercapturic acid. However, when doses exceeding safe margins of paracetamol are ingested, the normal metabolising routes of conjugation with glucuronide and sulphate become saturated, causing increased metabolism through the cytochrome P450 pathway. This increases the formation of NAPQI, leading to decrease in intracellular glutathione and subsequent hepatocellular necrosis (Figure 15.1).

There are three phases of clinical presentation. Phase 1 occurs with 12–24 hours following ingestion when patients present with gastrointestinal symptoms of nausea, vomiting and anorexia. Patients may display little evidence of liver injury until phase 2 (24–48 hours), in which the patient may exhibit elevations in aminotransferase, bilirubin and prolonged prothrombin. Right upper quadrant pain, hepatic encephalopathy, and renal impairment may sometimes be present. Phase 3 occurs in days 3–10 post ingestion when the onset of overt acute liver dysfunction is seen and when clinical and laboratory abnormalities peak.

The risk and severity of hepatic injury may be indicated by the serum paracetamol level obtained 4 hours after ingestion (Figure 15.2), however plasma paracetamol

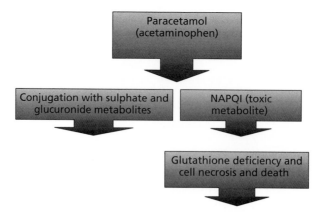

Figure 15.1   Paracetamol (acetaminophen) metabolism post overdose.

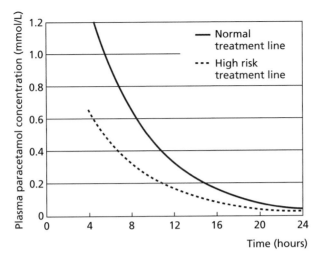

Figure 15.2 Guidelines for N-acetylcysteine treatment based on serum paracetamol concentration. Reproduced with permission from Ryder and Beckingham (2001).

concentrations cannot be used to assess the risk of hepatotoxicity after a 'staggered overdose', or in patients who present at more than 24 hours post ingestion. Individuals at high risk include those who are malnourished, chronic alcohol consumers and patients taking enzyme-induced drugs, such as anti-epileptic therapy, who are more susceptible to hepatotoxic damage.

Treatment is primarily aimed at replacing the glutathione reserves of the liver cells with N-acetylcysteine (NAC). NAC provides almost a 100% protection if given within 8 hours of ingestion. Those patients who present more than 15 hours after ingestion have a greater risk of developing hepatotoxicity because of the reduced efficacy of NAC (Greene et al., 2005). Nevertheless, although this is unlicensed in these situations, the consensus is that NAC should be started even if the patient presents several days post ingestion (Schiano and Black, 2004). Poor prognostic signs after a paracetamol overdose include hepatic encephalopathy, raised INR/PT, acidosis and renal failure. Chapter 13 outlines the management of ALF.

Non-steroidal anti-inflammatory drugs

The incidence of NSAID-induced hepatotoxicity is varied and ranges from 3.7–9.0/100 000 users. Associated risk factors are liver injury, older age, renal disease and alcohol excess (Norris, 2006). Most of the drug reactions are idiosyncratic but may cause hepatitis, cholestatic, granulomatous and autoimmune changes. NSAIDs should be avoided in patients with pre-existing liver disease due to the high risk of precipitating renal failure.

Statins (3-hydroxy-3-methyglutaryl coenzyme A (HGM-CoA) reductase inhibitors)

Statins are frequently prescribed for the treatment of hyperlipidaemia. Asymptomatic elevation of aminotransferases (greater than three times ULN) occurs in approximately 1–5% of exposed patients. This is primarily dose related and tends to occurs within the first few months of therapy. Therefore periodic monitoring of liver enzymes is recommended with discontinuation of the statin therapy in patients with persistent elevations in liver function tests (Norris, 2006).

It is commonly believed that use of statins is contraindicated for patients with ALF or advanced chronic liver disease. However, Bhardwaj and Chalasani (2007) propose that several recent studies and current expert opinion fully endorse the use of statins if clinically indicated in patients who have non-alcoholic fatty liver disease (NAFLD) and other chronic liver diseases.

Halothane

Halothane-associated liver damage has been recognised since the 1960s, and is associated with two types of liver injury that present as either mild, with raised serum aminotransferases, or ALF usually within 2 weeks of surgery (Sherlock and Dooley, 2002). The risk of liver injury is uncommon after a first exposure and ranges from 1/35 000 to 1/10 000 anaesthetics administered. Risk factors linked to halothane hepatoxicity include obesity, female sex, advancing age and repeated halothane exposure (risk increases to 7/10 000) (Norris, 2006). Underlying liver disease is not a risk factor.

Manifestations of halothane-induced liver injury may include serum aminotransferase levels increased by 25–250 times the ULN, with minimal elevation of serum ALP, and a high bilirubin level. The presentation of a fever, skin rash and esosinophilia implies an immune allergic reaction to halothane. Twenty percent of the halothane is biotransformed by the P450 cytochrome metabolism to an unstable toxic metabolite which may result in cellular injury and hepatic necrosis (Schiano and Black, 2004).

Isoniazid

Since the 1950s, isoniazid has been used for the treatment of both active and latent infections of *Mycobacterium tuberculosis* (Fountain et al., 2005), and is one the most important causes of drug-induced liver injury. Isoniazid is associated with two types of liver injury. The most common type occurs in 10–20% of patients, usually in the first few months of treatment. The patients are normally asymptomatic with a transient mild elevation of aminotransferases (Norris, 2006), and treatments can normally be continued with careful monitoring. Therefore serum aminotransferases should be monitored before treatment is started, and after 4 weeks of drug therapy. If increased serum aminotransferases are found, patients should have their liver function tests monitored weekly, with the cessation of treatment if the levels continue to rise (Sherlock and Dooley, 2002).

Overt isoniazid hepatitis occurs in approximately 1% of patients. Clinically the symptoms are those of acute viral hepatitis, which usually occur within the first 3 months of therapy; however this can be delayed by up to 12 months (Mahl and O'Grady, 2006). The drug must be stopped immediately, and the patients closely monitored, as the mortality for clinically jaundiced patients is 10% (Norris, 2006).

Other antitubercular therapies, such as rifampin and pyrazinamide, have additionally been associated with hepatotoxicity. As monotherapies this is usually because of a hypersensitivity reaction; however hepatoxicity is increased when these therapies are given in either combination or with isoniazid.

Amanita phalloides *mushroom poisoning*

Amanita phalloides (death cap) and *Amanita verna* (destroying angel) are fungi associated with severe hepatic injury. Toxicity is due to amatoxins which interfere with mRNA synthesis leading to hepatic necrosis. As little as three mushrooms can be fatal, and cooking does not destroy the amatoxins (Norris, 2006). Symptoms occur 6–24 hours after ingestion and can mimic gastroenteritis with nausea, stomach cramps, vomiting and watery diarrhoea. This is followed by a latent phase which lasts for 24–48 hours, where clinical symptoms improve but overt liver damage occurs. Patients can rapidly progress to ALF from massive hepatocellular necrosis (Schiano and Black, 2004).

Herbal and Chinese remedies

Every culture has explored the use of plants for medicinal purposes, therefore it is not surprising that 8–50% of people in western Europe and the USA have used some form of complementary therapy, with even higher usage reported in developing countries (Langmead and Rampton, 2001). However, both herbal and Chinese remedies are predominately unregulated, and as their use has expanded so has the acknowledgement of the toxic properties of many of these products, which may include both acute and chronic hepatotoxicity, veno-occlusive disease, cholestasis and cirrhosis (Skoulidis et al., 2005). Consequently there is growing support for the regulation of the use of herbal and Chinese medicines, to both maximise safety and to ensure appropriate usage.

Herbal-induced hepatotoxicity is often difficult to diagnose as, firstly, all other causes of liver diseases need to be ruled out and, secondly, patients frequently self-medicate, and fail to disclose use of herbal remedies. Therefore it is imperative to ascertain the use of herbal or Chinese herbal remedies whilst obtaining the patient's drug history. Some of the commonly known herbal hepatotoxins are identified below.

Chinese herbal remedies

Ma-Huang (Ephedra sinica)
Ma-Huang is derived from the plants of the *Ephedra* species, one of the oldest medical plants known and is commonly marketed in the west as a slimming aid and energy level enhancer (Chitturi and Farrell, 2000). Increasing use of herbal ephedra has led to a number of reports of serious adverse events which include hypertension, palpitations, tachycardia, stroke, seizures, acute hepatitis and ALF (Skoulidis et al., 2005).

Jin Bu Huan (Lycopodium serratum)
Jin Bu Huan has been used over centuries for sedative, analgesic and antispasmodic properties. However, several cases of acute and chronic hepatitis, fibrosis and steatosis have been reported (Chitturi and Farrell, 2000).

Herbal remedies

Germander (Teucrium chamaedrys)
Germander has been used for more than 2000 years for relieving fever, abdominal disorders and for its purported weight loss, choleretic and healing properties (Larrey and Pageaux, 1995). However, it has also been associated with both acute hepatitis and ALF. The presenting symptoms of abdominal pain and jaundice usually develop within 3–18 weeks of germander consumption, which is taken in forms such as herbal teas or capsules. Histology reveals a non-specific hepatocellular necrosis (Norris, 2006). Discontinuation of the treatment can normally see resolution of symptoms and recovery within 2–6 months; however there have been several reported fatalities. Reappearance of symptoms occurs rapidly upon germander re-exposure (Norris, 2006).

St John's wort (Hypericum perforatum)
St John's wort is a popular herbal remedy commonly used for the treatment of depression and anxiety. St John's wort is thought to enhance the activity of cytochrome P450 enzymes, therefore affecting the metabolism and efficacy of concomitant medications which include immunosuppressant therapies (Pak et al., 2004).

A study of renal transplant recipients found patients receiving 2 weeks of St John's wort therapy had a decrease in tacrolimus drug levels by more than 50%, which necessitated a 75% increase in immunosuppressive therapy to maintain therapeutic concentrations of tacrolimus (Mai et al., 2003). Similar findings have been demonstrated in transplant recipients receiving cyclosporine therapy.

Therefore the use of St John's wort should be discouraged post liver transplantation due to the increased risks of acute graft rejection.

Khat (Catha edulis)

Khat (*Catha edulis*) is an evergreen shrub, native to East Africa and Southern Arabia, in which the fresh leaves contain the pyrrolizidine alkaloids cathine, cathidine and cathinone (Brostoff et al., 2005). As cathinone has a structure similar to amphetamine, khat is commonly chewed to attain a state of stimulation (Al-Harbori, 2005). Whilst an uncommon cause of hepatotoxicity, khat has been associated with numerous health problems such as hypertension, acute coronary vasospasm, myocardial infarction, gastrointestinal problems and psychosis.

Herbal remedies for treatment in liver disease

The most researched herbal treatment for liver diseases is milk thistle (*Silybum marianum (L) Gaertneri*), its active constituents are collectively known as silymartin. Milk thistle has been reported in numerous case reports and uncontrolled studies for its use in hepatic failure due to *Amanita phalloides* mushroom poisoning, alcoholic liver disease, acute viral hepatitis and cirrhosis with varying results (Langmead and Rampton, 2001). The recommendations from a Cochrane review of 18 randomised control trials using milk thistle for alcoholic and/or hepatitis B or C virus liver diseases, suggests that there is a lack of evidence to support or refute any benefits, primarily due to the poor methodological quality of the studies. Therefore Rambaldi et al. (2005) advocate the need for further adequately conducted trials. In addition it is imperative to remember the liver's susceptibility to serious and sometimes fatal adverse events in patients taking herbal remedies (Langmead and Rampton, 2001).

The use of herbal supplements by patients with chronic liver disease remains high with up to 39% of patients reporting usage. Whilst there have been several studies exploring the benefits of herbal remedies, the data have been criticised for being either conflicting or weakly studied, consequently the use of herbal preparations necessitates further clinical trials before recommendations for their use can be made (Levy et al., 2004). Furthermore Pak et al. (2004) suggest that herbal usage can potentially increase prescription drug non-compliance, as patients may replace conventional therapies with herbal remedies to avoid prescription costs and drug side effects.

Chapter summary

Drug-induced liver injury is a common problem with over a 1000 implicated drugs, with a vast array of symptoms ranging from mild elevation of liver biochemical tests to ALF (Schiano and Black, 2004). The mainstay of management is firstly a high index of clinical suspicion and secondly the withdrawal of the agent. Whilst most patients will recover spontaneously, some patients will continue to deteriorate with varying degrees of severity and therefore each presenting problem should be supported with the appropriate treatment and, where indicated, transferred to a unit with transplantation facilitates. It is paramount always to ascertain a detailed drug history from patients that includes prescribed medications, OTC and both herbal and Chinese remedy usage. Additionally it is vital that all health care professionals have an understanding of the known hepatotoxic agents and to closely monitor and recognise the signs of drug-induced hepatotoxicity.

Illustrative case study

A 48-year-old gentleman of Somalian origin presented with a 1-week history of jaundice, pale stools and dark urine. The patient had no fever or night sweats, or any past medical history of note. He denied a previous history of intravenous drug use, blood transfusions, current medication, elevated alcohol consumption and was a non-smoker. The patient was heterosexual, and married with three children and had been resident in the UK for 10 years, with no foreign travel during this period. The patient, however, admitted to chewing khat (*Catha edulis* leaves) with an increased usage over the last 3 years, and was currently chewing two bunches per day.

It was noted on physical examination that the patient was clinically jaundiced, with no lymphadenopathy or stigmata of CLD. Laboratory investigations demonstrated a normal haematological profile, and a bilirubin of 76 µmol/L, ALP 161 IU/L, ALT 1152 IU/L, GGT 184 IU/L, albumin 33 g/L, and total protein 73 g/L. His remaining liver screen was negative for viral hepatitis and autoimmune antibodies, with normal ferritin and caeruloplasmin levels. An ultrasound scan showed a normal liver, spleen and hepatic and portal veins. Within 30 days of cessation of his daily khat consumption, the patient's liver function tests returned to within normal ranges.

References

Al-Habori M (2005) The potential effects of habitual use of *Catha edulis* (Khat). *Expert Opinion on Drug Safety* 4(6):1145–1154

Bhardwaj SS, Chalasani N (2007) Lipid-lowering agents that cause drug-induced hepatotoxicity. *Clinics in Liver Disease* 11(3):597–613

Brostoff JM, Plymen C, Birns J (2005) Khat – a novel case of drug induced hepatitis. *European Journal of Internal Medicine* 17:383

Chitturi S, Farrell GC (2000) Herbal hepatotoxicity: an expanding but poorly defined problem. *Journal of Gastroenterology and Hepatology* 15:1093–1099

Erlinger S (1997) Drug-induced cholestasis. *Journal of Hepatology* **26**(suppl 1):1–4

Fountain FF, Tolley E, Chrisman CR, Self TH (2005) Isoniazid hepatotoxicity associated with treatment of latent tuberculosis infection. *Chest* **128**:116–123

Greene SL, Dargon PI, Jones AL (2005) Acute poisoning: understanding 90% of cases in a nutshell. *Postgraduate Medicine* **81**:204–216

Langmead L, Rampton DS (2001) Review article: herbal treatment in gastro-intestinal and liver disease – benefits and dangers. *Alimentary Pharmacology and Therapeutics* **15**:1239–1252

Larrey D, Pageaux GP (1995) Hepatotoxicity of herbal remedies and mushrooms. *Seminars of Liver Disease* **15**:183–188

Levy C, Seeff LB, Lindor K (2004) The use of herbal supplements for chronic liver disease. *Clinical Gastroenterology and Hepatology* **2**:947–956

Mahl T, O'Grady J (2006) *Liver Disorders*. Health Press Limited, Abingdon

Mai I, Stormer E, Bauer S, Kruger H, Budde K, Roots I (2003) Impact of St Johns wort treatment on the pharmacokinetics of tacrolimus and mycophenolate acid in renal transplant patients. *Nephrology, Dialysis, Transplantation* **18**:819–822

McFarlane I, Bomford A, Sherwood R (2000) *Liver Disease and Laboratory Medicine*. ACD Venture Publications, Kent

Navarro V, Senior J (2006) Drug related hepatotoxicity. *New England Journal of Medicine* **353**:731–739

Norris S (2000) Drug- and toxin-induced liver disease. In: O'Grady JG, Lake JR, Howdle PD (eds) *Comprehensive Clinical Hepatology*. Mosby, St Louis

Norris S (2006) Drug and toxin induced liver disease. In: Bacon BR, O'Grady JG, Di Biscegie AM, Lake JR (Eds) *Comprehensive Clinical Hepatology*, 2nd edn. Mosby, St Louis, pp. 497–516

O'Grady JG (2006) Acute liver failure. In: Bacon BR, O'Grady JG, Di Biscegie AM, Lake JR (eds) *Comprehensive Clinical Hepatology*, 2nd edn. Mosby, St Louis, pp. 517–536

O'Grady JG, Alexander GJM, Hayllar KM, Williams R (1989) Early indications of prognosis in fulminate hepatic failure. *Gastroenterology* **97**(2):439–445

Pak E, Esrason KT, Wu VH (2004) Hepatotoxicity of herbal remedies: an emerging dilemma. *Progress in Transplantation* **14**(2):91–96

Rambaldi A, Jacobs BP, Gluud C (2005) Milk thistle for alcoholic and/or hepatitis B or C virus liver diseases. *Cochrane Database of Systematic Reviews*, Issue 2. Art. No.: CD003620. DOI: 10.1002/14651858.CD003620

Ryder SD, Beckingham IJ (2001) ABC of diseases of liver, pancreas, and other biliary system. Other causes of parenchymal liver disease. *British Medical Journal* **322**:290–293

Schiano TD, Black M (2004) Drug induced and toxic liver disease. In: Friedman LS, Keefe EB (eds) *Handbook of Liver Disease*, 2nd edn. Churchill Livingstone, Philadelphia, pp. 103–123

Sherlock S, Dooley J (2002) *Diseases of the Liver and Biliary System*, 11th edn. Blackwell Publishing, Oxford

Skoulidis F, Alexander GJM, Davies SE (2005) Ma Huang associated with acute liver failure requiring liver transplantation. *European Journal of Gastroenterology and Hepatology* **17**:581–584

Watkins PB, Seeff LB (2006) Drug induced liver injury: summary of a single topic research conference. *Hepatology* **43**(3):618–631

Pregnancy-related liver disease

16

Suzanne Sargent and Michelle Clayton

Introduction

Pregnancy-related liver disease is usually divided into three definitive areas: normal hepatic changes that occur during pregnancy, liver diseases specific to pregnancy and pregnancy in patients with pre-existing hepatic diseases. Whilst liver disease is uncommon during pregnancy, jaundice is reported in approximately 1 in 1500–5000 pregnancies, and is attributed to both viral hepatitis and intrahepatic cholestasis (Van Dyke, 2006). This chapter will provide an overview of the most common liver diseases specific to pregnancy as well as examining pregnancy in pre-existing liver conditions and post liver transplantation.

Normal changes during pregnancy

During pregnancy, women experience physiological, hormonal and physical changes that are necessary for fetal growth and development (Bacq et al., 1996). Plasma volume increases during pregnancy by approximately 40%, which leads to increased cardiac output and heart rate, peaking at 32 weeks (Rahman and Wendon, 2002). This increase in plasma volume leads to haemodilution which, in conjunction with the hormonal and physical changes, can cause alterations in many standard biochemical and haematological tests as demonstrated in Table 16.1.

Table 16.1   Normal changes in liver function tests during pregnancy. Adapted from Van Dyke (2006). Please refer to Chapter 2 for further information on liver function tests.

Laboratory test	Changes seen during pregnancy
Gamma-glutamyltranspeptidase (GGT)	25% lower during early pregnancy
Alkaline phosphatase (ALP)	Increases 2–3-fold during third trimester due to increased maternal bone turnover and leakage of placental ALP into maternal circulation
Serum albumin	Serum levels decrease due to increase in plasma volume
Alanine and aspartate aminotransferases (ALT/AST)	Not normally changed during pregnancy but may increase during labour due to secondary leakage from contracting uterine muscles
Globulins	Values increase
Prothrombin time (PT)	Unchanged
Bile acids	Increase 2-fold due to decrease in hepatic bile transportation
Total and free bilirubin	Lower due to haemodilution and low albumin concentration (reduced protein transportation)

The blood flow to the liver usually accounts for 38% of cardiac output, however whilst the overall cardiac output is increased during pregnancy, the blood flow to the liver is reduced to 28% of the total cardiac output, with the excess blood volume being shunted through the placenta (Sherlock and Dooley, 2002).

In addition, physical findings that are normally associated with chronic liver disease can also occur during pregnancy, both spider naevi, of the chest, face and neck, and palmar erythema are seen in up to 60% of women during normal pregnancy; these usually disappear after delivery (Knox and Olans, 1996).

Liver diseases specific to pregnancy

Liver disease is a rare complication of pregnancy and can be caused by a wide variety of conditions, some of which are discussed below. Whilst some of these complications are considered to be non-severe, some diseases specific to pregnancy can be fatal and may lead to tragedy for both mother and baby (Shames et al., 2005).

Hyperemesis gravidarum

Hyperemesis gravidarum (HG) is an idiopathic syndrome of severe nausea and vomiting that predominately occurs during the first trimester of pregnancy. The condition occurs in 1–20 patients per 1000 pregnancies. In some cases, the nausea and vomiting are so severe they can lead to dehydration, electrolyte disturbances or nutritional deficiencies, which may necessitate hospitalisation (Benjaminov and

Heathcote, 2004; Maroo and Wolf, 2004). Risk factors for HG include young age, obesity, no previous pregnancies, tobacco use and twin gestation (Van Dyke, 2006). Up to 25% of hospitalised patients with HG will have abnormal liver enzymes as demonstrated in Table 16.2, which normally resolve with the resolution of vomiting and dehydration. Total parenteral nutrition may be necessary in severe cases but fetal outcomes do not differ from those of the general population (Benjaminov and Heathcote, 2004; Van Dyke, 2006). However, mean birth weight of the offspring is reduced in those women who are severely affected by HG (Sherlock and Dooley, 2002).

Cholestasis of pregnancy

Intrahepatic cholestasis of pregnancy (ICP) has been noted as early as the first trimester of pregnancy but 80% of afffected women present in the third trimester. Pruritis is usually one of the first clinical signs, affecting the palms of the hands, soles of the feet and in some cases generalised itching all over the body. ICP leads to fetal distress, premature delivery and stillbirth if untreated (Kroumpouzos, 2002). Up to 25% of women affected by ICP suffer with jaundice which resolves post partum (Maroo and Wolf, 2004). Worldwide variation in geographical incidence of ICP is marked, with certain hotspots including Chile and Scandinavia. In Chile rates vary between 14 and 24%, with the highest rate reported in Araucanian Indians (Kroumpouzos, 2002). The overall prevalence in the UK is 0.7%, although the incidence of ICP in women of Indian and Pakistani descent in the UK is twice that of Caucasian women (Abedin et al., 1999). There is also a suggestion that seasonal variations occur, with ICP being higher in the winter months. Many suggestions have been postulated to account for these variations including genetic traits, dietary factors and climate (Coombes, 2000; Kroumpouzos, 2002).

Both oestrogen and progesterone play a part in ICP. Oestrogen interferes with bile acid secretion across the hepatocyte membrane (this is why pruritus can also occur in some women taking oral contraceptives). Progesterone is implicated due to its metabolites which inhibit hepatic glucuronyltransferase; this in turn reduces the ability to clear oestrogen from the hepatocytes, thus intensifying the effects (Kroumpouzos, 2002). Recently there has been interest in hepatocanalicular lipid transporter dysfunction that is caused by genetic variations (Van Dyke, 2006; Wasmuth et al., 2007). Elevation of bile acids is considered to be the most appropriate laboratory parameter for the diagnosis of ICP. Levels greater than 40 µmmol/L are associated with a higher risk of fetal complications which include increased preterm delivery, intrapartum fetal distress and intrauterine fetal death (Glanz et al., 2004).

The main focus of treatment is to ameliorate the pruritus and to reduce bile acids. To date there have been a number of drugs used, including guar gum, activated charcoal, S-adenosylmethionine (SAMe) and ursodeoxycholic acid (UCDA). A Cochrane review (Burrows et al., 2001) concluded that there was insufficient evidence to recommend any of the above alone or in combination for the treatment

Table 16.2 Results of laboratory tests in pregnancy associated liver disease. Reprinted from Maroo S, Wolf J (2004) The liver in pregnancy. In: Friedman LS, Keeffe E (eds) *Handbook of Liver Disease*, 2nd edn. p. 273; with permission from Elsevier. (PT = prothrombin time; PTT = partial thromboplastin time)

Condition	Aminotransferases	Bile acids	Bilirubin	Alkaline phosphatase	Uric acid	Platelets	PT/PTT	Urine protein
Hyperemesis gravidarum	1–2×	Normal	<85.5 µmol/L (<5 mg/dL)	1–2×	Normal	Normal	Normal	Normal
Intrahepatic cholestasis of pregnancy	1–4×	30–100×	<85.5 µmol/L (<5 mg/dL)	1–2×	Normal	Normal	Normal	Normal
Acute fatty liver of pregnancy	1–5×	Normal	<171 µmol/L (<10 mg/dL)	1–2×	↑	±↓	±↑	±↑
Pre-eclampsia/eclampsia	1–100×	Normal	<85.5 µmol/L (<5 mg/dL)	1–2×	↑	±↓	±↑	↑
HELLP	1–100×	Normal	<85.5 µmol/L (<5 mg/dL)	1–2×	↑	↓	±↑	±↑
Hepatic rupture	2–100×	Normal	±↑	↑	Normal	±↓	±↑	Normal

of cholestasis in pregnancy, and that further trials are required. However in reality most women do receive UCDA as it is considered to be the best currently available therapy to relieve pruritis and to reduce bile acids (Saleh and Abdo, 2007). UDCA is a naturally occurring bile acid which protects the bile ducts from injury from hydrophobic bile acids. The excretion of hydrophobic bile acids and other hepato-toxic substances from hepatocytes is improved when using UDCA (Kumar and Tandon, 2001). It additionally restores the ability of the placenta to transfer bile acids, thus reducing the delivery of bile acids to the fetus, which is associated with an improvement in fetal prognosis (Serrano et al., 1998; Sentilhes et al., 2006).

It is important to ensure that women who develop jaundice due to ICP have regular assessment of their clotting profiles. This is important to ensure that vitamin K-dependent coagulopathy in the mother does not occur due to interfer-ence in bile flow leading to malabsorption of vitamin K. Vitamin K should be administered to these women near the time of delivery to reduce postpartum haemorrhage. Due to deranged clotting this is usually administered via the intra-venous route (Van Dyke, 2006).

In relation to the fetus, increased antenatal surveillance and maternal bile acid measurements are necessary to reduce the incidence of stillbirth and other recog-nised fetal complications (Sentilhes et al., 2006; Van Dyke, 2006). Early delivery of the fetus at 36–37 weeks is recommended to prevent these (Van Dyke, 2006). ICP can recur in subsequent pregnancies so mothers need to be informed of this risk and also that they have a greater risk of developing pruritus if prescribed oral contraceptives (Van Dyke, 2006).

Pre-eclampsia/eclampsia

Both pre-eclampsia and eclampsia are rare but potentially fatal complications of pregnancy and are implicated in some liver diseases associated with pregnancy. Pre-eclampsia occurs in 5–7% of pregnancies, normally during the second and third trimester, and is characterised by a triad of hypertension, proteinuria and peripheral oedema, with an associated maternal mortality of up to 14% (Longo et al., 2003; Benjaminov and Heathcote, 2004). Hypertension in pre-eclampsia is defined as an elevation of 30 mmHg (systolic) or 15 mmHg (diastolic) above the value in the first trimester or any value above 140/90 mmHg recorded on at least two occasions, at least 4 hours apart (Knox and Olans, 1996; Heneghan, 2000; Longo et al., 2003). Severe pre-eclampsia consists of a systolic blood pressure >160 mmHg or diastolic pressure >110 mmHg, with significant proteinuria (at least 1 g/L) with or without evidence of other organ failure (Longo et al., 2003). Eclampsia is marked by seizures and coma in addition to pre-eclampsia (Benjaminov and Heathcote, 2004).

The aetiology of pre-eclampsia is unknown, but proposed mechanisms involve inappropriate vasoconstriction, vasospasm, abnormal placenta development, abnormal epithelial reactivity, activation of coagulopathy and decreased synthesis of nitric oxide (Maroo and Wolf, 2004). Risk factors for pre-eclampsia include pre-existing hypertension, extremes of child bearing age, first pregnancy and multiple gestations (Benjaminov and Heathcote, 2004).

Signs and symptoms of pre-eclampsia primarily depend on the severity, and range from epigastric pain, right upper quadrant pain, headaches, blurred vision, oedema, nausea and vomiting and proteinuria. In severe cases oliguria, respiratory distress, congestive cardiac failure and cerebral oedema may occur (Heneghan, 2000; Maroo and Wolf, 2004). Liver function tests are abnormal in 20–30% of cases as demonstrated in Table 16.2 and probably reflect hepatic dysfunction resulting from vasoconstriction of the hepatic vascular bed. The abnormalities normally resolve after delivery (Rahman and Wendon, 2002).

Maternal mortality largely results from abruptio placentae, hepatic rupture and eclampsia (Longo et al., 2003). Maternal morbidity associated with pre-eclampsia is the consequence of the multi-organ involvement of the disease and end-organ damage. The most significant consequence relates to cerebral involvement. Risk factors to the fetus are related to prematurity, low birth weight, fetal growth retardation and placental abruption (Maroo and Wolf, 2004).

Treatment for pre-eclampsia is dependent on both the severity and gestational age at diagnosis. Delivery of the infant is the preferred treatment for eclampsia and near-term pre-eclampsia. Other management strategies are controversial and include antihypertensive therapy, antiplatelet drugs, anticonvulsant therapy, magnesium sulphate and bed rest (Rahman and Wendon, 2002; Maroo and Wolf, 2004). In severe pre-eclampsia, intensive monitoring and correction of coagulopathy or thrombocytopenia should continue for up to 72 hours after delivery due to the susceptibility to seizures, haemorrhage and other complications (Rahman and Wendon, 2002).

Acute fatty liver in pregnancy

Acute fatty liver of pregnancy (AFLP) is a rare but significant complication of pregnancy, which may lead to acute liver failure and maternal and fetal death. Its incidence is 1 in 900–6000 pregnancies (Van Dyke, 2006) and is more common in first pregnancies, multiple births and those women carrying a male fetus (Maroo and Wolf, 2004).

It was first described in 1934 and termed acute yellow atrophy of the liver in pregnancy; this has been revised to AFLP due to the accumulation of microvesicular fat within the hepatocytes (Figure 16.1, Plate 16) (Knox and Olans, 1996). This fatty infiltrate leads to the liver being unable to maintain normal function and the development of hypoglycaemia, coagulopathy and hepatic encephalopathy with modest rises in ALT. Elevations of uric acid and renal insufficiency are common (Van Dyke, 2006). AFLP usually manifests itself at 30–38 weeks' gestation, initially with non-specific symptoms including malaise, fatigue, headache, nausea with or without vomiting and pain in the right upper quadrant or epigastric area (Jamerson, 2005). Jaundice and dark-coloured urine often present several days after the non-specific symptoms (Treem, 2002). About 50% of women with AFLP also have pre-eclampsia.

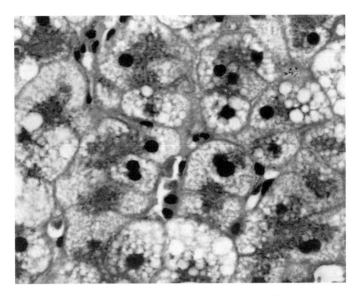

Figure 16.1 Liver biopsy demonstrating changes in acute fatty liver of pregnancy. Reproduced with permission from Sherlock S, Dooley J (2002) *Diseases of the Liver and Biliary System*, 11th edn, Blackwell Publishing. For a colour version of this figure, please see Plate 16 in the colour plate section.

Delivery of the fetus is required to resolve AFLP; therapeutic support of the mother may include intensive care management of the liver failure. Postpartum haemorrhage is common for those women who have developed coagulopathy. Maternal and fetal mortality range from 5–20% (Van Dyke, 2006).

Research into AFLP suggests that both the mother and fetus may have abnormalities in beta-oxidation of fatty acids. The more common abnormality is related to long chain 3-hydroxyacyl-CoA dehydrogenase (LCHAD). Therefore it is recommended that women who develop AFLP and their offspring are genetically tested for fatty acid oxidation deficiencies (Van Dyke, 2006). Women also need to be informed that AFLP can recur in subsequent pregnancies, as there is a 20% risk of recurrence in the general maternal population; however those mothers identified with a fatty acid oxidation deficit may be at a higher risk (Browning et al., 2006).

Haemolysis, elevated liver enzymes and low platelets syndrome

Haemolysis, elevated liver enzymes and low platelets (HELLP) syndrome is well described as a complication of severe pre-eclampsia related liver dysfunction. HELLP is characterised by microangiopathic haemolytic anaemia, thrombocytopenia and elevated liver function tests. It occurs in white multiparous women usually over the age of 25 years. It is common in the last trimester of pregnancy and up to 2 days post partum (Maroo and Wolf, 2004). Initial symptoms are vague and non-specific, including nausea, vomiting and right upper quadrant pain and tenderness. A high index of suspicion is important, including for those women who have already delivered.

Pre-eclampsia is a prerequisite for HELLP syndrome to develop. The diagnosis of HELLP is based on blood tests in women suspected of having pre-eclampsia. The prevention of end-organ damage is paramount as fibrin deposits have been found in the periportal sinusoids leading to ischaemic hepatocyte necrosis on liver biopsies of patients with HELLP syndrome (Van Dyke, 2006). As with AFLP expedient delivery is required, this may be supported with corticosteroids to improve lung maturity in the fetus. Corticosteroids have also been used to normalise some maternal biochemical changes and reduce hypertension (Matchaba and Moodley, 2004), however further research is required to validate these results.

Infant mortality is estimated at 10–60% (Maroo and Wolf, 2004), mainly due to intrauterine growth retardation and poor placental perfusion. Liver function in the mother again needs to be supported until resolution. Hepatic rupture in the mother is a rare but life-threatening event which can occur, therefore abdominal pain, hypotension and shock should be rapidly investigated. The recurrence of HELLP syndrome in women is estimated at 3–5% (Van Dyke, 2006). It is recommended that women who have had HELLP syndrome should be screened for procoagulant disorders.

A qualitative research study focusing on the experiences of women with HELLP syndrome reported that eight out of the nine women decided not to have another pregnancy due to their intense memories of HELLP syndrome and the strong fear of death they associated with pregnancy (Kidner and Flanders-Stepans, 2004).

There is evidence to suggest that HELLP syndrome and AFLP may clinically overlap in some pregnant women. Some of the features of HELLP, including proteinurea, oedema, thrombocytopenia, azotaemia and elevated creatinine, are also present in 50–100% of women with AFLP (Treem, 2002).

Hepatic rupture

Hepatic rupture is a devastating complication of pregnancy that occurs in 1/45000 to 1/250000 deliveries. Whilst 80% of cases are associated with pre-eclampsia or eclampsia, hepatic rupture is additionally associated with AFLP, HELLP syndrome, HCC, adenoma, haemangioma and hepatic abscess (Maroo and Wolf, 2004), trauma and cocaine abuse. The pathophysiology is not clear, but intraparenchymal haemorrhaging usually precedes the rupture (Benjaminov and Heathcote, 2004).

Patients typically present in the third trimester of pregnancy, or within 24 hours of delivery, with a sudden onset of severe right upper quadrant abdominal pain, nausea, vomiting, which progresses to abdominal distension, falling haematocrit and hypovolaemic shock (Heneghan, 2000; Maroo and Woolf, 2004). A diagnostic paracentesis demonstrates blood in the peritoneal cavity; however diagnosis is usually made with a CT scan, ultrasonography, MRI or angiography (Benjaminov and Heathcote, 2004).

Treatment consists of emergency caesarean section with volume resuscitation, surgical drainage and packing of the liver or, in some cases, hepatic embolisation or liver transplantation (Van Dyke, 2006). Maternal mortality rates have been reported as 50–75%, which is primarily caused by haemorrhaging. Fetal mortality is reported as 60–70%, and correlates with prematurity (Maroo and Wolf, 2004).

Pregnancy in pre-existing liver disease

Amenorrhoea and infertility are common in patients with end-stage liver disease, affecting up to 50% of patients (Heneghan, 2000). Amenorrhoea is thought to be related to hypothalamic pituitary dysfunction and not related directly to the liver disease. Nonetheless pregnancies do occur and for those who do conceive this is often a reflection of the degree of underlying hepatic function (Mahl and O'Grady, 2006).

Pregnancy in cirrhosis

Cirrhosis is not a contraindication to pregnancy and, despite some assumptions, it does not necessarily have an effect on patients with compensated cirrhosis and mild portal hypertension, despite the expansion of blood volume and increased intra-abdominal pressure. Therefore pregnancy should be planned for a period of time when the liver disease is well compensated (Benjaminov and Heathcote, 2004; Mahl and O'Grady, 2006). Known maternal complications that arise in nearly half of cirrhosis-affected pregnancies with significant portal hypertension include:

- Variceal haemorrhage
- Hepatic failure
- Hepatic encephalopathy
- Splenic artery aneurysm
- Malnutrition (Benjaminov and Heathcote, 2004)

Variceal bleeding primarily occurs in up to 24% of pregnancies in patients with known cirrhosis and portal hypertension and carries a maternal mortality of 20–50% (Benjaminov and Heathcote, 2004). Consequently patients should be aware of the risks and screened accordingly.

Treatment of variceal bleeding in pregnancy is similar to that in non-pregnant patients and primarily consist of endoscopic and pharmacological therapies as described in Chapter 4. However the use of vasopressin for the treatment of variceal bleeding should be avoided, due to the risk of inducing labour (Van Dyke, 2006). There are also some reports of TIPS being used successfully in the second and third trimester.

Wilson's disease

Prior to the introduction of the copper-reducing chelating agents such as penicillamine, successful pregnancies in Wilson's disease (WD) were rare due to reduced fertility, menstrual irregularities and the consequences of severe hepatic dysfunction. However, there have now been over 100 reported successful pregnancies, although pregnancy remains rare in patients who have cirrhosis (Heneghan, 2000; Ferenci, 2006).

Treatment must be continued throughout pregnancy due to the risk of acute liver failure if it is stopped. Patients should be advised to continue taking penicillamine, as this is not known to be harmful to the mother or baby (Van Dyke, 2006). In addition, improvements in the manifestations of liver disease have been reported and are a reflection of both the fetal demand for copper and a four-fold increase in the maternal circulation of caeruloplasmin (Heneghan, 2000).

Autoimmune hepatitis

Fertility in female patients with autoimmune hepatitis can be affected due to liver cirrhosis and hypothalamic pituitary dysfunction (Benjaminov and Heathcote, 2004). Nevertheless, pregnancies can occur in patients with well controlled autoimmune hepatitis, as menstruation returns. However the risk of unsuccessful pregnancy is high, with reported incidences in the range of 23–50% (Maroo and Woolf, 2004).

One of the primary concerns with pregnancy in autoimmune hepatitis patients relates to the pharmacological therapies commonly used for treatment. Whilst corticosteroids are generally considered safe, there are concerns regarding the potential teratogenic effect of azathioprine; however several studies in patients with autoimmune hepatitis, inflammatory bowel disease, and renal and liver transplant recipients have shown this to be generally safe with no adverse outcomes noted in either mother or baby (Heneghan et al., 2001). Approximately 1.2% of azathioprine is excreted in breast milk, and therefore it is only classified as 'probably safe' for use during breast feeding (Benjaminov and Heathcote, 2004). Cessation of pharmacological therapy is associated with disease relapse (Maroo and Woolf, 2004).

Patients need careful monitoring during pregnancy and for several months post partum as up to 43% of women with autoimmune hepatitis experience a flare-up of their disease within 6 months of delivery (Heneghan et al., 2001; Van Dyke, 2006).

Hepatitis B and C

The global incidence of hepatitis B and hepatitis C, modes of transmission and treatments are discussed in detail in Chapter 9. This section will therefore primarily discuss the risks and incidences of vertical transmission during pregnancy.

Pregnant women who are in close contact with carriers of hepatitis B virus (HBV) must be vaccinated, as both the vaccine and immunoglobulin are considered safe to be administered (Sherlock and Dooley, 2002).

The presence of hepatitis B surface antigen (HBsAg) in pregnancy is believed not to pose additional risks for the pregnancy or its outcome (Benjaminov and Heathcote, 2004). However, some retrospective data have demonstrated that women who are HBsAg-positive, have an increased risk of antepartum haemorrhage, diabetes mellitus and threatened preterm labour (Tse et al., 2005).

The incidence of transplacental transmission of HBV has not been reported. However, vertical transmission at the time of delivery is common (Van Dyke, 2006). If the mother is HBsAg-positive, the risk of infection is estimated at 25%, however if the mother is both HBsAg- and HBeAg-positive, the chronic infection rate is increased to 90% (Maroo and Woolf, 2004; Van Dyke, 2006).

Babies born to HBV-positive mothers, regardless of antigen status, should be vaccinated at birth and additionally given hepatitis B immunoglobulin. Further vaccination should then be given at 1 and 6 months of age. This combination therapy is 85–95% effective in preventing transmission (Maroo and Wolf, 2004; Van Dyke, 2006). With proper immunoprophylaxis, breast feeding of infants by chronic HBV carrier women poses no additional risk of viral transmission (Hill et al., 2002). For mothers with a high viraemia (HBV DNA of 1.2×10^9), it has been suggested that additional treatment with the antiviral therapy, lamidivine, during the third trimester of pregnancy may provide better protection against vertical transmission, when compared with active and passive vaccination of the neonate alone (Van Dyke, 2006).

Hepatitis C virus (HCV) does not adversely affect the pregnancy nor does pregnancy affect the course of the infection. However, pregnancy is contraindicated during HCV treatment or for at least 6 months after discontinuation due to the teratogenic effects of ribavirin. Vertical transmission of hepatitis C is uncommon, with an approximate incidence in 1–8% of births. However, high viral loads and co-infection with human immunodeficiency virus (HIV), spontaneous membrane rupture >6 hours before delivery, and fetal scalp monitoring are linked to a higher risk of transmission. There is no current treatment available to prevent viral transmission, and in addition the type of delivery (vaginal vs. caesarean section) appears to have no effect on transmission rates (Maroo and Wolf, 2004; Benjaminov and Heathcote, 2004). Breastfeeding has not been linked with transmission of the virus; however, mothers need to be aware of the increased risk if cracked or bleeding nipples occur, and should be encouraged to use alternative methods of feeding during this time.

Antibodies to HCV pass through the placenta, and the values may remain positive for 6 months in the infant. It is therefore recommended that babies born to HCV-positive mothers should be PCR tested at 3, 6 and 18 months of age. Those infants who remain positive after 6 months or 18 months are deemed to be chronically infected (Sherlock and Dooley, 2002; Maroo and Wolf, 2004).

Pregnancy post liver transplantation

Approximately 11% of patients who have had liver transplants are of reproductive age, and whilst amenorrhoea and infertility are common in women with liver cirrhosis (Nagy et al., 2003), liver transplantation allows for the return of normal menstrual patterns in up to 90% of patients of child-bearing age within a few months of transplantation (Heneghan, 2000). Pregnancies after liver transplantation are considered high risk due to the high incidence of hypertension, pre-eclampsia and premature delivery, and therefore should be followed carefully both by transplant clinicians/hepatologists and obstetricians (Jain et al., 2003; Van Dyke, 2006).

It is generally advised that conception should be postponed for at least 6–12 months post liver transplantation as this ensures that both the transplanted organ is functioning properly, and immunosuppressive therapy is stabilised. In addition the incidence of graft rejection after 12 months is significantly reduced (Benjaminov and Heathcote, 2004; Armenti, 2006).

Immunosuppressive therapy should be continued, but monitored carefully (Sherlock and Dooley, 2002). Although most immunosuppressive therapies are potentially teratogenic, few fetal abnormalities have been described (Van Dyke, 2006). Recognised side effects of immunosuppressive therapies are discussed further in Chapter 18.

Tacrolimus crosses the placenta and therefore is found in fetal blood and also in breast milk; it is reported to cause transient renal impairment and hyperkalaemia in the newborn. Therefore it is recommended that mothers do not breastfeed their babies (Heneghan, 2000; Jain et al., 2003). Data currently remain limited for newer therapies such as mycophenolate mofetil (MMF) (Bejaminov and Heathcote, 2004).

Several centres had reported successful outcomes in pregnancies in liver transplant recipients with favourable outcomes of no maternal deaths related to pregnancy or graft loss (Christopher et al., 2006). Delivery by caesarean section is significantly higher than in the normal population (40–46% in transplant patients vs 26%) (Nagy et al., 2003; Armenti, 2006); in addition only 70–78% of babies achieve the normal birth weight, which has been linked to developmental delay and cognitive impairment. Furthermore 35% of all births in post liver transplant patients were premature (Jain et al., 2003; Armenti, 2006). Other reported complications relating to pregnancy in liver transplant recipients are chronic hypertension, anaemia, elevated serum creatinine levels, diabetes and biopsy-proven graft rejection (Nagy et al., 2003).

Whilst successful pregnancy post liver transplantation is achievable, it is imperative that the pregnancies are recognised as high risk and close monitoring is undertaken. Some studies have demonstrated that pregnancies planned at least 2 years after liver transplantation, with stable graft function, can result in excellent maternal and neonatal outcomes when there is a good coordination of specialist care (Nagy et al., 2003).

Chapter summary

The development of liver disease during pregnancy is rare; however it is not without significant risks for both mother and baby. Vigilant antenatal surveillance and proactive management can reduce the risks identified, however there may be increased incidence in subsequent pregnancies, which needs to be conveyed to those affected.

Many women with chronic liver disease find difficulty in achieving a pregnancy due to reduced fertility. Those that do, need careful monitoring of their liver disease and also consideration of potential harm to the fetus due to prescribed medication; this is also a consideration for those patients who have had a liver transplant. Joint care between hepatologist and obstetrician is paramount for beneficial outcomes for mother and baby whatever the underlying cause of the liver disease.

Illustrative case study

A 35-year-old woman presented at 33 weeks of gestation with a 4-day history of abdominal pain, nausea, vomiting, oedema, visual disturbances and headaches. She had no significant medical history and the pregnancy had been relatively uncomplicated. On examination she was hypertensive with a blood pressure of 195/110 mmHg, her other vital signs were within normal range. She had mild ankle oedema and slight abdominal tenderness in the right upper quadrant, there was no evidence of hepatic encephalopathy, or history of itching and she was alert and orientated.

Her initial laboratory investigations demonstrated a WBC of $14,100 \times 10^9$/L, platelet count 37×10^9/L, haemoglobin 8 g/L, bilirubin 60 μmol/L, albumin 28 g/L, AST 400 IU/L, ALP 700 IU/L, and elevated INR (1.8) and serum lactate acid dehydrogenase. Her renal function demonstrated an elevated creatinine of 125 μmol/L, with a urine output greater than 0.5 mL/kg. Urinalysis at the time demonstrated a moderate proteinuria and blood. There was no evidence of infection. She was commenced on intravenous labetalol and magnesium sulphate infusions for management of her hypertension and seizure prophylaxis.

Further laboratory investigations demonstrated that her INR had increased to 2.0 and her platelet count had decreased to 25×10^9/L, with a positive haemolysis screen. A full hepatitis and virology screen were negative. An ultrasound scan showed increased brightness within the liver and patent vessels.

After being given a diagnosis of HELLP syndrome and correction of her clotting abnormalities with fresh frozen plasma and platelets, the patient underwent an emergency caesarean section. After successful delivery of a healthy 2300 g boy, the patient was transferred to a tertiary liver intensive care unit for further management. Initially the patient's AST increased to 800 IU/L returning to normal parameters within 48 hours. The platelet count was maintained >50 × 10⁹/L with support, until resolution of her thrombocytopenia. The patient was later transferred to the ward and discharged from hospital.

References

Abedin P, Weaver J, Egginton E (1999) Intrahepatic cholestasis of pregnancy: revalence and ethnic distribution. *Ethnicity & Health* **4**(1–2):35–37

Armenti VT (2006) Pregnancy after liver transplantation. *Liver Transplantation* **12**(7):1037–1039

Bacq Y, Zarka C, Brechot JF, Mariotte N, Vol S, Tichet J, Weill J (1996) Liver function tests in normal pregnancy: a prospective study of 103 pregnant women and 103 matched controls. *Hepatology* **23**(5):1030–1034

Benjaminov FS, Heathcote J (2004) Liver disease in pregnancy. *American Journal of Gastroenterology* **99**:2479–2488

Browning M, Levy H, Wilkins-Haug L, Larson C, Shih V (2006) Fetal fatty acid oxidation defects and maternal liver disease in pregnancy. *Obstetrics & Gynecology* **107**(1):115–120

Burrows RF, Clavisi O, Burrows E (2001) Interventions for treating cholestasis in pregnancy. *Cochrane Database of Systematic Reviews* Issue 4. Art. No.: CD000493. DOI: 10.1002/14651858.CD000493

Christopher V, Al-Chalabi T, Richardson PD, Muiesan P, Rela M, Heaton ND, O'Grady JG, Heneghan MA (2006) Pregnancy outcomes after liver transplantation: a single centre experience of 71 pregnancies in 45 recipients. *Liver Transplantation* **12**:1138–1143

Coombes J (2000) Cholestasis in pregnancy: a challenging disorder. *British Journal of Midwifery* **8**(9):565–570

Elias E (2007) Liver disease in pregnancy. *Medicine* **35**(2):72–74

Ferenci P (2006) Wilson disease. In: Bacon BR, O'Grady JG, Di Bisceglie AM, Lake JR (eds) *Comprehensive Clinical Hepatology*, 2nd edn. Mosby, Philadelphia, pp. 351–365

Glanz A, Marschall HU, Mattsson LA (2004) Intrahepatic cholestasis of pregnancy: relationships between bile acid levels and fetal complication rates. *Hepatology* **40**(2):467–474

Heneghan MA (2000) Pregnancy and the liver. In: O'Grady JG, Lake JR, Howdle PD (eds) *Comprehensive Clinical Hepatology*. Mosby, London

Heneghan MA, Norris SM, O'Grady JG, Harrison PM, McFarlane IG (2001) Management and outcome of autoimmune hepatitis. *Gut* **48**:97–102

Hill JB, Sheffield JS, Kim MJ, Alexander JM, Sercely B, Wendel GD Jr (2002) Risk of hepatitis B transmission in breast fed infants of chronic hepatitis B carriers. *Obstetrics & Gynecology* **99**(6):1049–1052

Jain AB, Reyes J, Marcos A, Mazariegos G, Eghtesad B, Fontes PA, Cassiarlli TV, Marsh JW, De Vera ME, Rafail A, Starlz TE, Fung JJ (2003) Pregnancy after liver transplantation with tacrolimus immunosupression: a single center's experience update at 13 years. *Transplantation* **76**(5):827–832

Jamerson P (2005) The association between acute fatty liver of pregnancy and fatty acid oxidation disorders. *Journal of Obstetric, Gynecologic, and Neonatal Nursing* **34**(1):87–92

Kidner M, Flanders-Stepans M (2004) A model for the HELLP syndrome: the maternal experience. *Journal of Obstetric, Gynecologic, and Neonatal Nursing* **33**(1):44–53

Knox T, Olans L (1996) Current concepts: liver disease in pregnancy. *New England Journal of Medicine* **335**(8):569–576

Kroumpouzos G (2002) Intrahepatic cholestasis of pregnancy: what's new. *Journal of the European Academy of Dermatology and Venereology* **16**(4):316–318

Kumar D, Tandon R (2001) Use of ursodeoxycholic acid in liver disease. *Journal of Gastroenterology and Hepatology* **16**:3–14

Longo SA, Dola CP, Pridijan G (2003) Preeclampsia and eclampsia revisited. *Southern Medical Journal* **96**:891–899

Mahl T, O'Grady J (2006) *Liver Disorders*. Health Press Limited, Abingdon

Maroo S, Wolf J (2004) The liver in pregnancy. In: Friedman LS, Keeffe E (eds) *Handbook of Liver Disease*, 2nd edn. Churchill Livingstone, Philadelphia

Matchaba P, Moodley J (2004) Corticosteroids for HELLP syndrome in pregnancy. *Cochrane Database of Systematic Reviews* Issue 1. Art. No.: CD002076. DOI: 10.1002/14651858.CD002076.pub2

Nagy S, Bush MC, Berkowitz R, Fishbein TM, Gomez-Lobo V (2003) Pregnancy outcomes in liver transplant recipients. *Obstetrics and Gynaecology* **102**(1): 121–128

Rahmen TM, Wendon J (2002) Severe hepatic dysfunction in pregnancy. *Quarterly Journal of Medicine* **95**:343–357

Saleh M, Abdo K (2007) Consensus on the management of obstetric cholestasis: national UK survey. *BJOG* **114**:99–103

Sentilhes L, Vespyck E, Pia P, Marpeau L (2006) Fetal death in a patient with intrahepatic cholestasis of pregnancy. *Obstetrics and Gynaecology* **107**(2 part 2):458–460

Serrano M, Brites D, Larena M, Monte M, Bravo P, Oliveria N, Marin J (1998) Beneficial effect of ursodeoxycholic acid on alterations induced by cholestasis of pregnancy in bile acid transport across the human placenta. *Journal of Hepatology* **28**:829–839

Shames BD, Fernndez LA, Sollinger HW, Chin T, D'Alessandro AM, Knechtle SJ, Lucey MR, Hafez R, Musat A, Kalayoglu M (2005) Liver transplantation for HELLP syndrome. *Liver Transplantation* **11**(2):224–228

Sherlock S, Dooley J (2002) *Diseases of the Liver and Biliary System,* 11th edn. Blackwell Science, Oxford

Treem W (2002) Mitochondrial fatty acid oxidation and acute fatty liver of pregnancy. *Seminars in Gastrointestinal Disease* 13(1):55–66

Tse KY, Ho LF, Lao T (2005) The impact of maternal HBSAg carrier status on pregnancy outcomes: a case control study. *Journal of Hepatology* 43:771–775

Van Dyke RW (2006) Liver diseases in pregnancy. In: Bacon BR, O'Grady JG, Di Bisceglie AM, Lake JR (eds) *Comprehensive Clinical Hepatology,* 2nd edn. Mosby, Philadelphia, pp. 487–496

Wasmuth H, Glantz A, Keppeler H, Simone E, Bartz C, Rath W, Mattsson LA, Marschall H-U, Lammert F (2007) Intrahepatic cholestasis of pregnancy: the severe form is associated with common variants of the hepatobiliary phospholipids transporter ABCB4 gene. *Gut* 56(2):265–270

17
Hepatobiliary malignancies

Nikie Jervis

Introduction

The aim of this chapter is to provide an overview of the three most common liver-related cancers occurring in the adult population of the UK: primary liver cancer (hepatocellular carcinoma, HCC), bile duct cancer (cholangiocarcinoma) and secondary liver cancer (metastatic disease). Additionally it will provide a brief examination of current management therapies and the psychosocial issues that can impact upon the delivery of holistic nursing care.

Hepatobiliary malignancies are amongst the most common and fatal cancers worldwide. Although previously thought to be rare in the UK, a review of the incidence rates over the last 20–30 years shows an alarming upward trend, with predictions of further rises.

Despite improving cancer survival statistics, it is still widely presumed that a diagnosis of cancer means death. It is a sad reality that for a number of reasons, people do die of cancer, or related illnesses; however improvements in diagnostics and treatments are lengthening survival periods. Curative therapies are now being offered and, more importantly, achieving their aim.

Providing care for someone diagnosed with cancer can be complex, not only due to the physical manifestation of the disease but also because of the emotional and social consequences. Uncertainty and fear can surround a cancer diagnosis, not only for the patient but also their families and, to some degree, the health care professionals involved in providing their care.

Definition

Cancer has a number of definitions. It is a group of diseases rather than one specific illness, however two main characteristics are common to all:

- Uncontrolled growth of cells arising from 'normal' tissue
- The ability of these abnormal cells to invade and/or spread to other sites (Souhami and Tobias, 1998)

There has been an enormous amount of work carried out globally to determine the cause(s) of cancer and it is generally accepted that there are external and internal factors involved, usually in combination.

Normal cells grow in an organised and predetermined way, they have a defined purpose, size and lifespan. Cancer cells do not: they divide as normal cells (mitosis) but, due to an alteration or mutation of their DNA, they ignore limitations, continuing to grow beyond their 'normal' boundaries. Left untreated, cancer cells breach normal restrictions, such as adjacent cells and structures, invading them and continuing to grow, surviving longer than their non-cancerous counterparts. Some cancers attract their own blood supply, gaining an ongoing supply of oxygen and nutrients for further growth. At a certain point of growth or cell volume their ability to spread to other sites of the body may become evident. Some of the cancer cells split from the site of origin and travel via the blood stream or lymphatic system to other parts of the body, where they settle and grow: these are metastases.

External factors that may lead to the development of cancer are called carcinogens, e.g. tobacco. These can 'trigger' cancer development by interfering with cellular DNA, which in turn can lead to alterations in the cell's normal growth pattern and behaviour. Viruses may also have this effect.

Internal factors are thought to be linked to the body's ability to tolerate exposure to certain carcinogens, its ability to repair any damage caused to cellular DNA and/or 'genetic susceptibility'. The latter is thought to be a genetic predisposition to cancer development that is activated by exposure to a particular trigger and may, in part, explain familial clusters where no direct hereditary link can be found.

Caring for someone with cancer can be complex, but by understanding both the objective (epidemiology, aetiology, diagnosis and treatments) and subjective (individual and social context) knowledge available regarding hepatobiliary malignancies, effective and appropriate care can be implemented.

Primary liver cancer

Hepatocellular carcinoma (HCC) is one of the most common cancers worldwide, both in incidence (fifth) and mortality (third), with 80–90% of HCCs forming on

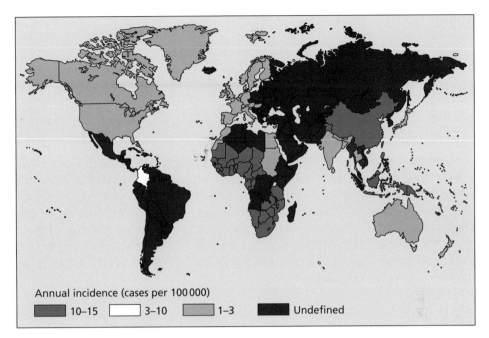

Annual incidence (cases per 100 000)

| ▓ 10–15 | ☐ 3–10 | ▓ 1–3 | ▓ Undefined |

Figure 17.1 Worldwide distribution of hepatocellular carcinoma. Reproduced with permission from Beckingham IJ, Krige JE (2001) ABC of diseases of liver, pancreas, and biliary system. Liver Tumours. *British Medical Journal* **322**:477–480.

the background of liver cirrhosis (Llovet and Beaugard, 2003). Traditionally seen as a cancer of the east or sub-Saharan regions, where viral hepatitis is endemic, HCC is increasing in incidence in the west, and is 'now one of the leading causes of death among patients with cirrhosis in Europe' (Fattovich et al., 2004) (Figure 17.1).

A recent study, commissioned by the British Society of Gastroenterology (BSG, 2006), found an alarming 350% increase in the overall incidence of cirrhosis in the UK, over the last 20 years, with a 900% rise in the under 45s. The study also reports a twofold increase in the incidence of HCC over the last decade. Ryder (2003) proposes that 1500 deaths occur per year due to HCC, with a predicted rise of 40–70% over the next 10 years. Contributory factors to both increases in cirrhosis and subsequent cancer development include viral hepatitis (B and C), alcohol consumption, non-alcoholic fatty liver disease (NAFLD) and haemochromatosis.

Viral hepatitis

The link with viral hepatitis has been well established over the years, particularly the correlation between hepatitis B virus (HBV) infection and HCC development

(Beasley, 1988). Hepatitis B is a DNA virus, with a mutation rate ten times higher than that of other DNA viruses. The virus binds itself to the liver cell's DNA, disrupting normal cell activity and growth, precipitating destruction and mutation. Early effective treatment of HBV can help to reduce the incidence of HCC development, by reducing viral load. This is discussed further in Chapter 9.

Carcinogenesis is linked, in this instance, with viral replication rather than cirrhosis per se. In endemic areas of the world 90% of HCC patients are HBV-infected and it worth noting here that not all of these patients have progressed to cirrhosis.

In patients with hepatitis C virus (HCV) no direct causal link has been established. However, there is an identified correlation, with several studies reporting evidence of HCV in up to 75% of patients with HCC (Bruix et al., 1989; Di Bisceglie et al., 1991; Nishioka et al., 1991). It has been suggested that the trigger is related to viral interference with the cell's central protein, thereby interrupting natural processes. HCV is thought to have a slow progression to cirrhosis (estimated 20–30 years post exposure), and tumour development is rare amongst the non-cirrhotic cohort of this group.

Alcohol

Reflected in health care statistics and much publicised in the media is the UK's growing incidence of excessive alcohol consumption, especially within the younger population (under 45s), which can lead to cirrhosis, and the development of liver cancer.

For patients with pre-existing liver disease, even drinking within the recommended guidelines can increase the risk of cirrhosis and HCC. Seemingly paradoxical, those who become abstinent following excess alcohol consumption, may be at greater risk of HCC development. This may be due to the cellular regeneration process of attempted repair, with cellular disruption occurring, or simply because continued imbibing results in a shorter lifespan, therefore the individual may die of the complications of alcoholic hepatitis/cirrhosis before HCC develops.

Metabolic liver diseases

There is a growing incidence reported in western countries of non-alcoholic steatohepatitis (NASH). NASH may be linked with diet, obesity (>60%), type 2 diabetes (~50%) and/or hypercholesterolaemia, it can lead to cirrhosis, and incidences of HCC have been reported.

Haemochromatosis also carries a higher risk of HCC development than other liver diseases. The risk is higher (7–9%) in untreated patients, where iron overload disrupts normal hepatocyte function. However the risk can be reduced (to 1–3%), though not negated, by venesection (Ryder, 2003).

Bile duct cancer

Bile duct cancer or cholangiocarcinoma (CCA) is the second most common primary cancer to occur within the liver. The incidence of CCA is rising significantly and is not purely attributable to the clarity of definition and coding, nor better diagnostics. The increased incidence is reportedly equal to mortality, with most recent figures reporting a tenfold increase over the last decade (1998 mortality rate = 1000 in England and Wales alone) (Khan et al., 2002; Gores, 2003; BSG, 2006).

Unlike HCC, CCA has no clearly identifiable causal link, though presence of a pre-existing biliary pathology may be associated with an increased risk.

- Primary sclerosing cholangitis (PSC) is evident in 30% of all newly diagnosed CCAs, and the most commonly associated risk factor occurring in the UK
- Cystic abnormalities also carry an increased lifetime risk of CCA, such as choledochal cysts which have a malignant transformation incidence of 5%, and Caroli's disease (life-time risk of ~7%, half that of PSC)
- Bile duct adenomas, papillomas and intraductal stone disease may also predispose to cholangiocarcinoma development
- Other factors include thorotrast exposure (a radiological agent not used in over 50 years, but with an indeterminate long-term adverse consequence) and smoking (increases risk in people with PSC). Chronic typhoid and liver flukes have also been identified as associated risks in certain parts of Asia, where CCA is relatively common

The prognosis for CCA is usually poor, invariably due to late presentation, with an expected survival range of 3–18 months. The prognosis can usually be inferred from symptoms and stage of disease at presentation (approximately 10–20% already have peritoneal involvement at time of diagnosis).

Secondary liver cancer

The liver is one of the commonest sites of the body for metastatic disease to be found. Primary sites may include breast and upper gastrointestinal tract, amongst others.

Colorectal cancer affects upwards of 30 000 people each year in the UK, and the incidence is rising. However, the mortality rate is reducing, in part due to primary disease management but also due to the improvements in secondary disease treatment, such as advances in surgical techniques and chemotherapy treatments (Bentrem et al., 2005; Ruan and Warren, 2005).

Up to 50% of those diagnosed with colorectal cancer will develop secondary disease, either simultaneously (synchronous disease) or subsequently (metachronous disease). Liver resection, as a potentially curative treatment, is now of widely acknowledged and proven benefit (Heriot and Karanjia, 2002).

Diagnosing hepatobiliary malignancy

Symptoms

Hepatobiliary cancers can be 'silent' diseases: there may be either no symptoms evident or, where present, they are mild or vague, possibly attributed to other health factors, such as underlying liver disease, other illnesses and/or treatments (e.g. HBV patient undergoing antiviral therapy). Mild and/or non-specific symptoms can include malaise, increasing lethargy, slight nausea or reduced appetite. Weight loss may be insidious.

Symptom occurrence is rare in early stage disease and detection at this point may occur incidentally, for example, as a result of a routine health screen or during investigation for another health matter. Abnormalities in liver function may be noted, even though the eventual diagnosis may not be initially suspected. More specific symptoms tend to be related to either an acute event, decompensation or advanced disease.

Approximately 5–15% of HCCs present following spontaneous rupture of the tumour, left untreated this is associated with a 1-month mortality rate of 90%, with no 'survivors' at 1 year.

Jaundice is rare and, usually, a very late sign of malignant disease for both HCC and colorectal liver metastases (CLM), however, for CCA it may be one of the most common presenting signs. Jaundice, pruritis, dark urine and pale stools indicate an obstructed biliary tree. Where gallstones can be ruled out, unexplained jaundice should be investigated as a priority, with the differential diagnoses including CCA and pancreatic cancer.

Investigations

The patient history should always include family medical history where known.

Bloods tests should include a full blood count, liver and renal function, and chronic liver disease screen including virology and tumour markers.

Tumour markers are substances within the blood that may, if elevated beyond the normal value, raise the suspicion of malignancy. However false-positives and -negatives can occur: positives with benign disease and negatives where no tumour markers are secreted (occurs in subgroups of the population). In hepatobiliary malignancies, the tumour markers usually tested for are AFP (alpha-fetoprotein) Ca19.9, Ca125 and carcinoembryonic antigen (CAE):

- AFP is associated with HCC. Laboratories vary, but a 'normal value' is usually <20 ng/mL (<7 KU/L). However, levels of up to 500 ng/mL have been reported in benign conditions (chronic hepatitis, pregnancy) and normal results have been reported in up to 20% of HCC patients (Wagman et al., 2000; Ryder, 2003)
- Ca19.9 is associated with both biliary and pancreatic malignancy. The usual normal value is <37 KU/mL. It is elevated in more than 85% of people with

CCA, however it may also be elevated in hyperbilirubinaemia and severe liver injury

- CEA is associated with colorectal cancer. The usual normal value is <5 ng/mL. It may also be elevated in cholangiocarcinoma: 30% of people with CCA have an elevated CEA. In colorectal disease, a CEA level in excess of 50 ng/mL has been found to be positively correlated with a poor prognosis. However, elevated CEA has also been detected in inflammatory bowel disease, chronic lung disease, biliary obstruction and liver injury
- Ca125 is usually associated with primary gynaecological or peritoneal malignancy. It may also be elevated in cholangiocarcinoma (40–50%), though this may be due to the presence of peritoneal involvement. The usual value is <35 kU/mL. Benign conditions which may be associated with an elevated Ca125 include menstruation, pregnancy and endometriosis

Radiological investigations

Radiology is essential to hepatobiliary malignancy diagnosis but reliability may be dependent upon equipment, operator and interpreter expertise.

Ultrasonography is the primary radiological investigation as it is not expensive and is non-invasive, with a reported sensitivity of 60–90% (dependent on size of lesion). In combination with AFP monitoring, the sensitivity for HCC detection can rise to 95%. It is also useful to help differentiate between malignant and benign causes of biliary obstruction.

CT can be used to confirm presence of lesion (Figure 17.2), if it is uncertain on ultrasonography. CT has a greater specificity for smaller lesions, with the potential

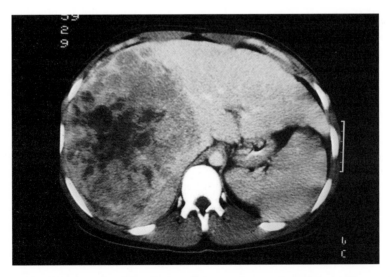

Figure 17.2 CT scan of a large hepatocellular carcinoma. Reproduced with permission from Beckingham IJ, Krige JE (2001) ABC of diseases of liver, pancreas, and biliary system. Liver Tumours. *British Medical Journal* **322**:477–480.

advantage of examining for the presence of extrahepatic disease. In addition CT may be more accurate for diagnosing and staging CCA as there may be greater clarity for examining the hilar region of the liver as well as adjacent vascular structures. CT may be the preferred technique in the diagnosis/staging and surveillance for CLM as it allows for full body imaging, thus facilitating primary and secondary site assessment.

Magnetic resonance imaging (MRI) can be utilised if there is still uncertainty following ultrasonography and CT. Magnetic resonance angiography and venography offer non-invasive modes of imaging, which can be of additional assistance where surgical intervention or interventional radiology is proposed.

Magnetic resonance cholangiopancreatography (MRCP) may also be of use in CCA, though endoscopic assessment may be preferred as it would allow for concurrent stent insertion if clinically indicated (preferably following CT scanning).

Positive emitron tomography (PET) may be useful in the assessment of secondary disease where traditional axial imaging may be indeterminate. PET assesses cell activity, the metabolic rate, therefore highly active cells such as cancer cells will be highlighted as 'hot spots'. However, inflammatory tissue as well as cells with a high metabolic rate (e.g. in the gut) will also be highlighted. PET is useful in CLM as it will help identify any extrahepatic sites of tumour occurrence, however its use in CCA is currently debatable (Khan et al., 2002) and it is rarely contributory in HCC diagnosis.

Laparoscopy, although still under discussion, is increasing in usage as both a diagnostic and therapeutic approach to hepatobiliary cancer management. Intraoperative ultrasonography can be utilised during laparoscopy to further advance tumour staging. Laparoscopic examination may also be used as a precursor to resection following examination, or to facilitate biopsy/node sampling to confirm diagnosis where curative resection or palliative surgery may not be possible.

Endoscopic investigations

Endoscopic retrograde cholangiopancreatography (ERCP) can image the biliary tree directly and also assess for pancreatic involvement if the origin of cancer has not been determined. Cytology brushings may be obtained and/or palliation of jaundice by stenting may be performed, although as a diagnostic tool it is preferred that stenting occurs after axial imaging has taken place. (Stenting may cause a localised inflammatory response that may obscure or complicate accurate diagnosis.)

Endoscopic ultrasound may allow for closer examination of the adjacent vascular structures in CCA and pancreatic disease, lymph node examination and/or sampling and distal bile duct/pancreatic head assessment. Tissue sampling for histological examination may also be obtained during this procedure, as well as differentiation between biliary and pancreatic origin of a tumour.

Upper and lower gastrointestinal tract endoscopy may also be carried out if diagnosis is equivocal. CCA can mimic CLM both clinically and radiologically, therefore clinical history and thorough evaluation are vital. It is important to identify the primary tumour, if present, to enable treatment specification.

Cancer surveillance

HCC surveillance is advocated in high-risk groups to improve early diagnosis, with the aim of early intervention and potential cure. The consensus for HCC appears to be ultrasonography and AFP every 3–6 months in patients who have:

- HBsAg positive
- HBV and HCV cirrhosis
- Alcohol-related cirrhosis (particularly those abstinent)
- Haemochromatosis
- NASH

Some hepatologists recommend that all cirrhotic patients are offered surveillance (Wagman et al., 2000; Llovet and Beaugard, 2003; Ryder, 2003).

For CCA and CLM there is no such consensus, this may be due to the current lack of evidence-based supportive literature and/or cost factors.

Treatment options

Successful, appropriate treatment of cancer is dependent upon accurate staging and careful patient selection. Accurate pretreatment staging not only informs treatment choices, but may also offer prognostic indicator information.

For most cancers the tumour/node/metastasis (TNM) staging system is used, however for HCC this provides an incomplete picture as it fails to assess underlying liver disease. Although primary and secondary liver cancers share the same anatomical site, they have a different histology, biology and history. So where TNM may be useful in secondary disease, it has limited value in primary liver cancer.

As a result a number of alternative systems have been proposed: the Okuda system (Okuda et al., 1985), the French classification (Chevret et al., 1999), BCLC (Barcelona Clinic Liver Cancer)(Llovet et al., 1999), CLIP (Cancer of the Liver Italian Programme, 2000) and CUPI (Chinese University Prognostic Indicator) (Leung et al., 2002). All incorporate additional information related to underlying liver disease and the patient's general health condition, however they vary in depth of information (Grieco et al., 2005; Levy and Sherman, 2005)

Careful patient selection is highly influential upon treatment outcomes, for each of these three malignancies: underlying liver function, stage of disease, modality of treatment suitable, treatment intent, co-existing pathologies and, most importantly, patient choice may determine what can or cannot be done to help treat the cancer.

At present the only treatment option that can be offered with potential curative intent is surgery.

Liver resection

Liver resections include hemi-hepatectomy (extended or formal), non-anatomical, segmentectomy, wedge resection and/or metastectomy. Hepatocellular carcinomas less than 25% are currently suitable for successful resection (due to either underlying liver disease and/or disease extent); the 5-year survival rate range is 30–70%. However, where early detection of tumour is identified, the survival figure can rise to >90%. Additional prognostic indicators include volume of residual liver and extent of resection.

Surgical interventions of CCA include partial liver resection and/or excision of the extrahepatic biliary tree. The 3-year survival rate from current data is 40–60%, with 5-year figures reported as 9–30%. However, this may be due to the reported high recurrence rate (50–70%). The origin of the disease appears to be significantly influential on outcome figures, extrahepatic CCA fares better than intrahepatic origin CCA.

Where curative resection cannot be performed for CCA, palliative surgical procedures may be performed, e.g. a biliary 'bypass' operation, which may alleviate biliary and/or duodenal obstruction, resulting in improved quality of life.

For patients with CLM, the surgical procedures are as for HCC. Approximately 7500 people per year in the UK will develop CLM, of which 50% may be staged as potentially suitable for liver resection. However, up to a third of these will be found to be inoperable at laparotomy. For those who do proceed to liver resection, 5-year survival rates are 40–50% and are rising. When contrasted with a 5-year survival of <1% for untreated disease, the benefit is clearly identifiable. The recurrence rate for CLM is high, with up to 60% of resected patients developing new or recurrent disease, however, unlike CCA patients, people with recurrent CLM may undergo further surgery, provided they are appropriately staged as suitable. Operative risk, survival and recurrence figures are equivalent to those of first time resection.

Liver transplantation

Liver transplantation is only suitable for those with HCC. However availability is limited due to an increased demand and a decreased number of donor organs (see Chapter 18). Five-year survival, of patients transplanted with HCC, is reportedly above 60%, although with recurrence rates estimated at 30–40%, this figure may decrease to around 20%.

There is a current debate regarding transplantation criteria and whether the criteria of tumour size currently used in the UK should be expanded. Emerging data from the Far East suggests that it is the biology of the disease rather than size per se that influences survival. A highly proliferative tumour carries a greater risk than tumour volume; for example a 7 cm indolent tumour may carry a lower risk of recurrence than three 1 cm highly active tumours. Macrovascular invasion and a grossly elevated AFP have been found to be significant predictive indicators of disease recurrence and/or death (Lee et al., 2004; Pawlick et al., 2005; Moray et al., 2007).

Palliative (non-curative) treatments

Transarterial chemoembolisation

Transarterial chemoembolisation (TACE) is a treatment for HCC, which takes advantage of the dual blood supply to the liver by the portal vein and hepatic artery. Chemotherapy is delivered directly into the tumour's blood supply via the hepatic artery. Mixed with the chemotherapy are particles (usually a lipiodal mix) that will also provide temporary arterial occlusion. The aim of this treatment is to destroy liver cancer cells by the direct installation of chemotherapy, with the secondary effect of arterial occlusion, which interrupts oxygen and nutrient delivery. It is not offered as a curative therapy, but may be offered as a holding treatment, to patients awaiting transplantation to help keep them within transplant criteria. Co-existing portal vein occlusion may be a contraindication, depending on cause and extent.

Response rates vary and there is some debate as to whether it is the cytotoxic or embolisation effect that has the greater anti-tumoural result. Around 30% of patients will show objective tumour response with no tumour progression, 30% will show no objective tumour response, but neither will there be evident progression and the final third will have no objective tumour response and evidence of tumour progression. There is a 2-year survival rate of 20–80%, with influential factors including response to and/or tolerance of cytotoxic therapy.

TACE can be repeated, usually at 6–8-week plus cycles, dependent on the chemotherapy drug and dosage used. A consideration where doxorubicin is used is the life-time dose limitation, that may restrict how often this therapy can be given.

A further consideration in patients with pre-existing viral disease is that the chemotherapy may re-activate quiescent disease; prophylactic therapy with appropriate antivirals is recommended (Johnson, 2005; Marelli et al., 2006, 2007).

Radio-frequency ablation

Radio-frequency ablation (RFA) is primarily used for HCC and CLM. A probe is inserted directly into the tumour, via the percutaneous, laparoscopic or open laparotomy approach and a predetermined 'burn' is delivered to the tumour. Limitations of this treatment include size and position of the tumour(s), including proximity to blood vessels and the diaphragm.

Long-term response rates are yet to be fully evaluated, but early initial results show a potential benefit over percutaneous injection therapies; survival benefit is yet to be seen (Camma et al., 2005; Pacella et al., 2005).

Percutaneous ethanol/acetic acid injection (PE/AI)

Percutaneous ethanol/acetic acid injection (PE/AI) is used for HCC and utilises a direct target approach, where either ethanol or acetic acid is injected, via the percutaneous route, into the tumour. The limitations of this treatments include size, number and position of the lesion(s) and periprocedural pain. As a palliative procedure PE/AI has a reported 5-year survival of less than 50% (Andriulli et al., 2006).

Systemic chemotherapy

Systemic chemotherapy has a less than 10% response rate in HCC, and is thought to be related to liver cancer's apparent drug resistance to cytotoxic therapy. As with TACE, prophylactic antiviral therapy should be considered pretreatment in patients with pre-existing viral disease to prevent reactivation/exacerbation. Chemotherapy has also been utilised post transplantation, where histology has indicated vascular or perineural invasion, however there is limited data regarding efficacy and there are no results from randomised controlled trials to evaluate this.

CCA appears to be slightly more chemoresponsive, with a partial response rate of 10–50%, dependent upon cytotoxic drug/regime used and stage of disease at time of treatment instigation. Gemcitabine as part of a combination regime has been reported to show favourable results, with an associated symptom control benefit. Jaundice, or rather hyperbilirubinaemia, can preclude chemotherapy as a treatment option. Unless optimal biliary drainage is achieved and the bilirubin level is less than twice the upper limit of normal (ULN), most oncologists would be reluctant to proceed with therapy. As a postsurgical adjuvant therapy, chemotherapy for CCA is as yet of unproven benefit; further evidence is required.

It is in the group of patients with CLM that chemotherapy has proven most beneficial, as evidenced in the reported improved survival rates (up by between 4 and 13%) in the Improving Outcome Guidance in Colorectal Cancer Manual update (NICE, 2004).

Photodynamic therapy

Photodynamic therapy (PDT) is a treatment that utilises a photosensitising agent, administered systemically, activated by a laser. The laser is attached to an endoscopic probe, that is inserted via ERCP. The agent attacks the cancer cells by causing necrosis. Initial studies, as reported in the NICE guidance (2005), suggest a survival benefit of approximately 4 months when compared with stenting alone, with a significant symptom improvement.

Radiotherapy

Radiotherapy has limited efficacy due to radiation hepatitis. However, it is useful in primary colorectal cancer and for the palliative treatment of bony metastases in HCC, CCA and CLM.

Whilst other therapies, such as tamoxifen and trialled therapies such as yttrium-labelled microspheres, have shown some benefits, further studies are required before these are widely adopted.

Nursing management

The perioperative mortality rate for liver resection at major specialist centres is less than 5%, with complications occurring in about 30% (including routine post-operative incidences, e.g. wound infection).

In patients without significant cirrhosis, up to 80% of the liver can be safely resected, due to its capacity for regeneration or rather hypertrophy with maintained functionality. However, in selected patients there may be concerns about potential for peri-/postoperative liver failure.

Postoperative considerations following liver resection include:

- Shock +/- haemorrhage: the liver is a highly vascular organ and carries a subsequent high risk of bleeding post surgery. Added to this is the potential for an impaired liver to develop a coagulopathy peri-/postoperatively. Therefore careful observation and monitoring +/- infusion of blood products +/- vitamin K administration are necessary
- Hepatic insufficiency: transient liver enzyme abnormality and the development of a degree of post-surgical ascites are not unexpected in the immediate postoperative phase. However, severe or prolonged abnormality is unusual and may indicate liver failure, particularly in patients with previously identified liver disease. Liver failure may be due to decompensation of pre-existing liver disease or to 'small-for-size' remnant liver – in either instance immediate identification and appropriate intervention are required to prevent further deterioration or death. Intensive therapy unit (ITU) admission with organ support interventions should be instigated. The incidence is less than 1%, however if liver failure does occur the mortality rate is significantly higher
- Bile leak: this can occur from the cut surface of the liver or from biliary anastamotic sites. These may be treated conservatively, endoscopically with stenting, radiologically by drain insertion or surgically. Careful observation and drain surveillance are required, with early cholangitic and/or septic symptoms reported and acted upon
- General postoperative care: effective, appropriate analgesia, prevention of infection, management of nausea/vomiting/ileus and early mobilisation are of paramount importance

In general the postoperative liver resection stay, for an uncomplicated procedure, should not exceed 7–10 days.

Chemotherapy drugs target rapidly dividing cells, such as cancer cells, and alter their ability to grow and duplicate. However, there are other cells within the body that naturally divide and grow rapidly (though in these instances the rate of growth and duplication is controlled), for example, hair. Common side effects related to cytotoxic therapy – whether given systemically or targeted (e.g. TACE) are:

■ Alopecia (hair loss) is common with doxorubicin (TACE-HCC) but less likely with gemcitabine (CCA). If alopecia is going to occur it usually starts around the second week post treatment. Hair loss may be minimal (i.e. hair thinning) or extreme (where the individual may even lose their eyelashes, eyebrows and nasal hair, all hair is affected). However chemotherapy-related alopecia is reversible and hair usually starts to regrow once treatment stops

■ Gastrointestinal disturbances range from mouth ulceration to nausea/vomiting to diarrhoea/constipation. The lining of the gastrointestinal tract is composed of rapidly dividing cells and therefore may also be affected by chemotherapy. Oral hygiene is important, although dental intervention is not advised during treatment. Symptom control/management techniques can help prevent or alleviate gastrointestinal tract disturbances; anti-emetics, natural remedies such as peppermint, chamomile or ginger may be given. Avoid or treat constipation with dietary alterations +/– mild laxatives

■ Haematological alterations. There is a certain period post chemotherapy administration when there will be a fall in the full blood count, potentially resulting in anaemia, thrombocytopenia and neutropenia. This is called the 'nadir period' – it usually self-resolves and the full blood count will be back within 'normal' range by the next dose of chemotherapy or within 5–7 days. However, in some people the drop is severe and if it is either symptomatic or prolonged, further intervention may be necessitated

  ■ Anaemia may be treated with iron supplements and/or transfusion, depending on the severity of drop of haemoglobin

  ■ Thrombocytopenia: bruising and/or spontaneous bleeding may occur if thrombocytopenia is severe or the platelet count falls below 30×10^9/L. Supportive therapy and infection-control protocol adherence are vital; wounds and scratches may take longer to heal

  ■ Neutropenia: if this is severe and/or associated with a fever or signs of infection, admission to hospital may be required for intravenous antibiotics or the administration of haemopoietic growth factor (HGF). HGF can help promote the neutrophil count but its use is restricted to protocol-driven administration and is reserved for use in profound or sepsis-related neutropenia

■ Virus reactivation. Chemotherapy may trigger reactivation or exacerbation of existing viral disease. Prophylaxis should be administered prior to starting therapy where possible

- In women the menstrual cycle may become irregular or even stop. Hot flushes, vaginal dryness and/or a reduced sex drive may be experienced, all of which will have an emotional as well as physical impact. Effective contraception is essential as pregnancy during chemotherapy should be avoided: body fluids are cytotoxic and the drugs themselves may be teratogenic. Fertility may be affected; this may be drug dependent and if the patient is of child-bearing age, discussion regarding protecting fertility, including egg harvesting, should be facilitated
- In men sperm production may be reduced; this may resume post treatment but as stated above, discussion regarding fertility and preservation methods should be facilitated. The ability to achieve and maintain an erection and to ejaculate should not be impaired by chemotherapy, however, due to the emotional and physical impact of a cancer diagnosis and its treatment, dysfunction may occur
- Counselling and support can help and should be offered where available

Chapter summary

Hepatobiliary malignancies are amongst the most common, and fatal, cancers worldwide. This chapter has given a brief overview of the three most common – primary liver cancer, bile duct cancer and colorectal liver metastases. Despite their historical rarity in the UK, the incidence of these cancers is increasing and the care involved is complex and multi-disciplinary.

Cancer will probably affect most of us, at some point in our lives, whether directly or indirectly. How we deal with such exposure is influenced as much by societal portrayal and belief, as it is by our emotional and physical response. Cancer can be cured, but where cure is not possible the aim of treatment and care is to support the individual to live well, physically, emotionally and socially, until they die. An important message to give as health care providers is that even if we cannot cure, we can help.

Illustrative case study

A 66-year-old male presented to his GP with a 2-week history of increasing abdominal distension and discomfort. He had a past medical history of hypertension which was well controlled with medication, and had a hip replacement 6 years ago. He was a non-smoker, teetotaller, and had no history of any recreational drug usage.

The patient was heterosexual and had been married for 34 years and had two grown-up children, and had recently retired from a governmental administrative job. There was no history of any recent foreign travel or any history of any blood transfusions or blood products. There was no relevant family history to note.

On examination of the patient there was no evidence of jaundice, or stigmata of chronic liver disease and no palpable liver or spleen. The abdomen was noted to be dull on percussion with no 'shifting ascites'.

Further laboratory investigation revealed a negative hepatitis, chronic liver disease screen. His laboratory investigation revealed AST 59 IU/L, bilirubin 24 µmol/L, albumin 28 g/L and alpha-fetoprotein level 700 ng/mL.

An abdominal ultrasonography confirmed a small volume of ascitic fluid, with a small and heterogeneous shrunken liver, and a spleen 17.6 cm in length. There was no visible duct dilatation or calculi. It was however noted that there were two small focal lesions of less than 3 cm in diameter. This was confirmed by a CT scan of chest/thorax and abdomen, which additionally demonstrated that there was no vascular or lymphatic involvement or any other lesions.

The patient was diagnosed with cryptogenic cirrhosis and hepatocellular carcinoma. Diuretic therapy was commenced for his ascites and he was referred to a tertiary transplant centre for transplant assessment.

References

Andriulli A, De Sio I, Brunello F, Salmi A, Solmi L, Facciorusso D, Caturelli E, Perri F (2006) Survival of patients with early hepatocellular carcinoma treated by percutaneous alcohol injection. *Alimentary Pharmacology and Therapeutics* 23:1329–1335

Beasley RP (1988) Hepatitis B virus. The major etiology of hepatocellular carcinoma. *Cancer* 61(10):1942–1956

Bentrem DJ, Dematteo RP, Blumgart LH (2005) Surgical therapy for metastatic disease to the liver. *Annual Review of Medicine* 56:139–156

British Society of Gastroenterology (2006) Care of Patients with Gastrointestinal Disorders in the United Kingdom. A Strategy for the Future. Available at www.bsg.org.uk

Bruix J, Barrera JM, Calvet X, Ercilla G, Costa J, Sanchez-Tapias JM, Ventura M, Vall M, Bruguera M, Bru C, et al. (1989) Prevalence of antibodies to hepatitis C virus in Spanish patients with hepatocellular carcinoma and hepatic cirrhosis. *Lancet* 2(8670):1004–1006

Camma C, Di Marco V, Orlando A, Sandonato L, Casaril A, Parisi P, Alizzi S, Sciarro E, Virdone R, Pardo S, Di Bona D, Licata A, Latteri F, Cabibbo G, Montalto G, Latteri MA, Nicoli N, Craxi A (2005) Treatment of hepatocellular carcinoma in compensated cirrhosis with radio-frequency thermal ablation (RFA): a prospective study. *Journal of Hepatology* 42(4):535–540

Chevret S, Trinchet JC, Mathieu D, Rached AA, Beaugrand M, Chastang C (1999) A new prognostic classification for predicting survival in patients with hepatocellular carcinoma. Groupe d'Etude et de Traitement du Carcinome Hépatocellulaire. *Hepatology* **31**(1):133–141

Corner J and Bailey C (eds) (2001) *Cancer Nursing. Care in Context.* Blackwell Science, Oxford

Di Bisceglie AM, Order SE, Klein JL, Waggoner JG, Sjogren MH, Kuo G, Houghton M, Choo QL, Hoofnagle JH (1991) The role of chronic viral hepatitis in hepatocellular carcinoma in the United States. *The American Journal of Gastroenterology* **86**(3):335–338

Fattovich G, Stroffolini T, Zagni I, Donato F (2004) Hepatocellular carcinoma in cirrhosis: incidence and risk factors. *Gastroenterology* **127**(Suppl 1):S35–S50

Gores GJ (2003) Cholangiocarcinoma: current concepts and insights. *Hepatology* **37**(5):961–969

Grieco A, Pompilil M, Caminiti G, Miele L, Covino M, Alfei B, Rapaccini L and Gasbarrini G (2005) Prognostic factors for survival in patients with early-intermediate hepatocellular carcinoma undergoing non-surgical therapy: comparison of Okuda, CLIP and BCLC staging systems in a single Italian centre. *Gut* **54**:411–418

Heriot AG, Karanjia ND (2002) A review of surgical techniques for liver resection. *Annals of the Royal College of Surgeons England* **84**:371–380

Johnson PJ (2005) Non-surgical treatment of hepatocellular carcinoma. *HPB* **7**(1):50–55

Khan SA, Davidson BR, Goldin R, Pereira SP, Rosenburg WMC, Taylor-Robinson SD, Thillainayagam AV, Thomas HC, Thursz MR, Wasan H (2002) Guidelines for the diagnosis and treatment of cholangiocacrcinoma: consensus document. *Gut* **51**(suppl 6):Vl1–9

Lee K, Park J, Joh J, Kim S, Choi S, Heo J, Lee H, Lee D, Park J, Yoo B (2004) Can we expand the Milan criteria for hepatocellular carcinoma in living donor liver transplantation? *Transplantation Proceedings* **36**(8):2289–2290

Leung TWT, Tang AMY, Zee B, Lau YW, Lai PBS, Leung KL, Lau JTF, Yu SCH, Johnson PJ (2002) Construction of the Chinese University Prognostic Index for hepatocellular carcinoma and comparison with the TNM staging system, the Okuda staging system, and the Cancer of the Liver Italian Program staging system. A study based on 926 patients. *Cancer* **94**(6):1760–1769

Levy I, Sherman M (2005) Staging of hepatocellualr carcinoma: assessment of the CLIP, Okuda and Child-Pugh staging systems in a cohort of 257 patients in Toronto. *Gut* **50**:881–885

Llovet JM, Beaugard M (2003) Hepatocellular carcinoma: present status and future prospects. *Journal of Hepatology* **38**(Suppl 1):S136–149

Llovet JM, Brú C, Bruix J (1999)Prognosis of hepatocellular carcinoma: the BCLC staging classification. *Seminars in Liver Disease* **19**(3):329–338

Marelli ML, Stigliano R, Triantos C, Senzolo M, Cholongitas E, Davies N, Tibballs J, Meyer T, Patch DW, Burroughs AK (2007) Transarterial therapy for hepatocellular carcinoma: which technique is more effective? A systemic review of cohort and randomised studies. *Cardiovascular and Interventional Radiology* 30(1):6–25

Marelli ML, Stigliano R, Triantos C, Senzolo M, Cholongitas E, Davies N, Yu D, Meyer T, Patch DW, Burroughs AK (2006) Treatment outcomes for hepatocellular carcinoma using chemoembolisation in combination with other therapies. *Cancer Treatment Reviews* 32(8):594–606

Mok TSK, Yeo W, Yu S, Lai P, Chan HLY, Chan ATC, Lau JWY, Wong H, Leung N, Hui EP, Sung J, Koh J, Mo F, Zee B, Johnson PJ (2005) An intensive surveillance program detected a high incidence of hepatocellular carcinoma among hepatitis B virus carriers with abnormal alpha-fetoprotein levels or abdominal ultrasonography results. *Journal of Oncology* 23(31):8041–8047

Moray G, Karakayali F, Yilmaz U, Ozcay F, Bilezikci B and Haberal M (2007) Expanded criteria for hepatocellular carcinoma and liver transplantation. *Transplantation Proceedings* 39(4):1171–1174

National Institute for Clinical Excellence (2004) Improving Outcome Guidance in Colorectal Cancer. Manual Update. NICE, London

National Institute for Clinical Excellence (2005) Photodynamic Therapy for Bile Duct Cancer. NICE, London

Nishioka K, Watanabe J, Furuta S, Tanaka E, Iino S, Suzuki H, Tsuji T, Yano M, Kuo G, Choo QL, et al. (1991) A high prevalence of antibody to the hepatitis C virus in patients with hepatocellular carcinoma in Japan. *Cancer* 67(2): 429–433

Okuda K, Ohtsuki T, Obata H, Tomimatsu M, Okazaki N, Hasegawa H, Nakajima Y, Ohnishi K (1985) Natural history of hepatocellular carcinoma and prognosis in relation to treatment. Study of 850 patients. *Cancer* 56(4):918–928

Pacella CM, Bizzarri G, Francica G, Blanchini A, De Nuntis S, Pacella S, Crescenzi A, Taccogna S, Forlini G, Rossi Z, Osborn J, Stasi R (2005) Percutaneous laser ablation in the treatment of hepatocellular carcinoma with small tumors: analysis of factors affecting the achievement of tumor necrosis. *Journal of Vascular Interventional Radiology* 16:1447–1457

Pawlick TM, Delman KA, Vauthey JN, Nagorney DM, Ng IOL, Ikai I, Yamaoka Y, Belghiti J, Lauwers GY, Poon RT, Abdalla EK (2005) Tumor size predicts vascular invasion and histologic grade: implications for selection of surgical treatment for hepatocellular carcinoma. *Liver Transplantation* 11(9):1086–1092

Ruan DT, Warren RS (2005) Liver-directed therapies in colorectal cancer. *Seminars in Oncology* 32(1):85–94

Ryder SD (2003) Guidelines for the diagnosis and treatment of hepatocellular carcinoma (HCC) in adults. *Gut* 52(Suppl III):iii1–8

Souhami RL, Tobias JS (eds) (1998) *Cancer and its Management*, 3ʳᵈ edn. Blackwell Science, Oxford

The Cancer of the Liver Italian Programme (CLIP) investigators (2000) Prospective validation of the CLIP score: a new prognostic system for patients with cirrhosis and hepatocellular carcinoma. *Hepatology* **31**:840–845

Wagman L, Hoff PM, Robertson JM, Dwivedy S (2000) Liver, gallbladder and biliary cancers. In: Wagman L, Hoff PM, Robertson JM, Dwivedy S (eds) *Cancer Management: A Multidisciplinary Approach*, 4th edn. PRR, Melville

18
Liver transplantation

Wendy Littlejohn and Joanna Routledge

Introduction

Liver transplantation is an established and accepted treatment of choice for patients with acute and chronic end-stage liver disease (Didier et al., 2006). Since the first liver transplant was carried out in 1963 by Dr T Starzl there have been many advances in surgical techniques, organ perfusion solutions and the advent of cyclosporine as an immunosuppressive agent (Starzl et al., 1982). These have contributed to liver transplantation evolving from an experimental high-risk procedure to an accepted treatment modality, with a steady improvement in both patient and graft survival (Starzl et al., 1981). Current national survival rates at 1 year post transplant are 89%; however, these will vary from centre to centre (UK Transplant, 2008).

As survival outcomes have improved, liver transplantation is now available to a broader range of patients with more complicated conditions. The increase in demand has not been met with an equivalent increase in the numbers of livers available for transplantation (Figure 18.1) leading to increasing waiting times, deteriorating health and increased mortality on the waiting list.

This increased demand has resulted in a need to increase the donor pool and make the best use of available organs. Splitting livers to benefit two recipients has now become a national liver transplant standard (DoH, 2005) and the use of non-heart beating livers shows the potential to significantly increase the number of livers available for transplantation (Muiesan et al., 2005).

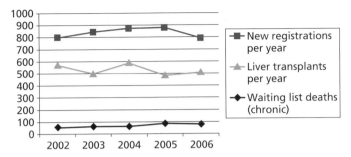

Figure 18.1 Numbers of UK listed transplant patients, annual liver transplants and the numbers of waiting list deaths in chronic disease patients 2002/3–2006/7 (UK Transplant, 2007).

Worldwide there are well-established and successful living related donation programmes both adult-to-adult and adult-to-child, which are currently being developed with the NHS in the UK.

Indications for liver transplantation

The indications for liver transplantation include most, if not all, of the hepatic diseases as discussed in previous chapters:

- Chronic hepatitis – viral, autoimmune
- Alcohol-related liver disease
- Non-alcoholic steatohepatitis
- Cryptogenic cirrhosis
- Toxin-/drug-induced hepatitis
- Cholestatic – primary biliary cirrhosis, primary sclerosing cholangitis, prolonged cholestasis, biliary atresia, familial cholestasis, cystic fibrosis, alagille syndrome, progressive familial intrahepatic cholestasis
- Metabolic – haemochromatosis, Wilson's disease, alpha-1-antitrypsin deficiency, storage diseases, hyperoxaluria
- Vascular – Budd-Chiari syndrome, veno-occlusive disease
- Primary hepatocellular carcinoma, hepatoblastoma
- Congenital abnormalities, urea cycle enzyme deficiency, familial amyloid polyneuropathy (Murray and Carithers, 2005)

Pretransplant assessment

It is important that potential candidates are referred early to specialist centres for liver transplant assessment, before they develop the complications of end-stage liver disease. This allows for the optimisation of their condition prior to transplantation. Late referrals with severe decompensation, malnutrition and development of associated syndromes carry a much higher risk and are more likely to develop postoperative complications and require longer recovery periods (Didier et al., 2006). Extensive physiological and psychosocial assessments are also necessary to ascertain the suitability of patients for transplant or to explore alternative therapies.

The transplant assessment has four main objectives, and is carried out by a multi-disciplinary team:

- Establish and confirm diagnosis
- Evaluate hepatic reserve/disease severity
- Evaluate anatomical structures and exclude contraindications
- Evaluate overall fitness of candidate to undergo liver transplantation

The routine tests and procedures which form the core of the assessment are outlined in Table 18.1. Further investigations or consultations may be added as indicated depending on the findings of the initial assessments. Potential candidates

Table 18.1 Laboratory investigations and diagnostic tests used for liver transplant assessment.

Routine blood tests
Full blood count, PT, INR, electrolytes, urea, creatinine, liver function tests, blood glucose, lipid profile, thyroid function tests, hepatitis serologies B and C, HIV, HTLV, EBV, CMV, Toxo, VZV, VDRL serologies, blood group

Diseases-specific blood tests
Anti-nuclear, anti-mitochondrial, anti-smooth muscle antibodies, ferritin, copper, caeruloplasmin, alpha-fetoprotein, HBV DNA, HCV RNA, HCV genotype, CA19–9, CEA, HIV DNA, CD4,T-cell count

Routine diagnostic testing
Chest radiograph, pulmonary function tests, arterial blood gases, electrocardiogram
(provided baseline for future reference, assess cardiopulmonary function, rule out any exsisting cardiopulmonary pathology)

Doppler ultrasound and CT scan
(assess liver configuration/contours, detect blood flows, evidence of portal hypertension, patency of vessels, detection and staging of lesions – size/position/invasion)

Endoscopy – staging and treatment of oesophageal varices

Liver biopsy – diagnostic, assess severity of disease

Consultations
Routine
Hepatologist, clinical transplant coordinator, anaesthetist, transplant surgeon, dietican, pharmacist, social worker
As required
Intensivist, alcohol and substance misuse specialist, cardiologist, haematologist, nephrologist, psychiatrist

should be assessed on their profile of complications, calculated prognosis and quality of life (Howdle, 2006).

Various tools have been used to grade severity of disease and determine prognosis; Child-Turcotte-Pugh classification, the prognostic model for end-stage liver disease (MELD), United Kingdom modified version of MELD (UKELD), and disease specific indices for primary biliary cirrhosis and sclerosing cholangitis (Christensen et al., 1984; Devlin and O'Grady, 1999; Wiesner et al., 2003), which help identify patients' needs and medical urgency for liver transplantation.

The recipients' understanding, willingness, motivation, previous medical compliance and their support systems must be evaluated. Issues of non-compliance and any form of addictive behaviour (alcohol/drug use) must be addressed before consideration for listing. A minimum period of 6 months of abstinence from alcohol must be achieved before transplantation and it is recommended to continue post transplant. Other substance abuse or dependence must also be addressed pre transplant as this is associated with relapse post transplant (Di Martini et al., 2001). Although tobacco is not a contraindication to transplantation, it is recognised as a major risk factor to the transplant patient, increasing risks of hepatocellular carcinoma (HCC) (Marrero et al., 2005) and vascular and arterial complications (Pungpapong et al., 2002). Smoking cessation is therefore recommended.

Extensive counselling and support are required by the patients to achieve this, along with proven abstinence monitoring and agreements of care between the patient and the transplant centre (Murray and Carithers, 2005). The use of written contracts has been advocated by several authors to reduce ambiguity (Gish et al., 1993).

The aim of psychosocial evaluation of the transplant candidate is to identify any factors that place the patient at high risk for poor outcomes post surgery, whether that is reduced life expectancy or quality of life. This assessment will initially be carried out by the transplant coordinator and social worker. Factors considered are outlined in Table 18.2.

Only through careful evaluation and analysis of the information obtained can the following be identified:

Table 18.2 Psychological evaluation of the transplant candidate.

Social support: family and friends, living environment, financial resources, employment, transportation, knowledge of social services/benefits available

Drug and alcohol and tobacco history: predict ability to maintain long-term abstinence and identify any risk factors for poor outcome. Assess the need for ongoing support

Psychiatric history: identification of mental illness which may affect compliance post transplant

Knowledge and understanding: assess level of knowledge about disease, transplant process. Identify an education strategy to ensure the patient can give informed consent

Coping mechanisms: identify coping strategies to chronic illness, frequent hospital admissions, attitudes to health, lifestyle changes and life-long immunosuppressant therapy and follow-up

Ability to collaborate effectively: assessment of behaviour during the evaluation, attitude to medications, illness. Adherence to medications, appointments, diet advice. Ability to report changes or deterioration in condition and to keep the team informed

- Severity of the disease and prognosis
- Clinical and biochemical indicators for transplantation
- Contraindications (absolute/relative) to liver transplantation
- Risk/benefit ratio of liver transplantation to the recipient
- Alternative treatment options that may prevent or delay transplantation
- Impact on quality of life
- Patients' preferences, goals and commitment
- Management plan (Howdle et al., 2006)

Contraindications to liver transplantation

There are relatively few absolute contraindications to liver transplantation and as more experience has been gained these have decreased in number.

Absolute contraindications include the following:

- AIDS
- Extrahepatic malignancy
- Advanced cardiopulmonary disease
- Uncontrolled extrahepatic sepsis
- Active alcohol/substance misuse
- Cholangiocarcinoma

Relative contraindications include the following:

- Multi-system organ failure
- HIV positivity
- Portal venous system thrombosis
- Pulmonary hypertension
- HBV DNA positivity
- Cachexia (under 70% of body weight)
- Morbid obesity (Didier et al. 2006)

Selection committee/minimal listing criteria

Once the transplant assessment is completed potential candidates are formally presented to the selection committee (which includes members of the transplant multi-disciplinary team) for discussion regarding the need and suitability for liver transplantation. The current criteria for listing are that a patient has a greater than 50% chance of being alive at 5 years post transplantation with a quality of life acceptable to the patient. If the chance is less than 50% transplantation should not be offered (Neuberger, 2001). The potential outcomes are:

- Suitable candidate – place on transplant list
- Suitable candidate too early – medical follow-up, reassess at later date
- Reversible current contraindications – treatment given, reassess and rediscuss

■ Absolute contraindication – declined for transplant, option of second
   opinion

Optimal selection of patients and timing of liver transplantation is crucial in
order to increase survival rates and decrease postoperative morbidity.

Pretransplant education

Education is critical to a successful outcome. It begins at the initial referral and
continues throughout the phases of assessment: listing, waiting time, transplant,
recovery and long-term follow-up, involving the potential recipient and family
members/carers (Ohler, 2003).

It is vital to establish a secure and trusting relationship with potential recipients
from the outset, to facilitate learning and achieve creditability. Education programmes can help alleviate fears, address misconceptions, help formulate questions, assist decision making, improve compliance, promote health and improve
coping mechanisms (Charlton and Ventura, 2006).

It is important to initially evaluate the patient's emotional state, physical health,
cultural needs, and level of knowledge, attitudes, abilities, readiness to learn and
learning style (Lipson and Dibble, 2005). This will help to provide individualised
patient education in order to enhance understanding (Zink et al., 2005).

Various teaching methods should be implemented over a period of time, and
information should be reinforced regularly to enhance and develop understanding
(Bernat and Peterson, 2006). The topics covered should include an overview of
liver transplantation, including risks and benefits, the assessment process and
allocation of organs, options of treatment for end-stage liver disease, the role of
the transplant team, waiting for an organ, recovery and postoperative complications, medications and follow-up. Talking to other patients regarding quality of
life changes can also increase understanding (Kizilisik et al., 2003).

Consent

Ensuring that patients are central to the decision-making process enables them to
make health care choices which are right for them. Patients need to be aware of
the choices open to them including the type of donor and type of transplant. This
ensures that the consent being sought is informed.

Waiting list management

Patients will be on the waiting list for variable periods of time depending largely
on donor availability, blood group and size. During the waiting time all patients

need to be regularly reviewed to ensure that they continue to meet criteria. Close monitoring ensures medical, pharmacological and nutritional treatments are optimised, and that any new problems are detected and treated. Patients deemed high risk at the time of listing will need to undergo a reassessment whilst on the waiting list to ensure their continued suitability (Neuberger, 2003).

An unknown proportion of patients are removed from the transplant list due to increased high risk, or they become unsuitable for transplant during the waiting period (Didier et al., 2006). Patients with end-stage liver disease have limited hepatic reserve and episodes of decompensation during the waiting time are common; the potential for renewed health is evident but recipients are also aware of the risk of death on the waiting list.

The waiting period can be extremely difficult and it is important to allow patients and families to express their feelings and concerns during this time. Each candidate's situation is unique but there are some typical stressors encountered by both the recipient and their family members (Brown et al., 2006):

- Lack of control – not knowing when the transplant will occur
- Deteriorating health – facing death
- Fear of dying before the organ is available
- Living life on hold – limitations
- Change in roles and lifestyle
- Financial concerns

It is important to build a relationship between the recipients and their transplant team, actively encouraging the recipient to play a part in their management through self-reporting changes in condition and compliance with diet and exercise. Providing honest information, reassurance and support for recipients throughout the transplant process will help them during the waiting time (Baker and McWilliams, 2003).

Allocation of organs

In the UK, each transplant centre is responsible for the assessment, transplantation and post-transplant care of referred patients, with each centre maintaining their own waiting list for patients with chronic liver disease.

A UK-wide national organ-sharing scheme is coordinated by United Kingdom Transplant (UKT) with each liver transplant centre responsible for abdominal organ retrieval in a given geographical zone. UKT maintains a national super-urgent waiting list for patients in acute liver failure as defined by O'Grady et al. (1993). This is discussed in more depth in Chapter 13.

When UKT is notified of an organ donor, priority is given to patients in acute liver failure on the super-urgent waiting list. If there are no super-urgent listed patients the liver is offered to the designated zonal team for one of their eligible chronically listed patients. If they are unable to utilise the organ (e.g. no suitable recipient, no intensive care bed, unsuitable organ), it will be offered to the other designated centres on a rotational basis. If unplaced it will be offered back to the zonal centre for private patients and then on to the other designated centres for their private patients and finally to Euro transplant for placement.

Many factors determine whether a liver is suitable for retrieval and transplantation, including medical, surgical and social history, cause of brain death, haemodynamic stability, laboratory data and serology. Details regarding the appearance, vascular anatomy, size and overall quality of the organ are conveyed to the implanting surgeon who will ultimately decide on the overall suitability of the liver. Transplant surgeons use their clinical skills and judgement in evaluating the condition of the liver available for transplant and matching it to the best recipient at that given moment (Adam et al., 2000) which is based on:

- Blood group – match
- Severity of liver disease – priority listed recipients
- Weight – donor to recipient +/– 20 kg
- Marginal grafts – better outcomes if given to fitter recipients
- HCC recipients
- Time and distance – non heart-beating livers, need short cold ischaemia time
- Date listed for transplant

The consequences of longer waiting lists and waiting times results in the allocation of organs to the sickest candidates with severely decompensated liver disease undergoing complex surgery. However, this will have an impact on postoperative recovery (Neuberger and James, 1999).

Liver transplant surgery

Conventional liver transplant involves the resection of the recipient native liver (hepatectomy), a short anhepatic phase where the native liver is removed (Figure 18.2, Plate 17), followed by implantation of a whole donor liver graft. Anastomosis of the inferior cava, portal vein and hepatic artery is performed (end-to-end donor to recipient) (Figure 18.3). The biliary connections involve either a primary duct-to-duct technique or require the performance of a hepaticojejunostomy. Figure 18.4 (Plate 18) shows the abdomen following the liver transplant with the new liver in situ.

The postoperative course of the patient will depend on the quality of the donor liver, the complexity of the surgery carried out and the clinical status of the recipient. The timely identification of potential complications is a critical factor in minimising morbidity and mortality; hence the nurse plays a key role in the monitoring and assessment of the patient (Table 18.3).

Complications in the critical care phase include primary non-function (PNF), which affects between 4 and 20% of liver transplant procedures. PNF is characterised by haemodynamic instability, coagulopathy, rising lactate and liver enzymes,

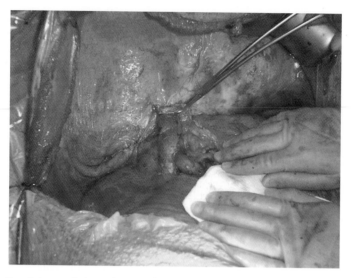

Figure 18.2 The abdomen during anhepatic phase of liver transplantation. For a colour version of this figure, please see Plate 17 in the colour plate section.

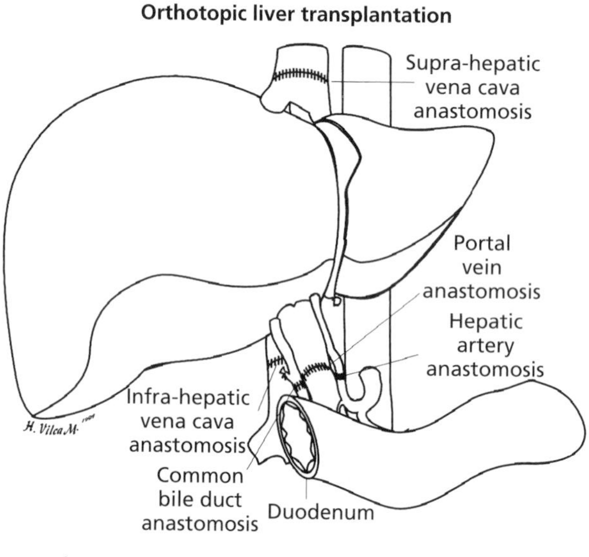

Orthotopic liver transplantation

Supra-hepatic
vena cava
anastomosis

Portal
vein
anastomosis

Hepatic
artery
anastomosis

H. Vilca M.

Infra-hepatic
vena cava
anastomosis

Common
bile duct   Duodenum
anastomosis

Figure 18.3 Diagram of anastomosis in liver transplantation. Used with permission from Hector Vilca-Melendez.

renal failure and poor bile output (Bezeizi et al., 1997), and results in the need for urgent re-transplantation. Additionally hepatic artery or portal vein thrombosis can also result in either re-transplantation or further surgery. Postoperative bleeding may require urgent re-exploration in theatre and can be the result of ongoing coagulopathy, inadequate haemostasis or slipping of a suture. Furthermore biliary complications, including anastomotic leaks, strictures and obstruction, are major

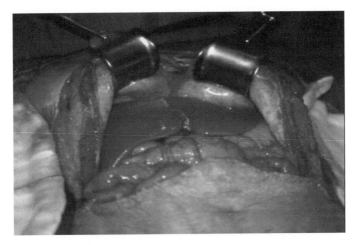

Figure 18.4   Abdomen following transplant with new liver in situ. For a colour version of this figure, please see Plate 18 in the colour plate section.

Table 18.3   Initial nursing management of the liver transplant recipient.

Ventilatory weaning and extubation
Haemodynamic monitoring and fluid management
Pain control
Wound assessment, monitoring of bleeding
Care of central and arterial lines, wound and biliary drains and urinary catheter
Laboratory tests including liver biochemistries, full blood count, serum lactate, blood gas analysis
Monitoring of psychological status
Care of the family

complications following liver transplant occurring in 15–20% of cases (Nemec et al., 2001; Eghtesad et al., 2005).

Infection is also a significant cause of morbidity and mortality in liver transplant recipients (Blair and Kusne, 2005). In the first month, many infections are related to the surgery and levels of immunosuppression. Opportunistic infections resulting from ongoing immunosuppression can occur such as cytomegalovirus (CMV), Epstein-Barr virus (EBV), herpes simplex virus (HSV) and varicella zoster virus (VZV). Most patients are treated with prophylactic antibiotics and antifungal medications; however those with elevated risk profiles for CMV are treated with antiviral therapy for 3 months following liver transplant.

Immunosuppressive therapy

Post-transplant immunosuppressive therapy consists of an 'induction' followed by a 'maintenance' regime. The induction will usually consist of high-dose steroids combined with a calcineurin inhibitor (CNI). The patient is converted to oral steroids after several days, which is then tapered. Maintenance immunosuppression continues with the CNI and complete withdrawal of the steroid within 6–12 months, with the exception of autoimmune-mediated liver disease. In stable patients lower therapeutic levels of CNI are usually permitted if tolerated.

Calcineurin inhibitors (CNI)

Calcineurin is believed to play a role in the production of cytokines, which are central to the graft rejection process. Cyclosporine and tacrolimus inhibit calcineurin and therefore inhibit cytokine production. The absorption of tacrolimus differs in that it is not dependent on the presence of bile and it is absorbed in the duodenum and jejunum. As the presence of food reduces the bioavailability of tacrolimus, it is advisable to take it on an empty stomach. Both cyclosporine and tacrolimus are metabolised by the cytochrome P450–3A enzyme in the gut and liver and therefore administration of medications that inhibit or induce this pathway may significantly affect the immunosuppression levels. Common groups of drugs which do this include calcium channel blockers, antifungal agents, macrolide antibiotics and prokinetic agents.

Most of the side effects of CNIs are dose dependent and are shown in Table 18.4. One of the major side effects, nephrotoxicity, is associated with CNIs and can be an acute or long-term problem resulting in renal failure in up to 20% of patients (Gonwa et al., 2001). Recent studies suggest that renal failure may be less of a problem with tacrolimus (Artz et al., 2004; Martins et al., 2004; Nankivell et al., 2004).

Sirolimus

Sirolimus (Rapamune, RAP) is structurally similar to tacrolimus but has a different mode of action. Sirolimus acts by inhibiting lymphocyte proliferation and inhibits the growth factors required for tissue repair, which can result in problems with wound healing, skin rashes and mouth ulcers. Metabolic side effects include increases in serum cholesterol and triglycerides and suppression of leucocytes, erythrocytes and platelets. Anaemia is especially problematic in patients with renal impairment.

Corticosteroids

Corticosteroids are an important component of most immunosuppressant regimens, and are used as a first-line treatment in the majority of cases for acute allograft rejection. Corticosteroids decrease the inflammatory response through

Table 18.4 Side effects of immunosuppressive drugs.

Tacrolimus	Cyclosporine	Azathioprine	Mycophenolate mofetil (MMF)	Corticosteroids
Renal dysfunction	Renal dysfunction	Anaemia	Nausea	Hypokalaemia
Hypertension	Hypertension	Thrombocytopenia	Vomiting	Hypertension
Hypomagnesaemia	Hypomagnesaemia	Leucopenia	Abdominal pain	Altered mood
Headache	Hyperkalaemia	Nausea	Marrow suppression	Lipid abnormalities
Tremor	Hirsutism	Diarrhoea		Cushinoid syndrome
Hyperkalaemia	Gingival hyperplasia	Alopecia		Gastric ulcers
Nausea, vomiting, diarrhoea				Myopathy
Post-transplant diabetes mellitus				Osteoporosis
				Fluid retention
				Cataracts
				Impaired wound healing

reduced production of cytokines (Donovitch, 2001). The side effects of steroid treatment are given in Table 18.4.

Antimetabolites

Azathioprine and mycophenolate mofetil (MMF) are antiproliferative immunosuppressive agents, which act on purine metabolism thus causing inhibition of either T-cells (azathioprine) or both T- and B-cell (MMF) activation. MMF is often used to facilitate dose reduction or withdrawal of CNIs in patients with renal dysfunction (Stewart et al., 2001). Gastrointestinal side effects may require dose reduction or withdrawal (Fung et al., 2005)

Antibody induction

Antibody induction can allow steroid reduction or even withdrawal after liver transplantation and can be especially useful in patients with hepatitis C, due to the relationship between steroid use and early recurrence of the disease in the allograft (Berenguer et al., 2006).

Antithymocyte globulin (ATG) is a polyclonal antibody preparation and causes depletion of T-cells. Profound lymphopenia occurs in most patients when ATG is administered. A 'first dose reaction' is seen in up to 80% of patients, which can be minimised by administering a combination of corticosteroids, paracetamol and an antihistamine prior to the administration of ATG.

Muromonab-CD3 (OKT3), a monoclonal antibody, binds to the CD3 molecule found on T-cells, resulting in an inactivation of T-cell receptors and a rapid fall in the numbers of lymphocytes. A release of cytokines into the circulation occurs when OKT3 is administered, which can cause reactions ranging from flu symptoms to pulmonary oedema and respiratory distress, often termed 'cytokine release syndrome' (Wilde and Goa, 1996). To overcome this, an antihistamine with adjunct paracetamol and corticosteroids are usually given prior to administration of OKT3.

IL-2 receptor antibodies

IL-2 receptor antibodies include basiliximab (Simulect®) and daclizumab (Zenapax®). Both drugs are similar in efficacy and action, resulting in a reduction in T-cell proliferation. In liver transplantation, IL-2 receptor antibodies are usually given when CNI reduction is important, for example in patients with renal dysfunction. The half-lives of both drugs are long so dosing is often weekly or fortnightly and several doses are usually required. Side effects are generally mild although occasional anaphylactic reactions have been reported (Baudouin et al., 2003).

Graft rejection

The control of rejection is an important factor in graft survival. Acute cellular rejection (ACR) occurs in up to 75% of liver allograft recipients, with the majority of episodes occurring within the first 90 days after surgery (Wiesner et al., 1993). Laboratory investigations show increasing transaminase, ALP and bilirubin levels. The patient may be asymptomatic or they may present with a fever and malaise with right upper quadrant tenderness on examination. A liver biopsy may be required to confirm the diagnosis. The first-line treatment consists of a 3-day course of 1 g of methylprednisolone (Wiesner et al., 1994); 70–80% of patients respond to this treatment (Adams and Neuberger, 1992). However, other agents may be required if the rejection episode is not responsive to steroids.

The incidence of chronic rejection has decreased in the past decade and currently occurs in less than 5% of patients (Martinez and Rosen, 2005), but may result in the need for re-transplantation.

Discharge planning and patient information

Effective planning is paramount to the successful discharge of the newly transplanted patient. An individualised care package is formed with close collaboration between the multi-disciplinary team, patient and their family. Specialist consultations may also be required prior to discharge, including diabetic nurses, for patients with new onset diabetes, hepatocellular oncology nurse specialists, clinical psychologists and psychiatrists. Communication channels between the transplant coordinator and the patient's GP will be maintained in order to discuss any further issues, such as complications which may necessitate hospital admission, coping mechanisms, ongoing educational needs or compliance issues. The transplant coordinator will maintain contact with the patient via telephone for the first few days post discharge and will then follow up in the clinic alongside the medical team.

Compliance

Non-compliance or non-adherence in the transplant patient is complex and multifactorial (Dew et al., 1996). Non-compliance is thought to be implicated in both acute and chronic rejection episodes and is responsible for up to 25% of late deaths (De Geest et al., 1998; Bunzel and Laederach-Hofmann, 2000). Many factors contribute to poor compliance, including inadequate social support (Gish et al., 1993), lack of motivation, denial about severity of illness or poor understanding, poor communication, depression and hopelessness (Krahn and Di Martini, 2005). These traits tend to be found more in those patients with either a chemical dependency or psychiatric disorder. Assessing non-compliance can be extremely difficult, as it can occur even when the patient has been sufficiently informed about the risks of their behaviour. Various strategies have been employed in order to increase patient compliance, such as simplifying medication instructions (Kiley et al., 1993), offering more frequent follow-up, including telephone follow-up and providing written reminders, however positive influence on therapeutic outcome is yet to be proven.

Quality of life following liver transplantation

Over the last two decades there has been a growing consensus not only to measure treatment success in terms of longevity but also to understand the influences of liver transplantation in transplant recipients. Consequently, assessing health-related quality of life (HRQoL) is considered imperative in the evaluation of efficacy, cost effectiveness and to understand both the impact of known post-transplant complications, and immunosuppressive therapy (Bravata et al., 1999). Consideration of patients' HRQoL could perhaps become increasingly important when prioritising organ allocation in view of shortages of donor organs and growing waiting lists.

Studies have predominantly focused on elective chronic transplant recipients, which have highlighted some specific health problems, such as fatigue, pain and complications of immunosuppressant therapy. However the vast majority of post-transplantation recipients report large gains in the QoL aspects most affected by physical health and psychological functioning (Bravata et al., 1999). Additionally HRQoL in patients transplanted for ALF is comparative to other liver transplant recipients regardless of the underlying aetiology (Sargent and Wainwright, 2006).

Long-term management in the liver recipient

Patients undergoing liver transplantation will require life-long follow-up. Transplant centre clinics or outreach clinics may take place locally, and will monitor liver and renal function, immunosuppression levels, identify any complications and continue health promotion and education. It is important for patients to attend age-appropriate health screening offered by primary care teams or GP practices.

Hyperlipidaemia

Hyperlipidaemia occurs in 16–66% of liver transplant recipients (Munoz, 1997) and may contribute to the development of cardiovascular disease, a known cause of morbidity and mortality in the transplant population (Massy et al., 1994). The cause is multi-factorial (Munoz, 1995), however increases in appetite as a result of immunosuppression and steroid therapy are thought to make a significant contribution to both hyperlipidaemia and to the development of post-transplant obesity, which has a reported incidence of 20–40% (Everhart et al., 1998). Tacrolimus appears less likely to cause hypercholesterolaemia than cyclosporine (Charco et al., 1999), therefore conversion to tacrolimus may improve hyperlipidaemia (Manzarbietia et al., 2001). It is essential to advocate a low-fat diet, exercise programmes and avoidance of alcohol and cigarettes (Kobashigawa and Kasiske, 1997). It may additionally be necessary to commence 3-hydroxy-3-methylglutaryl coenzyme A (HMG-CoA) reductase inhibitors (statins) (Imagawa et al., 1996).

Hypertension

Systemic hypertension develops in 55–85% of liver transplant patients within the first year of surgery (Stegall et al., 1995). Detection and treatment are important to reduce the risk of ischaemic heart disease, peripheral vascular disease and renal failure. Steroid withdrawal can be considered, if not already done (Everson et al., 1999), however in many cases, antihypertensive medication is required in order to achieve acceptable blood pressure control.

Diabetes

New-onset diabetes develops in approximately 15% of liver transplant recipients (Heisel et al., 2004) and the diabetogenic potential of the immunsuppressive drugs is thought to be a contributing factor (Marchetti, 2005). Risks are additionally linked to those who are obese, have alcoholic cirrhosis, or hepatitis C-related cirrhosis (Bigam et al., 2000; Baid et al., 2001; Tueche, 2003). Management of diabetes in liver transplant recipients is similar to that in the non-transplant population. Dietetic advice is discussed in Chapter 14.

Osteoporosis

Bone disease is a common problem in patients with chronic liver disease and post-transplant recipients (Hay, 1995). Patients often have low bone mass density prior to transplant due to factors such as malnutrition, immobility and deficiencies of calcium and vitamin D, which may be exacerbated post transplant. Both steroid therapy and increased immobility have been linked to rapid bone loss during the first 3–6 months post transplantation (McDonald et al., 1991). Treatment with calcium, vitamin D and hormonal supplements should be considered for patients both pre and post liver transplantation.

Malignancies

Malignancies are found to occur more frequently in transplant recipients, with an overall 3–5-fold increase in risk, when compared with the general population (Kinlen, 1985). In the immunosuppressed transplant patient the ability of the immune system to eliminate abnormal cells, which could become cancerous, is reduced and therefore potentially harmful cells have a greater chance of escaping detection and proliferating into a malignancy. Skin cancers, oropharyngeal malignancies and lymphomas are problematic for liver transplant recipients and patients transplanted for primary sclerosing cholangitis are considered high risk for the development of colonic cancers (Higashi et al., 1990) and should be screened accordingly.

Post-transplant lymphoproliferative disorder (PTLD) represents a common post-transplant malignancy (Penn, 2000). The term PTLD is used to describe a wide spectrum of lymphomas and lesions that may appear, depending on the transplanted organ and underlying disease. The symptoms are often non-specific and onset can present early, within 1 month of transplant, or after many years.

In order to facilitate detection of post-transplant malignancies, effective cancer screening is extremely important; in addition patients can be taught to self-examine and report any abnormalities or concerns. Minimising exposure to the sun is also imperative and patients should be counselled regarding their increased risks of skin cancer and the use of protective measures such as hats, protective clothing and the use of a high factor sunscreen.

Disease recurrence

Disease recurrence after liver transplantation has become more evident due to improved long-term survival. Re-transplantation represents a greater postoperative risk with higher mortality, therefore patients should be carefully counselled and must fully understand that liver transplantation does not guarantee freedom from the indicating disease. Re-transplantation for recurrent disease is also becoming a difficult ethical issue in light of the current donor organ shortage.

Chapter summary

Liver transplantation is now an established treatment option for patients with both acute and chronic liver disease, however the increased demand for donor organs has resulted in both longer waiting times and increased mortality for patients on the transplant list. Early referral, careful patient selection and a robust transplant assessment process are vital in order to optimise survival rates and decrease post-operative morbidity. Multi-disciplinary support of the patient and their family throughout the transplant process is also instrumental in ensuring an optimal outcome.

Illustrative case study

A 53-year-old gentleman was referred for transplant assessment with presumed alcohol-related liver disease. The patient reported previous alcohol consumption of two bottles of whisky per week over a 4-year period but had recently been abstinent for 6 months.

He presented with a history of lethargy, ascites and one episode of hepatic encephalopathy secondary to a urinary tract infection; the physical examination revealed a non-palpable liver, splenomegaly and minimal ascites. No other stigmata of chronic liver disease were noted.

A review of the blood tests supported the diagnosis of alcohol-related liver disease and a liver biopsy was planned to confirm the diagnosis. There was evidence of preserved renal function (creatinine 79 µmol/L, urea 1.9 mmol/L) and of improving synthetic function (albumin 35 g/L, INR 1.24).

Initially, it was considered too early to list for transplantation due to the possibility of some recovery in liver function as the period of abstinence increased. However a lesion in the liver was found on abdominal ultrasonography and CT scan.

The indication for transplantation was changed to HCC and the case was presented to the multi-disciplinary selection committee meeting, who accepted him for transplantation. During the waiting time the patient underwent two cycles of transarterial chemo-embolisation prior to being called in for transplant 11 months after listing.

The liver transplant procedure was uneventful but on day 9 post transplant a rising AST was noted from 40 to 110 IU/L. The tacrolimus level was also found to be low and subsequently the dosage was increased. A liver biopsy confirmed acute cellular rejection and methlyprednisolone 1 g was given intravenously for 3 days. By day 12 the AST had reduced to within normal levels and the patient was discharged 2 days later with an outpatient's appointment for the following week.

References

Adam R, Caillez V, Majno P (2000) Normalised intrinsic mortality risk in liver transplanation: European Liver Transplantation Registry Study. *Lancet* **356**: 621

Adams DH, Neuberger JM (1992) Treatment of acute rejection. *Seminars in Liver Disease* **12**:80–88

Artz MA, Boots JM, Ligtenberg G, Roodnat JI, Christiaans MH, Vos P, Moons P, Borm GF, Hilbrands LB (2004) Conversion from cyclosporine to tacrolimus improves quality of life indices, renal graft function and cardiovascular risk profile. *American Journal of Transplantation* 4(6):937–945

Baid S, Cosimi AB, Farrel ML, Schoenfield DA, Feng S, Chung RT, et al. (2001) Post transplant diabetes mellitus in liver transplant recipients: Risk factors, temporal relationship with hepatitis C virus allograft hepatitis, and impact on mortality. *Transplantation* 72:1066–1072

Baker MS, McWilliams CL (2003) How patients manage life and health while waiting for a liver transplant. *Progress in Transplantation* 13(1):47–60

Baudouin V, Crusiaux A, Haddad E, Schandene L, Goldman M, Loirat C, et al. (2003) Anaphylactic shock caused by immunoglobulin E sensitization after retreatment with the chimeric anti-interleukin-2 receptor monoclonal antibody basiliximab. *Transplantation* 76(3):459–463

Berenguer M, Aguilera V, Prieto M, San Juan F, Rayon JM, Benlloch S, et al. (2006) Significant improvements in the outcome of HCV infected transplant recipients by avoiding rapid steroid tapering and potent induction immunosuppression. *Journal of Hepatology* 44:717–722

Bernat JL, Peterson LM (2006) Patient-centred informed consent in surgical practice. *Archives of Surgery* 141:86–92

Bezeizi KI, Jalan R, Plevris JN (1997) Primary graft dysfunction after liver transplantation: from pathogenesis to prevention. *Liver Transplantation* 3:137–148

Bigam DL, Pennington JJ, Carpentier A, Wanless IR, Hemming AW, Croxford R, et al. (2000) Hepatitis C-related cirrhosis: a predictor of diabetes after liver transplantation. *Hepatology* 32:87–90

Blair JE, Kusne S (2005) Bacterial, mycobacterial and protozoal infections after liver transplantation – part 1. *Liver Transplantation* 11(12):1452–1459

Bravata D, Olkin I, Barnato A, Keefe E, Owens KL (1999) Health related quality of life after liver transplantation: a meta analysis. *Liver Transplantation and Surgery* 5:318–331

Brown J, Sorell JH, McClaren J, Creswell JW (2006) Waiting for a liver transplant. *Qualitative Health Research* 16(1):119–136

Bunzel B, Laederach-Hofmann K (2000) Solid organ transplantation: are there predictors for post transplant non compliance? A literature overview. *Transplantation* 70:711–716

Charco R, Cantarell C, Vargas V, Capderila L, Lazaro JL, Hidalgo E, et al. (1999) Serum cholesterol changes in long-term survivors of liver transplantation: A comparison between cyclosporine and tacrolimus therapy. *Liver Transplant Surgery* 5:204–208

Charlton M, Ventura K (2006) Education and the transplant patient. In: LaPointe Rudow D, Ohler L, Shafer T (eds) *A Clinician's Guide to Donation and Transplantation*. NATCO: Applied Measurement Professionals, Inc, Washington DC, pp. 549–558

Christensen E, Schlichting P, Fauerholdt L (1984) Prognostic value of Child-Turcotte criteria in medically treated cirrhosis. *Hepatology* 4:430–435

De Geest S, Abraham I, Moons P, Vandeputter M, Van Cleemput J, Evers G, Daenen, W, Vanhaecke J (1998) Late acute rejection and subclinical non compliance with cyclosporine therapy in heart transplant recipients. *Journal of Heart and Lung Transplantation* **17**:854–863

Department of Health (2005) National liver transplant standards (online). Available at http://www.dh.gov.uk/Publications policy and guidance (accessed 23/03/06)

Devlin J, O'Grady J (1999) Indications for referral and assessment in adult liver transplantation: a clinical guideline. *Gut* **45**(suppl 6):1–22

Dew MA, Roth LH, Thompson ME, Kormos RL, Grifith BP (1996) Medical compliance and its predictors in the first year after heart transplantation. *Journal of Heart and Lung Transplantation* **15**:631–645

Di Martini A, Day N, Dew M, Lane T, Fitzgerald MG, Magill J, Jain A (2001) Alcohol use following liver transplantation: a comparison of follow-up methods. *Psychosomatics* **42**:55–62

Didier S, Figueiro J, Bismith H (2006) Indications and patient selection. In: Bacon BR, O'Grady JG, Di Bisceglie AM, Lake JR (eds) *Comprehensive Clinical Hepatology*, 2nd edn. Mosby Elsevier, Philadelphia

Donovitch G (2001) Immunosuppressive medications and protocols. In: Danovitch GM (ed) *Handbook of Kidney Transplantation*. Lippincott Williams & Wilkins, Philadelphia, pp. 82–83

Eghtesad B, Kadry Z, Fung J (2005) Technical considerations in liver transplantation: what a hepatologist needs to know (and every surgeon should practice). *Liver Transplantation* **11**(8):861–871

Everhart JE, Lombardero M, Lake JR, et al. (1998) Weight change and obesity after liver transplantation: incidence and risk factors. *Liver Transplant Surgery* **4**:285–296

Everson GT, Trouillot T, Wachs M, Bak T, Steinberg T, Kam I, Shrestha R, Stegall M (1999) Early steroid withdrawal in liver transplantation is safe and beneficial. *Liver Transplant Surgery* **5**:548–557

Fung J, Kelly D, Kadry Z, Patel-Tom K, Eghtesad B (2005) Immunosuppression in liver transplantation: beyond calcineurin inhibitors. *Liver Transplantation* **11**:267–280

Gish RG, Lee AH, Keefe EB, Rome H, Concepcion W, Esquivel CO (1993) Liver transplantation for patients with alcoholism and end-stage liver disease. *American Journal of Gastroenterology* **88**:1337–1342

Gonwa TA, Mai ML, Melton LB, Hays SR, Goldstein RM, Levy MF, Klintmalm GB (2001) End stage renal disease (ESRD) after orthotopic liver transplantation (OLTX) using calcineurin based immunotherapy: risk of development and treatment. *Transplantation* **72**:1934–1939

Hay JE (1995) Bone disease after liver transplantation. *Liver Transplant Surgery* **1**:55–63

Heisel, O, Heisel R, Balshaw R, Keown P (2004) New onset diabetes mellitus in patients receiving calcineurin inhibitors: a systematic review and meta analysis. *American Journal of Transplantation* **4**:583–595

Higashi H, Yanaga K, Marsh JW, Tzakis A, Kakizoe S, Starzl TE (1990) Development of colon cancer after liver transplantation for primary sclerosing cholangitis associated with ulcerative colitis. *Hepatology* 11:477–480

Howdle PD (2006) History and physical examination In: Bacon BR, O'Grady JG, Di Bisceglie AM, Lake JR (eds). *Comprehensive Clinical Hepatology*, 2nd edn. Elsevier Mosby, Philadelphia

Imagawa DK, Dawson S, Holt CD, Kirk PS, Kaldas FM, Shackleton CR, et al. (1996) Hyperlipidemia after liver transplantation: natural history and treatment with the hydroxyl-methylglutanyl-coenzyme A reductase inhibitor pravastatin. *Transplantation* 6:934–942

Kiley DJ, Lam CS, Pollak R (1993) A study of treatment compliance following kidney transplantation. *Transplantation* 55:51–56

Kinlen LJ (1985) Incidence of cancer in rheumatoid arthritis and other disorders after immunosuppressant treatment. *American Journal of Medicine* 78:44–49

Kizilisik AT, Grewell HP, Shokouh-Amiri H, Vera SR, Hathaway DK, Gaber AO (2003) Impact of long term immunosuppressive therapy on psychosocial and physical well being in liver transplant recipients. *Progress in Transplantation* 13(4):278–283

Kobashigawa JA, Kasiske BL (1997) Hyperlipidemia in solid organ transplantation. *Transplantation* 63:331–338

Krahn LE, Di Martini A (2005) Psychiatric and psychosocial aspects of liver transplantation. *Liver Transplantation* 11(10):1157–1168

Lipson JG, Dibble SL (2005) *Culture in Clinical Care*. UCSF Publishing Press, San Francisco

Manzarbietia C, Reich DJ, Rothslein KD, Braitman LE, Levin S, Munoz SJ (2001) Tacrolimus conversion improves hyperlipidemia states in stable liver transplant recipients. *Liver Transplantation* 7:93–99

Marchetti P (2005) New onset diabetes after liver transplantation: from pathogenesis to management. *Liver Transplantation* 11(6):612–620

Marrero J, Fontana R, Fu S, Conjeevaram H, Su G, Lok A (2005) Alcohol, tobacco and obesity are synergistic risk factors for hepatocellular carcinoma. *Journal of Hepatology* 42:218–224

Martinez OM, Rosen HR (2005) Basic concepts of transplant immunology. *Liver Transplantation* 11(4):370–381

Martins L, Ventura A, Branco A, Carvalho MJ, Henriques AC, et al. (2004) Cyclosporine versus tacrolimus in kidney transplantation: are there differences in nephrotoxicity? *Transplantation Proceedings* 36(4):877–879

Massy ZA, Chadefaux-Vekemans B, Chevalier A, Bader CA, Drüeke TB, Legendre C, Lacour B, Kamoun P, Kreis H (1994) Hypercholesterolaemia: a significant risk factor for cardiovascular disease in renal transplant patients. *Nephrology, Dialysis, Transplantation* 9:1103

McDonald JA, Dunstan CR, Dilworth P, Sherbon K, Sheil AG, Evans RA, McCaughan GW (1991) Bone loss after liver transplantation. *Hepatology* 14:613–619

Muiesan P, Girlanda R, Wayel J, Vilca-Melendez H, O'Grady J, Bowles M, Rela M, Heaton N (2005) Single centre experience with liver transplantation from controlled non-heart beating donors: a viable source of grafts. *Annals of Surgery* 242(5):732–738

Munoz SJ (1995) Hyperlipidemia and other coronary risk factors after orthotopic liver transplantation: pathogenesis, diagnosis and management. *Liver Transplantation and Surgery* 1(Suppl 1):29–38

Munoz SJ (1997) Progress in post transplant hyperlipidemia. *Liver Transplantation and Surgery* 3:439–442

Murray KF, Carithers RL (2005) AASLD Practice Guidelines: evaluation of the patient for liver transplantation. *Hepatology* 41(6):1407–1432

Nankivell BJ, Chapman JR, Bonovas G, Gruenweald SM (2004) Oral cyclosporine but not tacrolimus reduces renal transplant blood flow. *Transplantation* 77(9):1457–1459

Nemec P, Ondrasek J, Studenik P, Hoki J, Cerny J (2001) Biliary complications in liver transplantation. *Annals of Transplantation* 6:24–28

Neuberger J (2001) Hope or efficacy in donor liver allocation? *Transplantation* 72(6):1173–1176

Neuberger J (2003) Management on the liver transplant waiting list. *Graft* 6(2): 93–97

Neuberger J, James OF (1999) Guidelines for selection of patients for liver transplantation in the era of donor organ shortage. *Lancet* 354:1636

O'Grady J, Schalm SW, Williams R (1993) Acute liver failure: redefining the syndromes. *Lancet* 342:273–278

Ohler L (2003) Patient education. In: Cupples S, Ohler L (eds) *Transplantation Nursing Secrets.* Hanley and Belfus, Inc, Philadelphia, pp. 305–311

Penn I (2000) Post transplant malignancy; the role of immunosuppression. *Drug Safety* 23:101–113

Pungpapong S, Manzarbeitia C, Ortiz J, Reich DJ, Araya V, Rothstein KD, Munoz SJ (2002) Cigarette smoking is associated with an increased incidence of vascular complications after liver transplantation. *Liver Transplantation* 8:582–587

Rodriguez A, Diaz M, Colon A, Santiago DEA (1991) Psychosocial profile of non compliant transplant patients. *Transplant Proceedings* 23:1807–1809

Sargent S, Wainwright S (2006) Quality of life following emergency liver transplantaton for acute liver failure. *Nursing in Critical Care* 11(4):168–176

Starzl TE, Iwatsuki S, Van Thiel DH, Carlton Garter J, Zitelli BJ, Malatack J, Schade RR, Shaw BW, Hakala T, Rosenthal JT, Porter KA (1982) Evolution of liver transplantation. *Hepatology* 2(5):614–636

Starzl TE, Klintmalm GBG, Porter KA, Iwatsuki S, Schroter GPJ (1981) Liver transplantation with the use of cyclosporine A and prednisolone. *New England Journal of Medicine* 305:266–269

Stegall MD, Everson G, Schroter G, Bilir B, Karrer F, Kam I (1995) Metabolic complications after liver transplantation, diabetes, hypercholesterolemia hypertension and obesity. *Transplantation* 6:105710–105760

Stewart SF, Hudson M, Talbot D, Manas D, Day CP (2001) Mycophenolate mofetil monotherapy in liver transplantation. *Lancet* 357(9256):609–610

Tueche SG (2003) Diabetes mellitus after liver transplant new etiologic clues and cornerstones for understanding. *Transplantation Proceedings* 35:1466–1468

UK Transplant (2007) Yearly statistics – Liver Transplants (online). Available at http://www.uktransplant.org

UK Transplant (2008) Transplant activity in the UK 2007/8 (online). Available at http://www.uktransplant.org (accessed 07/03/09)

Wiesner R, Edwards E, Freeman R, Harper A, Kim R, Kamath P (2003) Model for end stage liver disease (MELD) and allocation of donor livers. *Gastroenterology* 124:91–96

Wiesner RH, Ludwig J, Krom RA, Hay JE, Van Hoek B (1993) Hepatic allograft rejection: new developments in terminology, diagnosis, prevention and treatment. *Mayo Clinic Proceedings* 68:69–79

Wiesner RH, Ludwig J, Krom RA, Steers JL, Porayko MK, Gores GJ, Hay JE (1994) Treatment of early cellular rejection following liver transplantation eith intravenous methylprednisalone. The effects of dose on response. *Transplantation* 58(9):1053–1056

Wilde MI, Goa KL (1996) Muromonad CD3: a reappraisal of its pharmacology and use as prophylaxis of solid organ transplant rejection. *Drugs* 51(5):865–894

Zink S, Wertlieb S, Kimberly L (2005) Informed consent. *Progress in Transplantation* 15(4):371–377

Index